Dedication

This book is dedicated to my father, William George Whitaker, Jr., M.D. He was a highly regarded general surgeon and Chief of Staff at Piedmont Hospital in Atlanta, Georgia, for close to a decade. When he retired from active surgery, friends and colleagues endowed a William G. Whitaker, Jr., Chair of Surgery in his honor.

For over twenty years, I have been an outspoken advocate of alternative medicine, and I have often, almost routinely, criticized the excessive use of surgery that has become so common in modern conventional medicine. However, my father's style of medicine and my own were more similar than different. He was trained and worked in a different era, and he did what I have always endeavored to do—he cared for his patients.

His patients knew that he was genuinely concerned by the way he listened to their problems. He was a doctor in the truest sense of the word, not the faceless, robot healthcare provider of modern "government-controlled" medicine.

Though he often neither understood nor agreed with the style of medicine I had chosen, he frequently reminded me, almost like a mantra, that my primary responsibility was to take care of my patients.

I hope this book, a sincere effort to extend that caring, does just that.

angioplasty, carotid endarterectomies, and almost all cancer therapies is arguable.

On the other hand, there are reams of articles that support the scientific validity of lifestyle changes, a nutritional diet, regular exercise, herbal medicine, and vitamin and mineral supplementation. These approaches are neither taught in medical school nor used on a regular basis by practioners of conventional medicine.

Unfortunately, what drives the medical industry, like any business, is the bottom line. The problem with many excellent, safe, and beneficial therapies is that they cannot be structured into financial powerhouses.

In my opinion, we are rapidly headed for (if we have not already entered) an "allopathic dark age." Allopathic refers to the dominant medical system, which prescribes treatments centered against the disease. Dark ages in human culture are periods of time in which information is suppressed and progress takes steps backward, often due to governmental procedures that block new information and hinder progress. Individuals in the dark ages may even consider themselves enlightened, particularly if they are able to espouse the general, narrow dogma of the time.

A case in point is a newspaper column by Peter Gott, M.D. (Syndicated Newspaper Enterprises) in which he denounced the use of a valid alternative treatment for cardiomyopathy, a serious disorder of the heart muscle. I wrote Dr. Gott the following letter.

> Dear Dr. Gott,
>
> At first I was incredulous, then alarmed by your comments on coenzyme Q10.
>
> I have been practicing medicine in California for twenty years and have been dispensing, prescribing, and recommending coenzyme Q10 daily for over a decade. A health food store close to me has seven brands of high-quality coenzyme Q10, which are made in Japan.
>
> Coenzyme Q10 is not a "nontraditional" treatment of cardiomyopathy; it is the most powerful treatment of cardiomyopathy available. It increases the survival rate of cardiomyopathy patients tenfold compared to the combined therapy of ACE inhibitors, diuretics, and Lanoxin. No university centers are looking at coenzyme Q10, primarily because of the imposing procedures of the Food and Drug Administration. Per Langsjoen, M.D., a cardiologist in Tyler, Texas, has been prescribing and publishing information on coenzyme Q10 for years. He knows of no other efforts in this country.
>
> We are rapidly marching towards an allopathic dark age in which information not even remotely related to fact is "gener-

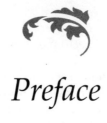

Preface

This is a book about alternative medical approaches to common diseases and health problems. It is primarily a listing of nutritional and natural remedies that may be overlooked by conventional physicians. You might reasonably ask yourself, why? The simple answer is that there is little money to be made in the use of natural remedies, regardless of how beneficial they may be for the patient. Conventional modern medicine generates over a trillion dollars a year by prescribing patented drugs and costly, often dangerous, invasive diagnostic and surgical techniques. There is an obvious place for these approaches: I use them myself and recommend them when appropriate, but conventional medicine should not exclude the use of safer, often more effective and far less expensive therapies.

The American public believes that the healthcare industry is scientific and follows a path that is ultimately beneficial for the patient or the ill individual. When I was in medical school, I passionately believed this to be true. I believed, as I walked the halls of my teaching institution's hospital, as I spent hundreds of hours memorizing diagnostic techniques and therapeutic interventions, that science was guiding the entire enterprise. Anything that was beneficial to the ill patient, such as acupuncture, vitamin E, or vitamin C, I believed, would be considered by this system, evaluated in an unbiased fashion, and incorporated for the benefit of men and women who trust physicians and the healthcare system to take care of them.

Is it possible that the system is impure, that it actively works against the dissemination of useful and helpful information that cannot be classified as a patented prescription drug or expensive medical technology? In fact, the Office of Technology of the United States Government stated several years ago that 80 percent of conventional medical therapies have no basis in science. The overwhelming majority of therapies for cancer and heart patients are offered with little more than "hope" and a big bill. Bypass surgery, taught in medical schools and popular in hospitals, has been scientifically disproven three times (discussed in full on pages 147). The scientific validity of

Before You Read On

- Do not self-diagnose. Proper medical care is critical to good health. If you have symptoms suggestive of any illness discussed in this book, please consult a physician, preferably a holistic medical doctor (M.D.), osteopath (D.O.), naturopath (N.D.), chiropractor (D.C.), or other natural healthcare specialist.
- If you are currently on a prescription medication, you absolutely must work with your doctor before discontinuing any drug.
- If you wish to try the natural approach, discuss it with your physician. Your physician may be unaware of all the natural alternatives; you may need to educate him or her. Bring this book along with you to the doctor's office. The natural alternatives being recommended are based upon published studies in medical journals, and references are provided if your physician wants additional information.
- Remember, although many natural alternatives, such as nutritional supplements and herbs, are effective on their own, they work even better if they are part of a comprehensive natural treatment plan which focuses on diet and lifestyle factors.

Contents

ated" to serve allopathic medical dogma. Doctors will become even more like robots, exhibiting no signs of independent thought. Your piece on coenzyme Q10 is testimony that perhaps you have already arrived.

For your reader with cardiomyopathy who inquired about coenzyme Q10, you need to set the record straight and inform her that she can get it at a health food store, if she so desires. To withhold this information from her is unreasonable, unethical, and will facilitate her demise, and potentially that of many others. However, since coenzyme Q10 is a nutrient, not a drug, it is not "politically correct" to mention anything positive about it, and the mention of health food stores is strictly forbidden.

What are you going to do?

One of the reasons why I am proud of this book is that it gives information on a wide scale that not only can help you but, in my opinion and as one of my goals, can help to prevent the dark age curtain from dropping completely.

Most of the products discussed in this book are available at health food stores. The gross sales of the nutritional supplement industry amount to approximately $4 billion per year, with 80 percent of those who run retail outlets working long hours, often for less than $35,000 per year. Compare that to pharmaceutical industry gross sales of $112 billion and the average physician's yearly income of $170,000. The drugs Zantac and Prozac by themselves will each gross more than the total business revenues of the entire nutritional supplement industry, while almost all nonallopathic traditions of healing, such as naturopathy, herbal medicine, nutritional supplementation, and homeopathy, are outside the mainstream, clustered in small, local health food stores and healing communities, and are under seige. The FDA, in apparent collaboration with allopathic medicine and the pharmaceutical industry, seems determined to keep these natural healing traditions out; if it succeeds, some of the best therapies for human ailments will be lost forever.

It is my hope that this book will provide the information you seek, and thus help to prevent the sounds of silence characteristic of all human dark ages.

Julian Whitaker, M.D.
May, 1994

Acknowledgments

All of us owe a great debt to Linus Pauling, whose courage, creativity, and originality have long inspired and guided me. He will be missed, but oh, what a life!

I want to thank Jeffrey Bland, Ph.D., Eric Braverman, M.D., Jack Dreyfus, Udo Erasmus, Ph.D., Karl Folkers, Ph.D., Alan Gaby, M.D., Patricia Hausman, L.N., Bill Lane, Per Langsjoen, M.D., Peter Langsjoen, M.D., John Lee, M.D., Michael Murray, N.D., Durk Pearson, Eugene Roberts, Ph.D., Billie J. Sahley, Ph.D., Mildred Seelig, M.D., Sandy Shaw, Morton Walker, D.P.M., Melvyn Werbach, M.D., Jonathan Wright, M.D., my colleagues at the American College for The Advance of Medicine and the American Preventive Medical Association, and all who have sought out natural methods of healing, often when it was dangerous to even speak about them. When all things are sorted out, they will be recognized as this century's true doctors. They sought to improve health with subtle, natural elements that are now being rediscovered and found to be far more effective than the "scalpel and drug" approach of the last fifty years.

I am grateful to my wife, Jutta, for her support and love, and to my children, Jay, Conrad, Louisa, and Max.

Thanks also to the staff of the Whitaker Wellness Institute. They are family to me. And a special thanks to Phillips Publishing, who took a chance and launched my newsletter *Health and Healing*. They took an even bigger chance by letting me "call it as I see it."

PART I

Real Healthcare Reform

Part 1 focuses on two primary topics: (1) our current healthcare system and (2) a comprehensive presciption for wellness. One problem with our current healthcare system is its focus on treating disease rather than promoting wellness.

The majority of our healthcare dollars—over $700 billion—is going towards the treatment of conditions that are largely preventable. Have you ever thought what might happen if more Americans discovered the preventive measures that would greatly reduce their risk of developing many common diseases? The whole healthcare system as it stands now would probably collapse, because it is fed not by people who are well and healthy, but rather by people who are sick.

The Whitaker Wellness Program, as outlined in Chapter 2, is a time-tested and proven method that I have used in my clinical practice for nearly twenty years. It is a program designed to help you take charge of your health care. It is a blueprint for healthful living.

1

The Non-Natural Roots of the Problem

Talk of healthcare reform is everywhere. It's the hottest political topic of the 1990s. The politicians in Washington are considering ideas from the right and left. State legislators are heatedly working on their own solutions.

For good reason. The cost of American medicine is careening wildly out of control, approaching $1 trillion annually. Yet the United States continues to rank below other Western nations in many key health indices, basic things such as life expectancy and infant mortality. Meanwhile a growing number of Americans are uninsured or find health care increasingly unaffordable.

National Task Force Politics

Unfortunately, it is not "healthcare" reform that our politicians are debating, it is the reform of "disease management." The National Task Force on Healthcare Reform established by the Clinton administration in 1993 should more accurately have been called the National Task Force on Disease Management Reform.

Let me explain. The combined influence of the pharmaceutical industry and of the United States Food and Drug Administration (FDA) has almost no wellness orientation. Our major medical policy and everything in our present healthcare system depends on people getting sick. The basic treatments covered by most medical insurance policies revolve around patented pharmaceutical drugs designed to suppress the symptoms of disease. When diseases get worse, as they tend to do when symptoms are suppressed, insurance covers the costs as doctors rely on patented machines and other expensive technology to calibrate the management of diseases. Surgeries, with drugs to assist and buffer their effects, are also covered.

A battle rages in Washington and in state legislatures among political parties, groups within the parties, big insurers and little insurers, and the American Medical Association and some of its specialty groups. Naturally, the self-interests of each group dictate different strategies for controlling the management of disease in this country.

Managing disease is a lucrative business. As long as people stay sick, they keep coming back for more. You and I may look at all the zeros in $1,000,000,000,000 and feel the weight of the cost involved. Special interest groups see only the benefits: inside that $1 trillion is a great deal of profit for them.

We do have a "healthcare" problem in the United States. A big one. Unfortunately, what we rarely hear from the people on the debating podiums, or from those who are writing legislation, is the underlying, fundamental problem, which is that our leaders haven't given enough consideration to what a system truly based on "health care" might mean. It is the system of disease care that needs reforming, not an economic shuffling of who pays for what.

The focus of our healthcare system is on disease rather than on health and this is at the center of our rising costs. Given these high costs, our relatively low health as a people is deeply disturbing. It would be one thing if Americans were getting their money's worth. But while the drug companies, doctors, insurance companies, and hospitals are pulling in substantial money, the medical approach promoted by these people is not necessarily helping us get well.

The Pharmaceutical Industry and Disease

The powerful effect that drug companies have on the disease orientation of medicine in the United States was clearly stated in a recent editorial entitled "The Addiction to Drug Companies" in the medical journal *Biological Psychiatry*. The editorial posited an unhealthy relationship between physicians and the drug suppliers.

> The overall influence of the [healthcare] industry is to emphasize drug treatment at the expense of other modalities: psychotherapy, social approaches, nutritional, herbal, and natural remedies, rehabilitation, general hygienic measures, non-patentable drugs, or other alternative approaches. It focuses attention on disorders that are treatable by drugs, and may promote over-diagnosis. It reinforces the practice of dealing with disease by treatment of symptoms, and diverts interest from prevention.[1]

Obviously, there is tremendous profit to be made by keeping the emphasis of our medical system away from prevention. In fact, the

Table 1.1 Rising Costs of Prescription Medications

Drug	1985 Price*	1991 Price*	% Increase
Premarin	$13.34	$33.09	148%
Inderal	19.61	44.74	128%
Synthroid	8.28	17.40	110%
Xanax	29.04	59.76	106%
Felden	114.70	219.90	91%
Procardia	27.31	51.78	90%
Ceclor	96.61	175.50	82%
Clinoril	50.08	86.11	72%
Dyazide	20.35	33.50	65%

*Average wholesale prices for 100-tablet package

Source: Families USA Foundation (*USA Today*, November 4, 1992)

pharmaceutical industry is the most profitable industry in America. Companies use a simple technique to secure this profit: They raise prices. Over the past few decades prices for prescription medication have skyrocketed at four times the rate of inflation. In 1993, with inflation at its lowest in years, this pattern continued to hold steady. General inflation (Producer Price Index) was at 1.5 percent, while the price of prescription drugs went up 6.4 percent. In the 12 years leading to 1992, the average prescription price went up 300 percent, from $6.52 to $22.50.[2]

Prices don't all go up at the same rate. In fact, on analyzing the data it becomes clear that two population groups have been targeted with increases: baby boomers and the elderly. Premarin, a hormonal drug used primarily by women around the time of menopause, is being prescribed more. Between 1985 and 1991 the price of 100 tablets rose 250 percent, from $13.34 to $33.09. See Table 1.1.

The elderly have been hit even harder. Eight of the ten drugs for which prices were raised in 1992 are used almost exclusively by the elderly: Tenex, Isordil, Catapres, Sinemet, K-Tab, Donnatal, Micro-K, and Hytrin. The ailments for which these are prescribed range from angina and hypertension to Parkinson's disease.

Is the classic economic scenario of supply and demand behind these increases? In fact, it seems to be the case, here in the United States, that all roads lead to higher profits for the drug companies. And higher costs to the consumer.

The pharmaceutical industry consists of many large, multinational companies. Most industrial nations have regulations which control pharmaceutical profits and limit what a company can charge for a drug in their country. How does the multinational drug company respond to these restrictions abroad? It charges more for its drugs in the United States.[3] Here, the method of regulation of pharmaceutical prices is that the drug companies set the prices for their products.

According to the laws of economics, free market competition would keep prices down. But the world of the pharmaceuticals is a different kind of place. There are several barriers to competition.

First, there are very few major players. Most of the power is in the hands of a few companies. Second, when a drug company develops a drug, it is granted a patent that can last up to twenty-two years when extensions are included. The company that developed the drug has exclusive marketing rights for the duration. When the patent expires, other drug companies are allowed to market the same drug as a "generic." At that point, the price of the original drug should come down. In fact, in many instances, the brand name drug will go up. Why? Doctors tend to continue with the higher-priced name drug because the pharmaceutical companies spend billions of dollars each year in search of that loyalty: about 22 cents on every dollar spent by drug companies goes for promotion and marketing, about $13,000 per doctor each year. This is more money than the companies spend on research and development of new drugs.[4]

A close analysis of the situation reveals that rather than price-cutting competition, the drug companies engage in competitive price escalation. Here is one instructive case. In 1977, the anti-ulcer drug Tagamet was introduced by Smith-Kline. Tagamet had a virtual lock on the market until Zantac was introduced in 1983. Glaxo, the company that introduced Zantac, cited improved tolerance and fewer side effects and charged a premium for their drug.

Smith-Kline, rather than lowering the price of Tagamet, increased it, and the price of the two drugs has continued to increase. When two new drugs came into this market, Pepcid (1986), marketed by Merck, and Axid (1988) by Eli Lilly, each followed Glaxo's lead, charging a premium rather than competing on price.

In short, the system seems to work like this. A new drug comes into a market with new claims. It charges more. The makers of older drugs take advantage of the differential and raise their price. Is it any wonder drug prices are skyrocketing?

The Industry and the Doctor

It is my belief that the drug industry has a much bigger hand in the crisis in our medical system than simply raising its prices. First, let me provide a historic note. In 1912, the American Medical Association (AMA) hadn't yet fully succeeded in convincing the American public that its disease-management approach was the road down which

American medicine should walk. The AMA made a quiet advance that year, establishing something called the Cooperative Advertising Bureau, a mechanism for sharing medical journal advertising revenues between the AMA and its chapters. It was intended as a way to control and increase advertising revenues by stopping conflicts between the AMA journal and the periodicals of its affiliates.

It was a smart organizing move by the AMA. Just three years later, in 1915, combined advertising dollars from these journals were dominating AMA revenues. The power of the pharmaceutical dollar in the AMA has not diminished, as the industry makes significant contributions to centers for medical education. The industry makes "charitable contributions" to major medical centers and funds endowed professorships and research positions knowing that this practice brings a return of profits both sooner and later.

Gifts and Educational Incentives

Most physicians receive little formal medical education on how drugs work. How then do they learn to distinguish between various drugs? In our present disease management system, most of the 550,000 prescribing physicians rely for their information on the over 45,000 representatives of the drug companies. This is such a tremendous educational responsibility that these "detail people" should be as well-educated as any "visiting professors," but less than one in twenty of these experts-by-default has had any formal training in pharmacology.

The educational settings are often exciting, far-off resort settings, with all expenses paid by the drug companies. The salespeople wine and dine and rationally and scientifically attempt to convince the doctor that their company's drug is the one they should be prescribing. Other environments favored by the detail people include major sporting events, elegant dinners, and celebrity performances.

This kind of relationship between the drug companies and the doctors they supply has been decried in a number of major medical journals. Some medical organizations have also put together panels to establish guidelines for professional conduct.

No Strings Attached?

In 1990, the American College of Physicians (ACP) authored a position paper to address the practice of drug companies influencing doctors by providing these extravagant "gifts" and stipends.[5] The ACP paper said that such incentives shouldn't be accepted if "acceptance might influence or appear to others to influence clinical judgment." The paper goes on: "A useful criterion in determining acceptable activities and relationships is: Would you be willing to have these arrangements generally known?"

A better requirement would be that doctors hand each and every patient an up-to-date list of any and all stipends or benefits the physician has received from any drug manufacturer. A process of real education—of patients—might then begin.

A 1992 article published in the *New England Journal of Medicine* addressed the question of gifts.[6] The author, Douglas Waud, M.D., noted that the term "gift" implies that no strings are attached. He believes that strings are always attached to the various perks and incentives packed into the multi-billion dollar pharmaceutical promotional budgets. So, writes Waud, the term "gift" in the ACP guidelines should actually read "bribe." He further confronted the ACP and the AMA for urging a policy that physicians "stick to bribes that are small enough to be swept under the rug."

Advertising Misleads Physicians

The extent to which drug advertising funds the activities of the American Medical Association and its affiliates has already been noted. Advertising dollars dominate their revenues.

To get a sense of this, take a look at a medical journal the next time you are in a doctor's office. You will see that much of the contents consist of advertisements from drug companies, including color pictures which suggest all the benefits of the drug being offered.

Now take a look at the page that follows the color picture and you'll see the fine print. Here are the contraindications and adverse effects of the drugs, the ways the drug might possibly make a patient sick. For the patient, these "thousand words" are clearly worth more than the picture.

Recall as you skim the journal that the money represented by these advertisements doesn't merely support the magazine. It also funds the political and media campaigns of organized medicine as represented by the AMA.

One can begin to grasp the extent of this inter-relationship by realizing how many of these magazines exist. More than one journal targets each specialty and sub-specialty. Other periodicals are devoted to news accounts. The same pattern exists: Like all magazines, these journals are vehicles for advertising and generate money which may be used politically to foster a limited view of medical care in our country. Many of these journals are sent free of charge to physicians and the publisher can boast a broad circulation to the advertiser, thereby increasing advertising rates.

These advertisements, with all the billions behind them, should be above reproach. This is not always so. The claims of the drug companies are often misleading.

In 1981 the FDA established a guideline which stated that "advertisements must present true statements relating to side effects, contra-indication, and effectiveness."[7] The FDA further stated that failure to do so would be considered false and misleading.

Has this helped? Unfortunately, the FDA's attention to the issue has made little impact. Misleading advertising abounds in medical journals. An expert panel recently judged that over 92 percent of all advertisements in a leading medical journal failed to comply with the FDA guidelines. A full 34 percent contained misleading or erroneous information.[7]

Patients may be reassured by the idea that most doctors make their decisions based on medical knowledge, not advertising. This claim has been studied and these studies conclude that doctors are more influenced by advertising than by scientific evidence.[8]

Another key factor influencing a physician's decision to choose a certain drug is the opinion of colleagues who will usually provide perspective based on professional experience. Unfortunately, the opinion your physician regards so highly may have been based instead on something the colleague learned at the golf course.

The FDA's Role

The FDA was developed with some specific public health concerns at stake. The first were the horrors of the meat-processing practices at the turn of the century. The agency's responsibilities were originally outlined in sections of the Public Health Service Act of 1908 and later in the Food, Drug, and Cosmetic Act of 1938.

Under these acts it was the FDA's mission to (1) "ensure that foods are safe, pure, and wholesome, are made or processed under sanitary conditions, and are honestly labeled and packaged; to carry on research and public education; to set regulations governing the definitions and standards of identity of foods, containers, and labeling; and to promote honesty and fair dealing in the interest of the consumer" and (2) "determine the safety and effectiveness of drugs and medical devices."[8]

The FDA's Agenda

The intent of Congress when it created the FDA was to create a governmental agency which would serve the public. I would rather suggest that it believes its mission statement reads: (1) to protect the interests of the drug industry and to promote a drug-oriented view of medical care; (2) to turn a blind eye to the chronic diseases promoted by the modern food industry; and (3) to wage war against the natural food industry, alternative health care providers and others who challenge the mainstream conception of the public health.

This agenda needs to be exposed and amended. The FDA, as with other government agencies and special-interest groups, has recently (reluctantly and belatedly) made some changes. It has come around to acknowledge the validity of the positions that nutrition-oriented doctors have held for decades. A new section of the FDA's agenda could be added: (4) will, upon adopting the positions of the alternative providers and natural products industry which it once deemed as quackery, show no learning curve, and continue to keep them as outsiders.

The FDA is charged with keeping the public safe. To define the public safety by ensuring that dietary supplements do not interfere with the sales of any drug currently on the market or in development is counterproductive to the needs of the ill patient.

The FDA and Dietary Supplements

Over the years, the FDA has limited the availability of dietary supplements. In 1973, FDA officials considered classifying all vitamin and mineral supplements that contained more than 150 percent of the U.S. Recommended Dietary Allowance (RDA) as drugs, with all the rules and regulations that accompany such a classification.

A massive consumer movement wanted to maintain the public's right to easy access to these common natural products. After much debate, Congress passed the Rogers-Proxmire amendment in 1976, which prevented the FDA from classifying nutrients as drugs unless specific drug claims were made.

This was a lesson. Clearly the *public* health would need to be protected by the actions of an involved public. Citizens would need to keep watch on their purported protector, the FDA.

The FDA has claimed that its role is ensuring public safety, yet the FDA has approved the sale of many dangerous drugs. According to a detailed report, of the 198 drugs that the FDA approved between 1976 and 1985, a staggering 52 percent proved to have "serious post-approval risks." The report was released by the General Accounting Office of the U.S. Government in 1990. Among the possible side effects were death and various disabling health disorders including liver damage; depression and psychological disturbances; severe allergic reactions; and other serious disorders.

Why would the FDA approve any potentially harmful drugs? FDA officials cite greater benefit over risk as the reason. A better answer may be found in the results of a Congressional investigation in 1989. Congress discovered that FDA officials had accepted bribes from drug manufacturers to speed their products through the agency's approval process. This particular investigation eventually led to the conviction of five companies and twenty-two individuals for corruption or fraud. What is even more alarming is that their activities and behavior were part of an ongoing collaboration between the FDA and the drug companies, and was not an aberration.

Let's assume the value in the FDA's assignment to regulate dietary supplements, but evidence of substantial danger exists. One way to evaluate this danger would be to compare it to that from drugs that have been approved by the FDA.

According to detailed analysis of all available data, there are over 10 million adverse reactions yearly from FDA-approved over-the-counter and prescription drugs. We are not talking about mild nausea or headaches. Between 60,000 and 140,000 people die each year from adverse drug reactions. Each year, more Americans die after taking prescription drugs than died in the entire Vietnam war. This constitutes a real "public health issue."

On the other hand, only a single death related to a vitamin supplement was reported in the United States by the American Association of Poison Control Centers (AAPCC) in 1990. One death. And there is good reason to question whether or not it was appropriately attributed to the supplement. In August, 1992, Citizens For Health obtained a copy of the case history. (Citizens for Health is a nonprofit organization which seeks to maintain the rights of consumers to have access to alternative medicine and dietary supplements. Chapters may be found in all fifty states, with a home base in Tacoma, Washington. For more information on Citizens For Health, call 1-800-357-2211.)

The case history for the vitamin-related death involved a 28-year-old man who suffered from severe paranoid schizophrenia. Medications at the time of his death included aspirin, Lovastatin (Mevacor), acetaminophen, Navane, Cogentin, Desipramine, and the vitamin, niacin. The cause of death was severe liver damage.

Reading the small print in the pharmaceutical ads reveals that Lovastatin as well as acetaminophen (e.g., Tylenol) and Navane (an antipsychotic drug) can cause the type of liver damage produced in this patient. As a precautionary measure, liver function tests every six weeks are recommended when patients are on Lovastatin and Navane. But no liver function tests were performed on the man for at least twelve months prior to his death.

The patient also had a history of "hoarding his medication" for up to ten days. He would then take them all at once. The manufacturer of Lovastatin recommends never taking a double dose of the drug even if a dose is missed. Why? Because the drug can cause serious liver damage. In fact, deaths and serious liver damage were reported in the early stages of the development of Lovastatin.

Given the known side effects of the drugs the patient was on, it is unlikely that the man's death was the result of niacin toxicity alone.

How the AAPCC could conclude the death was due to niacin alone is questionable and may reflect significant bias.

The FDA has used this purported vitamin-caused death and has inflated the figure many times over as the debate over dietary supplements and herbal products heated up again in 1992 and 1993.

On the *Larry King Live Show* (August 14, 1992), FDA spokesperson Mary Pendergast stated that vitamins were responsible for dozens of deaths each year in the United States. Dr. David Kessler, Commissioner of the Food and Drug Administration, made a number of misleading and false statements when he spoke to Congress at the Hearing on the Dietary Supplement Health and Education Act of 1993.

The fact of the matter is that more than 100 million Americans regularly use dietary supplements, and the rate of side effects is extremely low. Using the FDA's own data and according to all the available medical literature, dietary supplements are 2,550 times safer than over-the-counter drugs. Imagine the advertising campaign that a drug company could launch if some new drug were found to be this safe.

The evidence is simply not there to back up the FDA's concerns. The real public health danger is not the potential side effects of nutritional supplements and herbs. The danger lies in restricting the public's access to these useful agents.

FDA Dietary Supplement Task Force Report

In June of 1993, the FDA published a report from its Dietary Supplement Task Force. Included was a paper which served notice that the FDA wanted to dramatically change the rules around regulation of dietary supplements, entitled "Advanced Notice of Proposed Rule-Making for the Regulation of Dietary Supplements."

In these papers the FDA outlined its five major issue areas:

1. Health claims on supplements
2. The regulation of amino acids as drugs
3. Nutrient limits in dietary supplements
4. Nonessential nutrients (as determined by the FDA) would be viewed as "unsafe food additives"
5. Herbs should be viewed as drugs

One way to evaluate the FDA recommendations is to ask two questions which honorable regulators use to guide their work. Two types of danger exist from wrongful regulation. One such danger is to allow the sale of a product which is later shown to have substantial harmful effects. The history of drug regulation is full of stories of this type of mistake. For instance (as previously mentioned), over one-half of the drugs approved by the FDA since 1976 were later found to be much more toxic than previously thought; several had to be removed from the market. The magnitude of the toxic reactions to FDA-approved drugs has perhaps hindered the agency's capacity to trust that naturally-occurring, healthful substances exist which will not debilitate or cause the death of their users.

The question is: Does the public face a substantial risk if the FDA allows greater (rather than lesser) freedom of distribution for vitamins, minerals, amino acids, and herbal preparations? The answer, for each of these substances, is no.

The other guiding question is whether the regulating agency is withholding something from the public which could be beneficial. The facts suggest that the FDA is wrong to propose such restrictive rules. The public health certainly benefits from these agents and information to which the public has an inherent right would be limited by the FDA's proposed rules.

Point 1: Health Claims on Supplement Labels

The FDA has recommended that health claims for nutritional supplements be permitted only if the FDA finds "significant agreement" among qualified experts that such claims are scientifically valid. The concept of "significant agreement" is subjective. In practice, the FDA has the power to define what is a valid claim. Often, their decisions defy common sense.

The FDA has a mandate to safeguard the American public health; taken too far, the consumer's fundamental right to choice is usurped. FDA director David Kessler has stated (on the *Larry King Live Show*): "The American public does not have the knowledge to make wise health care decisions . . . The FDA is the arbiter of truth . . . Trust us. We will tell you what's good for you."

I would like to trust the FDA. When it comes to nutritional supplement regulation, the administration could start by including experts on its Task Force, leading scientists working with natural products, nutrition-oriented physicians and doctors who regularly heal people through the use of herbal products. But these people were not asked to participate, though their experience and expertise would be invaluable on such a committee. These are the people who have the clinical and practical experience on adverse effects. This omission is critical.

The FDA's position to date runs counter to the views of the leading scientists studying the value of nutritional supplements. Five specific supplement health claims which the FDA has reviewed were either denied or approved after prolonged denial.

1. *Folic Acid and Neural Tube Defects*   After an enormous amount of scientific evidence, the FDA did approve the claim that folic acid supplements can prevent certain birth defects. Initially the FDA rejected the claim and violated its own proposed stance. Significant scientific agreement existed long before the FDA would acknowledge it. Despite FDA disapproval, the U.S. Public Health Service, the U.S. Centers for Disease Control, and the American College of Obstetricians and Gynecologists began recommending folic acid. These major organizations suggested that all women of child-bearing age consume 400 micrograms of folic acid per day to protect against neural tube defects. Finally the FDA approved the claim.

It is sad to think that thousands of children were born with a birth defect which could have been prevented. The agency prohibited the public's access to what has been called one of the most exciting medical findings of the last part of the twentieth century.

2. *Calcium and Osteoporosis*   The FDA now allows claims which link supplemental calcium with prevention or slowing of the process of osteoporosis. Interestingly, research to deny this connection was not nearly as comprehensive as that on some other valid claims the FDA has rejected. I call this "the Tums claim." Could the fact that major drug companies were involved with calcium supplementation have played a role?

3. *Omega-3 Fatty Acids and Heart Disease*   The FDA disallowed a claim linking omega-3 fatty acids and prevention of heart disease, despite the fact that every professional conference on the subject had concluded that the public should be encouraged to increase consumption of omega-3 fatty acids to reduce the risk of heart disease and other related conditions. The cholesterol-lowering ability of omega-3 oils from cold-water fish or flax seeds had already been demonstrated in hundreds of carefully controlled studies.

One reason the FDA might take a stand against omega-3 oils, given their significant ability to reduce heart disease, could be in consideration of the fact that the treatment of high cholesterol and heart disease is highly profitable for the major drug companies.

4. *Antioxidants and Cancer Prevention*   Many scientists and physicians have started recommending higher intakes of antioxidants such as vitamin C, vitamin E, and beta-carotene to prevent cancer as well as heart disease. Why? The supporting evidence is simply overwhelming. One advocate for this claim, Dr. Gladys Block of the University of California at Berkeley, a leading expert on the association of antioxidants and cancer prevention, in comments submitted to the FDA, wrote: "Given the compelling evidence supporting the biochemical

mechanisms, the extensive and consistent epidemiological data (population studies) on the role of antioxidant intake and the inability of clinical trials to resolve the issue of benefits of dietary levels, the public good calls for permitting this health claim."

The FDA dismissed Dr. Block's petition, and that of others who supported her opinion. The FDA demands "significant agreement" on all health claims, yet even when significant agreement among leading experts exists, the FDA looks in another direction.

5. Zinc and Immune Function in the Elderly   The FDA has also studied the role of dietary supplements of zinc in improving immune function in the elderly, and concluded that the claim was not adequately supported. It is well-proven that zinc is critical to proper immune function in all people, and that most elderly, because of decreased intake as well as impaired absorption of zinc, are not getting enough to support good health. Depressed immune function in the elderly greatly increases the risk for infection and cancer.

Well-Accepted Benefits of Common Dietary Supplements

The FDA has repeatedly denied benefits from dietary supplements even when such benefits have significant confirmation in the medical literature. One of the most notable exclusions was the claim that vitamin C can help prevent and treat the common cold. Another was the beneficial role that vitamin E and other dietary antioxidants can play in preventing heart disease.

It has been over twenty years since Linus Pauling wrote *Vitamin C and the Common Cold*. In the book Pauling based his conclusions on several studies which showed that vitamin C was highly effective in reducing the severity of symptoms as well as the duration of the common cold. Since 1970, over twenty double-blind studies have been conducted designed to test Pauling's assertion.[9] Every study demonstrated that the group receiving the vitamin C had either a decrease in duration or symptom severity. Yet the clinical effect is still debated in the medical community.

The vitamin C studies have consistently demonstrated results superior to over-the-counter cold medications. Yet the FDA stance has prevented manufacturers of vitamin C products from making any health claims for their product. Meanwhile, the makers of over-the-counter common cold medications spend hundreds of millions of dollars trying to convince the American public that these products are the answer to the common cold when, in fact, numerous studies have shown them to be of little real value.

Numerous studies have also demonstrated the fact that an individual's level of antioxidants may be a more significant factor in determining the risk of developing heart disease than are cholesterol levels. Large-scale studies with vitamin E, vitamin C, and beta-carotene have shown that these antioxidants are capable of significantly reducing the risk of dying of a heart attack or a stroke. One study looked at 87,245 nurses. It concluded that nurses who took 100 IU of vitamin E daily for more than two years had a 41 percent lower risk of heart disease compared to nonusers of vitamin E supplements.[12] Another study involved 39,910 male healthcare professionals. The results were similar: a 37 percent lower risk of heart disease with the intake of more than 30 IU of supplemental vitamin E daily.[13]

These 1993 studies on vitamin E only confirm what people in the health food industry and nutritionally-minded physicians have known for more than fifty years. Vitamin E is good for the entire cardiovascular system. It is useful in both the prevention and in the treatment of heart disease.

Positive Side Effects

The tremendous range of benefits from so many of these supplements means that an individual who takes them for one concern may well gain value in other areas. I call these the positive side effects of nutritional supplements.

For instance, a person may take Vitamin C as a cancer prevention. Studies show that it will also help ward off heart disease and the common cold. The public health would be served in many ways. The individual's health would be better, and therefore miss fewer work days. Due to the immune support value of vitamin C, millions of dollars in lost productivity might be recovered. And the long-term costs associated with end-stage heart disease or cancer might be avoided.

Point 2: Amino Acids Regulated as Drugs

The FDA's "Report on Dietary Supplements" in 1993 included a recommendation that "amino acids be regulated as drugs." Why? Extensive analysis of the scientific literature demonstrated an excellent safety record. Over 500 human research studies involving the administration of single amino acids demonstrated that amino acid supplements are without side effects. Over 200 studies of L-tryptophan found no adverse effects.[12]

L-tryptophan is the amino acid that the FDA has apparently targeted in order to mount an attack against all amino acid supplements. As the FDA and others close to the issue know, the problem was not with the amino acid. The problem was contaminated batches from just one supplier of L-tryptophan.

What if, instead of a supplement manufacturer, a trumpet manufacturer made a mistake? A single batch of trumpets is found to cut the lips of those who play them. A government agency then confiscates all the trumpets, even those that don't cut the lip. After "careful review" it determines there is a health risk to all musicians. Trumpets are banned entirely and a study of all musical instruments is commissioned. The study concludes that musical instruments are safe. But the agency, stating that musical instruments "may not be safe," starts confiscating violins, flutes, guitars, oboes, pianos, and organs, all in the interest of the health of musicians.

For more than thirty years, L-tryptophan was used by thousands of people in the United States, safely and effectively, for insomnia and depression. In October 1989, some individuals taking this amino acid started reporting strange symptoms: severe muscle and joint pain, high fever, weakness, swelling of the arms and legs, and shortness of breath. The syndrome was dubbed EMS (eosinophilia-myalgia syndrome). Virtually all cases of tryptophan-induced EMS were subsequently traced to a Japanese manufacturer, Showa Denko. Of the six Japanese companies which supplied tryptophan to the U.S., Showa Denko was the largest. It supplied 50 to 60 percent of all the tryptophan being used here. Due to a change in manufacturing procedures, tryptophan produced by Showa Denko between October 1988 and June 1989 became contaminated with a substance now linked to EMS.

When the problems associated with tryptophan became known, the amino acid was immediately taken off the market, a responsible FDA response which gave the agency time to figure out the source of the problem.

There are numerous examples of contaminated foods and medicines causing health problems and even death. In most industries, once the problem of contamination is discovered and resolved, manufacturers are once again allowed to market their products. The products may be grapes, Perrier, Tylenol or hamburgers from Jack in the Box. The products are allowed back on the shelf. This is responsible public health policy.

Tryptophan, a very useful amino acid, has not been allowed back in health food stores, though the contamination issue has been resolved. Yet, while the FDA blocked the sale of tryptophan in dietary supplements, it allowed L-tryptophan to be added to infant formulas and formulas designed for intravenous feedings. Did this mean that this "unsafe" substance was only safe for sick people and babies? Of course not. The reason is a political one. The infant formula industry and intravenous food industries are both part of the FDA's "kitchen cabinet." The dietary supplement industry is not.

The Raid on Dr. Jonathan Wright

The FDA's public health stance on tryptophan eventually created a positive (although unintended) public health effect. A May 6, 1992, FDA raid on Dr. Jonathan Wright and the Tahoma Clinic which provided L-tryptophan to its patients gave the public a good view of the FDA, whose agents, accompanied by ten police officers clad in flak jackets and with guns drawn, broke down the door, flooded the office and terrorized everyone in it. In this image the mind-set of the FDA toward nutritional supplements was effectively captured.

Doctor Wright believed that his patients had the right to tryptophan. Ten months before the raid, in July of 1991, the FDA had seized uncontaminated L-tryptophan from Dr. Wright's clinic. Wright knew it was uncontaminated; he'd checked its source; the source wasn't Showa Denko. Dr. Wright, a leading nutrition-oriented physician for two decades, felt that the FDA's seizure of the L-tryptophan was unlawful and wrongful, so in August of 1991, Wright sued the FDA for his tryptophan on behalf of his patients.

Within a month after he filed suit, Dr. Wright's clinic came under surveillance by the FDA. FDA agents sifted through trash bins outside his office looking for evidence of wrongdoing and used aliases to pose as patients.

The May 6th raid was public confirmation that the agency was targeting nutritionally oriented physicians. Their intent was not to protect the public, but rather to destroy Dr. Wright. A truckload of items was seized. These included patient records; injectable, preservative-free vitamins, minerals, and glandular extracts; noninvasive allergy and sensitivity testing equipment; computer equipment; instruction and training manuals; and many other items including fifty dollars' worth of postage stamps. FDA agent, Victor Meo, from Seattle, was filmed giving the finger to the camera that was filming the looting of Dr. Wright's office.

When a licensed physician gets this treatment from his own government, one would conclude that he must be a major threat to society. But in a twenty-year career, no patient complaints were made to any governmental agency about Dr. Wright.

Since the FDA looted Dr. Wright's office, it has yet to file a single criminal charge against him. No patient or anyone else has stepped forward to testify against him. Yet the government continues to hold over a hundred thousand dollars worth of the property that it confiscated.

Over the last decade, twenty-five physicians who regularly employ nutritional and other natural therapies have faced raids. Many major suppliers of nutritional or herbal supplements have been similarly mistreated or harassed by the FDA in recent years.

Point 3: Dietary Supplement Limits

The FDA believes it is important to establish Dietary Supplement Limits, to limit the level of a given vitamin or mineral it deems safe. If a dietary supplement contains levels in excess of these guidelines, the FDA views the product as containing "unsafe food additives," which would give the FDA the right to seize the product.

The levels are referred to by the FDA as RDIs, or Reference Daily Intakes. With recent evidence about the need for supplementing nutrients, and the depleting effect of modern life on nutrient levels, a thoughtful re-assessment would consider recommendations for levels above those deemed safe in the past.

The RDIs proposed by the FDA are below Recommended Daily Allowance (RDA) levels. Originally, RDAs were designed to determine the required levels of essential nutrients to prevent nutritional deficiency. Substantial evidence exists that supports the notion that increasing the intake of specific nutrients may help to promote optimal health, and either reverse or prevent the development of many diseases. To limit the available level of any given nutrient would severely limit its potential benefits.

Point 4: Nonessential Nutrients as "Unsafe Food Additives"

Many nutritional substances exert benefit yet are not deemed "essential." The FDA would label these substances as unsafe food additives, and would not approve them for use in food or supplements.

The trace minerals chromium and selenium are two such agents. The National Academy of Sciences, the group that sets the RDAs, has established recommended intakes for these minerals, yet the FDA proposed regulations in 1990 and 1991 which sought to classify these trace minerals as food additives. So, despite the fact that both chromium and selenium are essential to human health, they would not be available for use as dietary supplements.

To illustrate the FDA's position, consider their attempt to block the sale of products containing gamma-linoleic acid (GLA), a type of fatty acid found in evening primrose, black currant, and borage oil.

The FDA declared GLA an unsafe food additive, then proceeded to seize inventory from companies supplying GLA products. The FDA's contention was that black currant oil was an unsafe food additive and was being added to gelatin capsules. To call safe food substances food additives when they are encapsulated sprung forth in the 1980s as a useful regulatory hook for nutritional supplements.

One company, Traco Labs, fought back. Traco's decision to sue the FDA, like that of Dr. Wright, was gutsy. Traco spent over a hundred thousand dollars on legal fees. The three judges assigned to the case reprimanded the FDA for its "Alice-in-Wonderland reasoning in an effort to make an end-run around law."[13]

When this attempt to limit the sales of GLA products failed, the FDA circulated a memorandum to Congress which included this statement: "(Regarding) evening primrose oil and related products, black currant oil and borage oil, all of which contain gamma-linoleic acid, this component poses serious health concerns related to convulsions, potential changes in blood clotting, and other tissue changes."

This statement is unfounded. In the legal case with Traco Labs, the FDA's own scientists and toxicologists testified as expert witnesses and reported no safety problems with any GLA product.

Point 5: Herbs as Drugs

Currently, herbal products are sold as "food supplements" and manufacturers are prohibited from making any therapeutic claims for their products. The Task Force on Dietary Supplements has recommended that the FDA regulate herbs as "new drugs." This would force manufacturers of herbal products to go through the standard drug-approval process, which typically takes ten to eighteen years and costs roughly $230 million. Because herbs cannot be patented, no manufacturer would have the incentive to spend this kind of money and herbs would effectively disappear from use.

European countries have different policies for herbs, which have made it economically feasible for companies there to research and develop herbs as medicines. In Germany, herbal products can be marketed with health claims if they have been proven to be safe and effective under the legal requirements for herbal medicines, which are identical to those of all other drugs. Whether the herbal product is available by prescription or over the counter is based upon its application and safety of use. Herbal products sold in pharmacies are reimbursed by insurance if they are prescribed by a physician.

The proof that a manufacturer in Germany is required to provide to illustrate the safety and effectiveness of an herbal product is far less complicated than the proof required by the FDA in the United States. In Germany, a special commission (Commission E) developed a series of 200 monographs on herbal products.[14] These are similar to the OTC (over-the-counter) monographs in the United States. An herbal product is viewed as safe and effective if a manufacturer meets the quality requirements of the monograph, or if the manufacturer can produce additional evidence of safety and effectiveness. This can include data from existing literature and anecdotal information from practicing physicians, as well as limited clinical studies.

A good illustration of the difference in regulatory policies for herbal products in the United States compared to Germany is *Ginkgo biloba*. In Germany, as well as in France, extracts of Ginkgo biloba leaves are registered for the treatment of cerebral and peripheral vascular insufficiency.[15] Ginkgo products are available by prescription and over the counter. Ginkgo extracts are among the top three most widely prescribed drugs in both Germany and France, representing a combined annual sales figure of more than $500 million. In contrast, ginkgo extracts identical to those approved in Germany and France are available in the United States as food supplements.

The FDA has rejected the idea of modeling an independent Expert Advisory Panel on Germany's Commission E. Other ideas to create a suitable framework for the marketing of herbal products in the United States have also been turned down.

The FDA is concerned about public safety. But as with other dietary supplements herbs are proving to be extremely safe. A June, 1992, article in the *Food and Drug Law Journal* included the results of an extensive review on herbal safety conducted by the Herb Research Foundation.[16] This foundation is a nonprofit organization composed of leading experts in the United States on naturally-derived drugs, pharmacology, and toxicology. The Herb Research Foundation's review was based on reports from the American Association of Poison Control Centers and the Centers for Disease Control. The review, published by the prestigious *Food and Law Review*, confirmed that there is no substantial evidence that toxic reactions to herbal products are a major source of concern.

There are numerous herbs in the environment that can cause significant toxicity. However, the herbs commonly used in the United States for health purposes are generally quite safe. When toxic reactions do occur, dosages far in excess of those commonly recommended are the reasons. Recent examples of over-dosage problems have been seen with comfrey root and chaparral.

Unfortunately, concern for public safety does not appear to be motivating the FDA's regulatory activism. How closely are their concerns linked to the concerns of drug companies who may be worried that more Americans are discovering the beneficial effects of herbs? Are they concerned that the market share currently claimed by some of their more popular drugs will fall?

Saw Palmetto versus Proscar

Proscar (*finasteride*) is an FDA-approved drug for the treatment of an enlarged prostate due to benign prostatic hyperplasia (BPH). This condition is extremely common. It affects more than half the men over forty years of age. Because the condition is common, the market for therapeutic agents to address it is potentially very lucrative. Merck, Proscar's manufacturer, has predicted sales will soon reach $1 billion annually.

BPH is characterized by symptoms of bladder obstruction which include increased urinary frequency, nighttime awakening to empty the bladder, and reduced force and caliber of urination. The anatomical cause of these symptoms is that an enlarged prostate will pinch off the flow of urine.

The saw palmetto (*Serenoa repens*) is a small scrubby palm tree native to the West Indies and the Atlantic Coast of North America from South Carolina to Florida. This tree has berries with a long folk history of use in treating conditions of the prostate. Recently, the therapeutic effect of the fat-soluble extract of saw palmetto berries has been shown to greatly improve the signs and symptoms of an enlarged prostate in clinical studies.[17] In fact, based on the results of the clinical trials, the fat-soluble extract of saw palmetto berries is much more effective than Merck's manufactured drug Proscar. (See Table 1.2.)

Proscar lacks overall effectiveness. It is effective in less than 50 percent of cases after patients have taken the drug for a full year (see the *Physician's Desk Reference*). In contrast, studies on the saw palmetto extract have shown it to be effective in nearly 90 percent of patients. The benefits are usually felt after four to six weeks.

Clearly, the saw palmetto extract is superior to Proscar. What must really chill the Merck company is that it is also significantly less expensive: only one-fourth the price.

These are the facts. Unfortunately, most men with BPH will never hear about the extract from the saw palmetto berry. Merck and the FDA are to thank for this. In 1990, Enzymatic Therapy, the company that introduced the extract in the United States, petitioned the

Table 1.2 Saw Palmetto versus Proscar In Treatment of Prostate Enlargement

	Saw Palmetto Extract	*Proscar*
Urine Flow	38% to 50% improvement	16% to 22% improvement
Residual Volume	42% improvement	No improvement
Overall Symptoms	88% to 92.5% improvement	Less than 50%
Decrease in nocturia	3.12 to 1.69 awakenings	No improvement
Complications	none	Decreased libido
		Ejaculatory disorders
		Impotence
		Urogenital birth defects

FDA to have saw palmetto approved for the treatment of BPH. The FDA rejected the application. The reviews of the saw palmetto extract published by the FDA in *New Developments* (March 5, 1990) presented the FDA's reasons for not allowing claims for prostate improvement.

In *New Developments,* the FDA recognized "statistically significant" improvement using saw palmetto for patients with BPH. Despite saw palmetto extract's clear superiority over Proscar (based on clinical trials), the FDA finally concluded that the data was not "clinically significant."

Because of this FDA judgment, manufacturers of the saw palmetto extract cannot mention the good news of this agent's value to those with BPH. Manufacturers are not allowed to provide information to physicians who treat patients with BPH. Proscar, meantime, continues to be approved and for sale without the cheaper, more effective competition. Instead of spending $75 a month for Proscar, men could be spending $15 a month for the saw palmetto extract. They could be getting better results.

To add insult to injury, men on Proscar must live with the drug's side effects, including decreased libido, ejaculatory disorders, and impotence. Is there any drug that can stimulate more marital problems than Proscar? In addition, women of child-bearing age are instructed not to even handle the drug or expose themselves to the semen of men on the drug as it has been shown to cause urogenital birth defects in offspring.

Why wouldn't the FDA approve an herbal treatment that was shown to be more effective than an approved drug, without the side effects? Why wouldn't it care to make the economic benefits of this treatment available? Why would the FDA continue to maintain sole approval of a drug that was less effective than an herbal treatment?

Numerous other such examples abound (and will be presented throughout this book) where an herb is more effective, less expensive, and safer to use than standard drug therapy. The FDA, in apparent collaboration with the drug companies, must find it profitable to keep us dependent upon manufactured, expensive drugs.

The Solution: Get Involved and Stay Involved

At the time of this writing, the Dietary Supplement Health and Education Act (SB 714 and HR 1709) sponsored by Senator Orrin Hatch from Utah and Congressman Bill Richardson from New Mexico was moving through Congress. The legislation provides for reasonable regulation of the supplement industry. It would also prevent the FDA from blocking truthful claims and labeling nutritional supplements as food additives.

Both foci of the bill are in the consumer interest. Of course there are cases where vitamin manufacturers have been out of line in their manufacturing practices and their health claims. Some have simply refused to follow good manufacturing practices. Allowing truthful claims will keep the FDA honest and will help improve the health and well-being of many Americans.

Over 60 percent of our senators and a clear majority of our representatives are sponsors of these bills. A tremendous public lobbying effort in cities and towns across the United States has slowly produced these positive signs over a year of hard work.

If the Hatch-Richardson bill passes through Congress, the bill will guarantee citizens continued access to all of the dietary supplements described in this book.

But regardless of the outcome of this campaign, citizens must stay vigilant. One piece of legislation will not guarantee our rights forever. Threatened drug companies will put their think tanks of lawyers and lobbyists to the task of unraveling these gains. They'll come out with a new strategy. Other battles will emerge.

The successful battle twenty years ago that defeated an attempt by drug companies to gain control of dietary supplements won because of citizen involvement. If the Hatch-Richardson bill passes in a shape which honors the intent with which it was conceived, it will be due to citizen involvement and activity.

Chapter Summary

The American healthcare system is potentially undermined by any alliance between the drug industry and the FDA. The drug industry uses its vast economic power to continue to promote a system of medicine focused on disease management. The industry is supported by the policies of an agency that was established to regulate it: the U.S. Food and Drug Administration, which has continually underestimated the health value of dietary supplements.

Consumers are aware. Physicians are realizing that all may not be as the drug companies paint it. Research upholds the concept of preventive health care, not merely disease management. A growing body of research makes clear that many dietary supplements and herbs are extremely useful in promoting health. Modeling our healthcare system on the idea of maintaining good health suggests a new role for the FDA. Rather than blocking the dissemination of information on dietary supplements, the FDA must help consumers make informed choices regarding their use.

Hopefully, by the time you are reading this book, the right to use nutritional supplements and herbal products will be protected by new legislation. The necessity of continuing citizen vigilance will not have ended. Only when the FDA has clearly embraced a new relationship toward dietary supplements will the agency be fulfilling its original mission: protecting the public interest. Only then will our medical system be a true free marketplace. Only then will we have a chance to move medicine from its role of disease management and focus instead on the support of health and wellness.

2
The Whitaker Wellness Program

For nearly twenty years, I have specialized in "how to keep you well." I use diet, exercise, vitamins, minerals, and herbs to treat patients with heart disease and other chronic, degenerative diseases.

The prevention and treatment of many common degenerative diseases often needs no more than vigorous lifestyle changes, some easy-to-follow dietary guidelines, and the appropriate use of nutritional supplements. Too much of modern medicine gravitates to the dramatic, the technological, the expensive, and the dangerous—and does not really promote health.

The Definition of Health

Have you ever tried to define health? You are probably thinking: "That shouldn't be too difficult." But just give it a try. You'll find it isn't easy. You may say: "You are healthy when you don't feel sick." Does this really define health? What about the so-called silent killers like heart disease, cancer, and strokes? A person may feel perfectly well and still be harboring a dangerous or even fatal condition. So you take another tack. "Health is freedom from disease." Now that sounds like a simple statement of fact. But does the mere absence of disease represent radiant health? I don't think so.

When the World Health Organization was asked to define health, they came up with a definition that really seems to work: "Health is a state of complete physical, mental, and social well-being, and not merely the absence of disease or infirmity."

This definition of health implies an active process with an ultimate goal of complete well-being or wellness. Do you know anyone who is radiantly healthy? Someone who has an abundance of energy, is good-natured, and looks fit? People who attain such high levels of wellness share common values. To them, health is their most valuable possession.

Most of us take our health for granted. But what would your life and the lives of those you love be like if your health was endangered? Don't make the mistake that many people make. Don't wait to realize how important your health is until after you have lost it. Instead, make health and wellness your top priority—today.

If you are currently in poor health, do not be disheartened. Over the years, I have seen thousands of patients get healthy. I have conducted hundreds of one-week and two-week workshops, where patients come for evaluation, second opinions, treatment, and education on the principles outlined in this chapter. Some come for "preventive medicine." Most come with serious diseases. Fortunately, my prescription for wellness assists people in regaining health, not only in preventing disease. This is a remarkable feature of a wellness orientation. Often the same steps that might be recommended for prevention can also reverse a disease process.

Using the Whitaker Wellness Program, you will be practicing true preventive medicine. From a doctor's standpoint, preventive medicine can be somewhat boring. If it is done well, the doctor has less to do. In fact, often, the doctor is no longer in the driver's seat. From your perspective, however, preventive medicine is likely to be the most valuable insurance policy you will ever have. Many of your friends and family will unfortunately succumb to degenerative diseases and "go under the knife." They will submit to a battery of drugs with a whole host of side effects. While you will, hopefully, be watching on the sidelines in a state of good health.

There are seven individual steps in my prescription for wellness. But this is not a program where each step depends upon the completion of the previous steps. In this plan, each step is an improvement in and of itself. None depends upon the others for its benefits. Yet, by following all the steps the benefits are compounded. The more of the steps you take, the healthier you will be. But even if you are successful at doing only one or two of the seven basic steps, you'll be better off than before. No matter what your health history or what your health condition is at present, each step is going to make a vital improvement in your life. So begin today to implement these steps. In a month's time you will find yourself gratified with a growing sense of well-being.

Step 1: Adopt a Healthy Lifestyle

If you want to be healthy, you have to live a healthy lifestyle. In our daily lives, achieving and maintaining health involves a process of learning to consistently choose a healthy alternative over a less healthy one. People who achieve a high level of wellness consistently make healthy choices. As a result, their lives are full of health, happiness, and vitality. Wellness-oriented individuals are those who:

Take personal responsibility for their health.
Have a positive mental outlook on life.
Eat nutritious foods and maintain ideal body weight.
Develop a healthy heart and circulatory system through good nutrition and physical activity.
Have high energy levels.
Handle stress and challenges well.
Balance the stresses of life with adequate rest and recreation.
Do not use alcohol, tobacco, or illegal drugs.

As a result of this healthy lifestyle, these individuals have a high resistance to disease. While all of these factors are important, I want to stress eliminating smoking and excessive drinking from your lifestyle. Smoking and alcohol abuse are two of the most detrimental things you can do to a human body.

Religion and Good Health   While I would be the last one to be considered a spiritual leader or advisor, I do know that individuals who follow a religious path tend to be healthier. According to many studies, people who practice a religion enjoy more good health.

In a recent survey of 1,473 people, Purdue University psychologist Kenneth Ferraro found that only 4 percent of people who went to church reported ill health, compared to 9 percent of those who did not. Only 26 percent of the "never attenders" reported excellent health, while 36 percent of the "weekly attenders" enjoyed excellent health.[1]

For the study, researchers looked at three aspects of religiosity: (1) frequency of attendance at church or synagogue; (2) the experiential aspect, or sense of feeling close to God; and (3) the specific creed or beliefs. Of these three factors, only active participation was found to make a big difference in the individual's health.

Why?

Researchers offered four possible explanations:

1. Religious people tend to avoid health-destructive behaviors like smoking, using drugs, or alcohol.
2. Religious activity provides a social network for coping and support that is quite different from our secular network.
3. Faith activates a special meaning and value system to help us make sense of the world and our lives.
4. Religious practice may modify our perception of the stress associated with physical suffering and give us hope.

I am not advocating any specific denomination; I am simply pointing out that people who pray and regularly participate in religious activities are apparently healthier. According to Fred Plummer, pastor of my church, Irvine United Church of Christ, regular religious activity provides our increasingly complicated lives with a much-needed source of balance. Interestingly, the ancient Arabic definition for the word "religion" was *balance*. Religion can help provide a balance between the inner and outer worlds.

I personally think that one of the big reasons people who practice religion are healthier has to do with the values that religion instills. In this enormously materialistic world we live in, we tend to view material possessions as higher in value than more admirable human traits such as honesty, compassion, loyalty, friendship, or fellowship. Most religions place these values in a larger perspective.

Smoking and Good Health   If you are a smoker, you absolutely must stop. Smoking is not a pleasure, it is a compulsive feeding of an addictive behavior, and is indeed the single most deleterious thing you can do to your health. It will increase the incidence of almost all degenerative diseases. Meantime, single-handedly, smoking will destroy your lungs.

SMOKING INCREASES YOUR RISK FOR:

> Cancer
> Heart disease
> Stroke
> Emphysema and bronchitis
> Other degenerative diseases

In my medical practice, I do not "help" people to stop smoking. I "help" them with the cravings and the discomfort once they have stopped. When that happens, I use whatever eases the discomfort. I use many tools, which include acupuncture, sedatives, nicotine patches or chewing gum, or any other "nonsmoking" aid. However, people have to stop smoking first before I become involved.

One tool is particularly useful. Most smokers would not light a cigarette if they knew there was an invisible man with a large stick right behind them who is there to bash them in the back of the head with their first puff. Sure, the refusal to feed the compulsive addiction would produce "discomfort." But a bash in the back of the head would be viewed as worse.

I recommend that smokers incorporate a nonviolent, negative incentive. Patients bet a substantial amount of money that they will not smoke for six weeks. (It is important to put a time limit on this program because most people feel that they can do anything for six weeks.)

For my staunch Republican patients, I suggest they bet $200 to $500 to be sent in their name to the Democratic general fund. For my Jewish patients, I will encourage them to bet from $200 to $500 to send to their least favorite organization, such as the PLO.

It is important that the amount of money they bet be within their capacity to pay, yet still be enough to inflict substantial pain. The agreement should be clearly articulated in writing, signed by the individual who plans to stop smoking, and signed by a witness.

The choices are then up to the individual. There are essentially three of them: (1) Not to smoke for the given time period; (2) to smoke and to send the money to their least desired "charity;" or (3) to smoke, deny it, and sell their soul to the devil. I generally do not allow individuals to sign the agreement until they have gone home and thought about it for at least one day.

At the end of six to eight weeks, most patients are well on their way to being nonsmokers. If they choose to smoke some at that time, fine—but they will always know they can stop again with a negative-incentive bet.

Alcohol and Good Health   Alcohol abuse has been identified as the greatest drug problem in the United States. It seriously affects the health of some 10 million people. While moderate drinking (no more than one or two drinks per sitting) has actually been shown to be associated with increased longevity, excessive drinking is strongly associated with five of our nation's leading causes of death:

Accidents
Cirrhosis of the liver
Pneumonia
Suicide
Murder

While there is no single effective treatment for alcoholism that will work successfully for everyone, studies have shown that most alcoholics can be rehabilitated. If you need help curbing your intake of alcohol, contact your local chapter of Alcoholics Anonymous, or ask your physician for a referral to a treatment center.

Also, as internationally known nutritionist Roger Williams has demonstrated for over thirty-five years, broad-spectrum nutritional supplementation can help reduce cravings and the amount of alcohol consumed. Although most of these studies were in animals, I have seen it do the same in humans.

Step 2: Become More Active

If the physiological benefits of physical activity could be put in a pill, you would have the most powerful anti-aging and health-promoting medication available. Research shows that for every single hour you exercise, you increase your longevity by two hours. Exercise improves just about everything about your constitution, from your mood to your intestinal function. Yes, believe it or not, exercise helps eliminate constipation. Just take a look at all the benefits of regular physical activity.

MUSCULOSKELETAL SYSTEM

> Increases muscle strength
> Increases flexibility of muscles and range of joint motion
> Produces stronger bones, ligaments, and tendons
> Lessens chance of injury
> Enhances posture, poise, and physique

HEART AND BLOOD VESSELS

> Lowers resting heart rate
> Strengthens heart function
> Lowers blood pressure
> Improves oxygen delivery throughout the body
> Increases blood supply to muscles
> Enlarges the arteries to the heart

BODILY PROCESSES

> Improves the way the body handles dietary fat
> Reduces heart disease risk
> Helps lower blood cholesterol and triglycerides
> Raises HDL, the "good" cholesterol
> Helps improve calcium deposits in bones
> Prevents osteoporosis
> Improves immune function
> Aids digestion and elimination
> Increases endurance and energy levels
> Promotes lean body mass, burns fat

MENTAL PROCESSES

> Provides a natural release from pent-up feelings
> Helps reduce tension and anxiety

Improves mental outlook and self-esteem
Helps relieve moderate depression
Improves the ability to handle stress
Stimulates improved mental function
Relaxes and improves sleep
Increases self-esteem

To achieve these benefits, exercise regularly. For exercise to be effective, it does not—and should not—feel like a burden. You do not have to become a "jock" to enjoy the benefits of regular physical activity. To help you make exercise a part of your life, focus on one key word: activity, not exercise.

Commit yourself to becoming more active—one day at a time. Choose from one to five of the activities in the following list. (Fill in your own preferred activity if it is not listed here. Do one activity for at least 20 minutes a day and preferably for an hour. Make it your goal to simply enjoy the activity. The important thing is to get your body moving enough to raise your pulse a bit above resting level.

Gardening	Tennis	Stationary bike
Bicycling	Jogging	Treadmill
Walking	Aerobics	Stairclimbing
Swimming	Dancing	Weight lifting
Golfing	Bowling	Heavy housecleaning

Walking may be the best choice for many people. Brisk walking is a great activity because it works the muscles of the lower body, the largest muscles in the body.

If you are going to walk on a regular basis, I strongly urge you to buy a pair of high-quality walking or jogging shoes. The technology used to improve the quality of these shoes has certainly made walking and slow jogging safer and more enjoyable.

And why not make your daily walk a social event? Locate one or two people in your neighborhood with whom you would enjoy walking. You will certainly be more regular if you have made a commitment to others than if you depend solely on your own motivation. Commit to walking three to five mornings or afternoons each week. Increase the exercise duration from an initial ten minutes to at least 30 minutes.

Once you can comfortably do 30 minutes of brisk walking, increase your pace. You can do this by walking for 5 minutes, then breaking into a slow trot for 5 minutes, and then alternating walking and slow trotting for the rest of the 30 minutes. This will obviously increase the distance you cover, as well as the amount of exercise. You can increase the intensity of this walking exercise by gradually increasing the amount of time you jog.

Step 3: Take a Multiple Vitamin-Mineral Formula

Vitamin and mineral supplements are an integral part of the treatments offered at the Whitaker Wellness Institute. However, they are not the main focus. All the supplements in the world cannot compensate for an unhealthy lifestyle, poor diet, and lack of physical activity. Supplements are just that—a supplement to the diet, physical activity, and lifestyle program. They are not the primary healing factors.

As our leaders in Washington are debating methods of cutting our "disease management cost," they would benefit from suggestions on how to prevent these diseases that are costing so much. One way that I see is to encourage Americans to take vitamin and mineral supplements.

Many people think of cost when they think of supplements. But the modest sum of $20 to $50 a month provides some remarkable health benefits.

Americans and Supplements

When we look in the mirror, we probably see ourselves as much more complex than the people who tempt us with junk food might want us to be. In fact, over 100 million Americans regularly take dietary supplements, despite the fact that many "experts" do not actively endorse the practice. Despite this professional stance, 98 percent of medical doctors take supplements themselves.

What has led so many of us to take it upon ourselves to start taking nutritional supplements? The best answer is that people are talking to each other. The nutrition movement is a popular, grass roots movement. One person begins taking supplements and begins to feel better. Some nagging health concerns begin to resolve. Maybe someone's energy increases. This person shares that experience with friends or family members. Some of these people start taking supplements. They benefit, and share the information. In this way, movements grow.

Most of us know that we are not getting all the nutritional value we need from our diets, or that we have nutritional habits that could be improved. We know that our lives are stressful, or that we are regularly exposed to conditions in our environment which strain our health. We talk to each other. We hear about taking supplements. It makes sense. Common sense. This exchange between friends provides the momentum which has led 100 million people to supplements.

A tremendous amount of research supports this common sense. The United States government has sponsored a number of comprehensive studies looking at the American diet. Among these are the Ten-State Nutrition Survey, HANES I and HANES II, and diverse

USDA nationwide food consumption studies. The results are conclusive: Most Americans consume a diet that is inadequate in nutritional value. In some selected age groups, for certain nutrients, just 20 percent of the individuals consumed nutrients at Recommended Daily Allowance (RDA) levels. Roughly 50 percent of the U.S. population shows at least marginal deficiencies.[2]

Using the RDA as the marker is inappropriate for many individuals, if it is health and not simply fear of disease that motivates us. Making good health the primary goal is the best way to become healthy!

Many experts, practical as they may be, tend to become somewhat theoretical and even idealistic when talking about supplements. Media accounts of expert debates over the use of supplements regularly include a comment that "people should be able to get all the nutrients they need from food." Therefore, they conclude, supplements are not necessary. Yet all available evidence shows that the chances of any one of us consuming a diet that even meets the RDAs are extremely rare; most Americans do not even come close. A vitamin and mineral supplement is an important aid to our nutritional habits.

The nutritional deficiencies most people have do not tend to show up as specific diseases. In our culture, diseases such as scurvy, which results from a lack of vitamin C, are extremely rare. But signs of a lack of proper nutrients do frequently show up in patient health profiles. Clues may be fatigue or lethargy. Some individuals may feel that they lack a sense of well-being, or find difficulty in concentration. Symptoms are often vague. Physicians who do not have a nutrition orientation may simply pass off such conditions as being all in the patient's mind, and consider them untreatable.

Many other physicians and researchers, however, do recognize that nutrition may be a significant factor. They use the term *subclinical* to refer to nutrient deficiencies which are marginal. Marginal vitamin C deficiency, for instance, is thought to be common. Laboratory diagnosis of such deficiencies usually involves detailed and expensive dietary analysis. The tests can be far more expensive than the cost of an annual supply of the lacking nutrient for which the patient is being tested.

The RDA and the Role of Nutrients

Since 1941, the Food and Nutrition Board of the National Research Council has established Recommended Daily Allowances (RDA) for vitamins and minerals. These RDAs have unfortunately provided a false framing to the debate over the nutritional needs of individuals.

The original goal of the guidelines was to reduce the incidence of diseases linked to severe deficiencies. These include scurvy, as noted above. Deficiency of niacin is linked to pellagra. Low vitamin B1 has been linked to beriberi.

The RDAs don't reflect modern scientific understanding of what levels promote optimum health. The RDAs were designed for groups, and we know that individuals vary widely in their nutritional requirements. The Food and Nutrition Board has stated simply: "Individuals with special nutritional needs are not covered by RDAs."[3]

In truth, a growing percentage of people fall into a "special nutritional needs" category—smokers, for instance, and drinkers; individuals who work or live in conditions where they are exposed to toxic chemicals; people whose lives are full of stress. Progressive thinkers are looking at the role of diets that are full of highly processed foods and food additives. The ambient chemicals in our industrialized society are also known to interfere with nutrient function.

How many of us are not in at least one of these categories?

The Food and Nutrition Board is only slowly acknowledging these realities, and now acknowledges that smokers need twice as much Vitamin C as nonsmokers. It hasn't yet looked at the uptake of other nutrients with which smoking interferes. Their recommendations were created 40 to 60 years ago; RDAs do not adequately take into consideration modern environmental and lifestyle factors, typical of most lives, which are known to destroy vitamins and bind minerals.

RDAs do provide an important public service in defining the levels of nutrients we need to prevent full-blown deficiency diseases. Yet the RDAs give no guidance about the "optimal" levels of nutrients a person should consume if the goal is health, and not merely the absence of major diseases. Common sense suggests that if optimal health is the goal, the level of intake of these nutrients should be higher.

A tremendous amount of scientific research, in fact, indicates that this is the case. Such research is especially clear on the so-called *antioxidant* nutrients. These include Vitamin C and Vitamin E, beta-carotene, and selenium. This growing body of research provides an important step in taking the realities of modern life into account when setting recommended nutrient levels. We still have much to learn regarding the optimum level of nutrients.

Vitamin and Mineral Formulas

While additional research will help us gain more specific understanding of what optimal nutrient levels may be, the evidence is clear that taking a well-designed vitamin-mineral formula is a sensible addition to our daily regimens.

Each of the vitamins plays diverse, important roles in human health. Vitamins work with enzymes as catalysts, speeding up the making or breaking of the chemical bonds that join molecules together. These chemical reactions are necessary for our body functions. The connection between vitamin intake and fatigue and lethargy is evident in the importance these substances have in energy production.

All totaled, there are thirteen known vitamins. Generally, they are classified into those which are water-soluble (vitamin C and the B vitamins) and those which are fat-soluble (vitamins A, D, E, and K).

A good multiple vitamin-mineral formula will also meet mineral needs. We know that optimal human nutrition requires twenty-two different minerals. Like vitamins, minerals play diverse roles. They are involved in the composition of our bones and blood. They are required to maintain normal functioning of our cells. And minerals function along with vitamins as components of body enzymes.

Taking a high-quality multiple vitamin-mineral supplement provides all of the known vitamins and minerals. It serves as a foundation upon which to build. Dr. Roger Williams, a premier biochemist, states that healthy people should use multiple vitamin and mineral supplements as an "insurance formula" against possible deficiency. This does not mean that a deficiency will occur in the absence of the vitamin and mineral supplement, any more than not having fire insurance means that your house is going to burn down. But given the enormous differences from person to person, and the varied mechanisms of vitamin and mineral actions, supplementation with a multiple formula seems to make sense.

The recommendations in Table 2.1 for the daily intake levels of vitamins and minerals are designed to provide an optimum intake range in selecting a high-quality multiple. In the Whitaker Wellness Program, additional levels of vitamin C, magnesium, and potassium are recommended.

There are a number of very good multiple vitamin and mineral formulas available at health food stores that are far superior to your standard one-a-day type multiple formulas available at pharmacies and drug stores. I recently took a stroll through our local health food store and found the following formulas to meet my satisfaction: Biovital (Enzymatic Therapy), Advanced Nutritional System (Rainbow Light), Source of Life (Nature's Plus), Multi-4-EF (Kal), and Mega Pak (Nature's Life).

At the Whitaker Wellness Institute, we use a formula called Forward, which I created specifically for my patients. For information on Forward and other products, call Healthy Directions at 1-800-722-8008.

Affordability   Many people ask whether they can afford to begin taking a multiple vitamin-mineral formula. They think not of their long-range health benefits, but of the immediate cost of taking supplements.

Table 2.1 Daily Optimal Supplementation Range for Adults

Vitamins	Daily Dosage
Vitamin A (retinol)	5,000 IU*
Vitamin A (from beta-carotene)	5,000–25,000 IU
Vitamin D	100–400 IU
Vitamin E (d-alpha tocopherol)	400–800 IU
Vitamin K (phytonadione) 6	60–300 mcg†
Vitamin C (ascorbic acid)	100–250 mg
Vitamin B1 (thiamin)	10–100 mg
Vitamin B2 (riboflavin)	10–100 mg
Niacin	10–100 mg
Niacinamide	10–30 mg
Vitamin B6 (pyridoxine)	25–100 mg
Biotin	100–300 mcg
Pantothenic acid	25–100 mg
Folic acid	200–400 mcg
Vitamin B12	200–400 mcg
Choline	10–100 mg
Inositol	10–100 mg

Minerals	
Boron	1–2 mg
Calcium	250–750 mg
Chromium	200–400 mcg
Copper	1–2 mg
Iodine	50–150 mcg
Iron	15–30 mg
Magnesium	250–500 mg
Manganese	10–15 mg
Molybdenum	10–25 mcg
Potassium	200–500 mg
Selenium	100–200 mcg
Silica	200–1,000 mcg
Vanadium	50–100 mcg
Zinc	15–30 mg

*IU = International Units

†mcg = microgram

Let me ask you this: How much are you currently spending on prescription and over-the-counter drugs each month? How much money could you save if you were able to get off these medications? My guess is that the amount is significant. Most prescription drugs are expensive. And what about surgical procedures? Replacement of ear tubes in a child can run from $1,500 to $2,000. Coronary bypass operations usually cost over $40,000. How much are your co-payments and deductibles costing you for preventable problems?

We need to ask an important question in this country. How much healthcare money would be saved if more Americans simply took a high-quality multiple vitamin and mineral supplement? Our views of health and disease are so clouded by the perspectives of the existing disease-management forces that this question may seem a little simple. Yet, results of recent studies indicate that by taking adequate levels of vitamin E, vitamin C, selenium, and magnesium the rate of heart disease could be reduced by 50 percent. This alone would result in savings of over $50 billion per year.

Fifty billion dollars buys a lot of multiple vitamin-mineral formulas. And this represents savings from just one health problem. Chances are you are already spending a lot on your healthcare needs. Any way you look at it, taking a multiple vitamin-mineral formula is going to reduce your healthcare costs.

Using money diverted from current or anticipated direct medical costs is just one way to pay for nutritional supplements. You can also support a good supplement program by using some of the money you are currently spending on things that rob you of health. According to *The 1992 Top-Ten Almanac* by Michael Robbins (Workman Publishing), the top ten items purchased in our grocery stores, ranked by dollar volume, are:

1. Marlboro cigarettes
2. Coca Cola Classic
3. Pepsi Cola
4. Kraft Processed Cheese
5. Diet Coke
6. Campbell's Soup
7. Budweiser beer
8. Tide detergent
9. Folger's coffee
10. Winston cigarettes

And we wonder why we are sick. Does your body run on caffeine and nicotine? The top ten list contains four caffeinated beverages and two brands of cigarettes.

A recent study demonstrated that men taking 400 milligrams or more of vitamin C per day had 50 percent less fatal heart attacks and lived six years longer than men taking 100 milligrams or less. (For reference, the RDA for vitamin C is 60 milligrams.[4] Will Marlboro cigarettes or Coke do that?

Antioxidants like vitamin E, beta-carotene, and selenium have also been shown to reduce your risk of heart disease and other degenerative diseases, including cancer and cataracts.[3] Can Budweiser do this?

The scientific evidence supporting the benefits of generous amounts of B-complex supplementation would fill a library. These nutrients, taken as a supplement, ensure that your metabolism is up to optimum function. Is this what you get from a Pepsi, a candy bar, or a chocolate chip cookie, which are loaded with sugars and oxidized fats?

We have been conditioned in this country to spend our money on items that rob us of our health. "Happiness" is swigging some dark, sugary cola that depletes your body of nutrients. And we believe it. Three of the top ten items are colas!

Frito-Lay recently launched a smaller corn chip. Their advertising budget for this product is close to $100 million. The nutritional value of the new chip is a net negative. Yet, through advertising you will come to view it first as "something new," and essential for you to try. Imagine, a $100 million earmarked to sell a fried corn chip with minus nutritional value.

Who, on the other hand, is going to spend that kind of money to convince you of the value of nutritional supplements? As detailed in Chapter 1, the FDA has determined that it is illegal for nutritional supplement manufacturers to "sell" you their products. If a vitamin company used the results of studies showing that vitamin C reduces heart disease to promote their product, the FDA would likely raid the company. With guns drawn, the FDA would seize the product on the grounds that the company was "making a drug claim" for the nutrient. It doesn't matter if the claim happens to be true.

We Americans pride ourselves on our intelligence and independence. But when it comes to junk food, we need to take a new look in the mirror. We are all too easily convinced by ad slogans. We rarely think of the money we are wasting. Then we wonder if we can afford nutrients that could possibly save our lives.

It is imperative that you free up some money to improve your health and prolong your life. A high-potency multiple vitamin-mineral supplement containing the recommended levels of nutrients may cost $20 to $30 for a month's supply, roughly a dollar a day.

Let's look at some of the ways this money can be freed up. One candy bar is 50 cents. A 9-ounce bag of potato chips is $1.59. Any convenience store or vending machine junk snack runs 75 cents to a dollar. That's almost three dollars, right there, and we're talking loose change. I know a lady who was hooked on one of the colas. She drank ten a day. It wasn't until she realized that she was spending almost $2,000 a year on soda that she had a desire to stop.

The bottom line is that anyone can afford nutritional supplements. In fact, you cannot afford to be without them. This is money well spent. The only risk is that you could increase your health, live with more vitality, and prevent future healthcare costs.

Many people find out that good health is addicting. They begin to respond to a different sort of advertising. This is the advertising campaign of their bodies and minds, responding to the health steps that have been undertaken. Choosing what is good for you becomes easier as you follow all the steps in the Whitaker Wellness Program.

Step 4: Take Extra Antioxidant Nutrients

The natural health movement has been far ahead of conventional medical opinion regarding the value of antioxidants. In recent years, increasing numbers of mainstream news accounts, and even public service advertising, have brought the terms *antioxidant* and *free radical* to general public attention. These terms are now in the vocabulary of most health-minded individuals.

I can recall the mixture of pleasure and distaste with which I greeted mainstream acceptance of this nutritional understanding. Pleasure, because it was good to see this knowledge reaching a broader audience. Distaste, because the "experts" continued to espouse an essentially political position that downplayed the importance of supplements to achieve appropriate levels of these nutrients. The FDA continues to refuse to acknowledge that antioxidant supplements can be good for our health.

Free radicals have been shown to be responsible for the initiation of many diseases, including heart disease and cancer, the two main killers of Americans.[5] Free radicals are molecules which are highly reactive. They bind to, and destroy, body components. The damage is called "oxidative." This is the process which makes us age.

The last thing a free radical wants to meet as it is going about its destructive business inside the body is an antioxidant. Antioxidant nutrients, which include selenium, beta-carotene, vitamin E, and vitamin C, are compounds which help protect us against free-radical damage. These agents are known to be effective against cancer, heart disease, and other degenerative diseases. Antioxidants are also thought to slow down the aging process.

Free Radicals

Efforts to discover an optimal level for antioxidant intake must take into account the two types of sources of free radicals. Normal metabolic processes like energy production, efforts to detoxify, and mechanisms which stimulate immune defenses spin off these agents. Many free radicals are a part of healthy cellular processes. Even the most pristine existence will produce free radicals.

However, the choices an individual makes and general environmental conditions can dramatically alter free-radical activity. A smoker inhales high levels of free radicals, which deplete key antioxidant nutrients like vitamin C and beta-carotene. Controllable contributors to free-radical activity are alcohol and fried foods. Other sources are difficult for us to control: solvents, formaldehyde, pesticides, air pollutants, and ionizing radiation.

Taken together, all these sources create what is called the free-radical "load." For individuals exposed to these factors, more antioxidant support is needed.

Taking supplemental antioxidants is a classic example of what Dr. Roger Williams meant when he said vitamins are an "insurance policy." As is evident from the list of factors producing free radicals, all of us living in the world today are at high risk, due to ambient environmental factors. The most cost-effective insurance policy, in this case, is to take additional vitamin C and vitamin E, along with your high-quality multiple vitamin-mineral formula. The known value of consuming adequate levels of these two vitamins is great. And how much is still unknown? In how many additional "undiscovered" ways are these vitamins essential to good health, or useful in effectively combating disease? Many significant health benefits are associated with these two amazing agents.

Vitamin C

The most publicized antioxidant vitamin is vitamin C. Numerous experimental, clinical, and population studies have shown positive results from increased vitamin C intake: reducing cancer rates; protecting against cigarette smoke and air pollution; boosting immunity; and increasing life expectancy.[6]

As is true of the many-faceted value of most nutrients, this vitamin is absolutely essential to our very being. The active tissues of the body respond particularly well to large concentrations of vitamin C. The level of vitamin C in the blood is about 0.5 milligram per deciliter, whereas in the adrenal and pituitary glands, the level is 100 times higher. In the liver, spleen, and lens of the eye it is concentrated by at least a factor of twenty. In order for these concentrations to be maintained in these tissues, the body has to generate enormous amounts of energy to pull vitamin C out of the blood against this tremendous gradient. By taking large amounts of vitamin C, you can assist your body in its attempt to concentrate vitamin C into active tissue, by reducing the gradient. Studies have shown that in order to increase the vitamin C content of some of these tissues (such as the lens of the eye), dosages of at least 1,000 milligrams at a time are required.

Lest we forget, human beings are unique; we lack the capacity to produce our own vitamin C. Almost all other animals are capable of manufacturing vitamin C upon demand. Other warm-blooded mammals manufacture large quantities of vitamin C each day. If we translated the amount these animals produce into human terms, it would be in the magnitude of 5,000 to 7,000 milligrams daily. When animals are under stress, they produce substantially higher amounts.

To debunk the myth that vitamin and mineral supplements only create "healthy urine," remember that many beneficial substances ingested by mouth are often excreted in the urine. For example, if you had a serious infection and were given an antibiotic which later showed up in the urine, does this mean that you didn't need the antibiotic?

Immune Function   Considerable biochemical evidence shows the vital role vitamin C plays in many immune mechanisms. It appears in high concentrations in white blood cells, particularly in lymphocytes, which points to the value of taking increased amounts of vitamin C during infections. If the vitamin is not replenished, a relative deficiency will ensue. Many positive clinical and experimental trials have shown its efficacy.

Collagen   Another essential process in which Vitamin C is critically important is the manufacture of collagen, the main protein substance in the human body. Collagen is critical for cartilage, tendons, and other connective tissue. Thus vitamin C is important in wound repair, in preventing easy bruising, and in healthy gums.

Some of vitamin C's known value in this regard has come from the understanding of scurvy. Symptoms of this disease, due to vitamin C deficiency, are extensive bruising, poor wound healing, and bleeding gums. Scurvy sufferers are marked by tendencies toward hysteria and depression, as well as infections.

Stress   Research shows that stress increases the amount of vitamin C excreted through the urinary tract. The causes of the stress can be physical, for example, cigarette smoke, pollutants, and allergens. Or the cause can be elusive, due to psychological, emotional, or other obscure physiological factors. Regardless of the cause of the stress, its effect on our bodies is the same. Increased vitamin C intake during such times can compensate for this loss.[7]

Other Associations   The list of conditions where increased vitamin C is recommended includes high blood pressure, hepatitis, diabetes, cataracts, high cholesterol levels, and allergies. Not surprisingly, considering its long list of benefits, increased vitamin C levels are also associated with increased life expectancy.

Optimal Levels   A highly politicized debate rages over the level of vitamin C that is required by humans. The RDA is 60 milligrams for adults. Dr. Linus Pauling and his followers believe that two to nine grams per day is optimal and that this amount should go up in times of stress.[8] The low RDA simply cannot be explained by even the most restrictive reading of the research on this vital nutrient.

In addition to eating foods rich in vitamin C—like broccoli, fruits, bell peppers, and other fresh vegetables—I recommend that my patients take an additional 5,000 milligrams of vitamin C daily, in divided doses (usually three), rather than all at once. Around my house, we keep an inexpensive bottle of 500-milligram tablets, and I simply take a half-handful several times during the day.

Vitamin C can cause gas and diarrhea if too large a dose is taken at first. These side effects will stop if the dosage is reduced, then built back up gradually, and divided into two or three doses a day. In fact, the most common method for gauging how much vitamin C you need is based on when you feel gastrointestinal symptoms. Some experts recommend taking an amount of vitamin C slightly below the level that causes these symptoms. This practice is referred to as taking vitamin C to "bowel tolerance."

Vitamin E

Vitamin E is required by most animal species, including humans. The vitamin was discovered in 1922 when rats fed a purified diet without vitamin E became unable to reproduce. When wheat germ oil, which contains high levels of vitamin E, was added to their diet, fertility was restored. For this reason, when vitamin E was originally isolated, it was called the "anti-sterility" vitamin.

Alpha-tocopherol is the chemical name for the most active form of vitamin E. The term *tocopherol* comes from the Greek words *tokos,* which means "offspring," and *phero,* which means "to bear." Hence, tocopherol literally means "to bear children."

Vitamin E functions primarily as an antioxidant in protecting against damage to cell membranes. Without vitamin E, the cells of the body would be quite susceptible to damage. Nerve cells would be particularly vulnerable. Severe vitamin E deficiency is quite rare, but there are a number of conditions where low levels of vitamin E have been reported. These include acne, anemia, some cancers, gallstones, Lou Gehrig's disease, muscular dystrophy, Parkinson's disease, and Alzheimer's disease.[9]

Vitamin E supplementation has been shown to exert a protective effect in many common health conditions, including heart disease, cancer, stroke, painful leg cramps, fibrocystic breast disease, cataracts, and viral infections.

The clinical applications of vitamin E are quite extensive. Some of the studies were discussed in Chapter 1. In addition, low vitamin E levels were shown, in a recent large population study in Europe, to be a far better predictive factor of heart disease than the factors most people associated with heart disease. High blood cholesterol was predictive 29 percent of the time and high blood pressure 25 percent of the time. But low levels of vitamin E in the blood was shown to be predictive of a heart attack almost 70 percent of the time.[10]

As an important antioxidant, vitamin E helps support many body functions. Vitamin E protects the lining of the artery wall from oxidized cholesterol particles. This protection stops the process of atherosclerosis. In fact, the antioxidant properties of vitamin E protect all cells of the body from free radicals.

I used to recommend taking an extra 400 IU of vitamin E daily. However, more recent studies have convinced me to increase my recommended dosage to 800 to 1,200 IU per day. Make sure the vitamin E is natural d-alpha-tocopherol. Vitamin E, even though it is fat-soluble, is extremely well tolerated. Even at these high doses it does not have side effects.

I also recommend consuming more polyunsaturated fats, like flax oil and fish oils. The more polyunsaturated fats consumed, the greater the risk that they will be damaged. Vitamin E prevents this damage. So as the intake of polyunsaturated fatty acids increases, so does the need for vitamin E.

Step 5: Take Extra Magnesium and Potassium

Magnesium and potassium are the most important minerals within the individual cells of the body. Of these two, magnesium may be the more important. Outside of the antioxidant nutrients, I believe that magnesium may be the most important nutrient for supplementation.

Magnesium and potassium, along with sodium and chloride, are electrolytes, mineral salts that can conduct electricity when they are dissolved in water. They are so intricately related they are most often discussed together in nutrition textbooks. Electrolytes are always found in pairs; a positive molecule like sodium or potassium is always accompanied by a negative molecule like chloride. Electrolytes function in the maintenance of:

Water balance and distribution
Acid-base balance
Muscle and nerve cell function
Heart function
Kidney and adrenal function

Magnesium and potassium are involved in many cellular functions including energy production, protein formation, and cellular replication. A deficiency of either magnesium or potassium is characterized by a host of symptoms. These include mental confusion, irritability, weakness, heart disturbance, problems in nerve conduction and muscle contraction, muscle cramps, loss of appetite, insomnia, and a predisposition to stress.

Magnesium and potassium deficiency are extremely common in the geriatric population and in women during the premenstrual period. Deficiencies are often the result of factors which reduce absorption or increase secretion. These include high calcium intake, alcohol, surgery, diuretics, liver disease, kidney disease, and the use of oral contraceptives.

Magnesium

The low magnesium levels in the diets of most Americans represent a clash between ideals and practical realities. Most conventionally trained dietitians point to the abundance of magnesium found in whole foods. Green leafy vegetables, seeds, whole grains, nuts, legumes, and tofu are all excellent magnesium sources. Because magnesium is so abundant, dietitians tend to assume that Americans are getting enough of this nutrient.

The realities don't match the ideal. Studies show that healthy adults average between 143 and 266 milligrams of magnesium per day. This is far below even the RDA, which has been set at 350 milligrams for adult males and 300 milligrams for adult females. A more precise method of establishing a recommended level, based on body weight (6 milligrams per kilogram of body weight), is recommended by many nutritional experts. This produces somewhat higher recommendations. Roughly 300 milligrams is appropriate for a person just over 100 pounds; nearly 550 milligrams would be recommended for a person who weighs 200 pounds.

Why, if magnesium is so abundant, are average daily intakes so low? A part of the answer is that commonly eaten foods which are very healthy are actually low in magnesium. Examples are fish and most of our favorite fruits. The rest of the answer is that most Americans are eating far too many processed foods, and too much meat and dairy products. Refining processes remove most of the magnesium, and dairy and meat are low in magnesium.

The health risks associated with low magnesium are many. Our susceptibility to many health problems increases. These range from insomnia, PMS, and menstrual cramps, to kidney stones, heart disease, and cancer. In two areas, the preventive value of adequate magnesium is widely accepted.

Kidney Stones   Magnesium helps prevent the formation of kidney stones, by increasing the solubility of calcium in the urine. Studies have shown that supplemental calcium prevents recurrence of kidney stones. Anyone who has passed a kidney stone, or even heard a story of the excruciating pain this usually causes, knows the value of prevention.

The Heart   I have noted the importance of magnesium, in general, in the body's energy production. For the heart, this relates to the ability of the heart muscle to contract. Very low levels of magnesium have been found in individuals who suddenly die of heart attacks. The magnesium deficiency may produce a spasm in the coronary arteries which in turn reduces the flow of blood and oxygen to the heart. Magnesium deficiencies increase susceptibility to high blood pressure. Conversely, supplementing magnesium has been shown to offer important protection against cardiovascular disease.[11]

Dosage   How much magnesium do I recommend? At least 1,000 milligrams of elemental magnesium. The best forms of supplemental magnesium are magnesium aspartate or magnesium citrate. Absorption studies indicate that magnesium is easily absorbed orally when it is bound to aspartate or citrate. In addition, both of these compounds may also help fight off fatigue. Aspartate feeds into the Krebs cycle, the final common pathway for the conversion of glucose, fatty acids, and amino acids to chemical energy (ATP). Citrate is itself a component of the Krebs cycle. Krebs cycle components such as aspartate, citrate, fumarate, malate, and succinate usually provide a better mineral chelate for minerals. In other words, minerals chelated to the Krebs cycle intermediates are better absorbed, utilized, and tolerated, compared to inorganic or relatively insoluble mineral salts. Magnesium chloride, oxide, or carbonate are the common mineral salt versions.[12]

   Several major suppliers of nutritional products offer magnesium bound to either aspartate, citrate, or other Krebs cycle intermediates: Solgar, TwinLab, and Natrol. Take additional magnesium from this source, in addition to your multiple vitamin-mineral formula, to achieve a total daily intake of 1,000 milligrams of elemental magnesium.

Potassium

Even physicians who scoff at most nutritional recommendations will warn their patients against eating too much salt. Most people now know that too much salt has something to do with heart disease.

   Unfortunately, such advice gives the patient only a part of the picture. Human physiology is complex and any patient needs an overall action plan for dietary changes and health. Studies which have associated salt with heart disease and cancer look at more than just salt. The critical concern is the potassium to sodium ratio (K:Na).

Most Americans have a potassium-to-sodium ratio which is less than 1:2. In simple English, people are ingesting twice as much salt as potassium. Numerous studies have shown that this skewed ratio in the American diet is a major contributor to cancer and heart disease. Reversing the ratio is protective against these killers and is known to be therapeutic against high blood pressure.[13]

Merely reversing the potassium-to-salt ratio in the American diet is not enough. A ratio of greater than 5:1 in favor of potassium is recommended by most researchers. And this may not yet be optimal. Most vegetables and fruits have a potassium-to-salt ratio of more than 50:1. If a diet high in fresh fruits and vegetables is analyzed, the K:Na ratio can go higher than 100:1.

How did this ratio in the American diet get so out-of-whack? First, let's look at "pass the salt": sodium chloride. Sodium as a naturally occurring constituent of food accounts for just 5 percent of the total salt we eat. In most cases, this is all of the sodium that the body requires.

"Hold the salt," then, is clearly a good recommendation. However, salt as a condiment still amounts to only another 5 percent of our total salt intake. Nearly half (45 percent) is added in the cooking of foods. And another, less visible, 45 percent is added in food processing.

The near-omnipresence of salt in the customary American diet requires a number of "defensive" strategies to keep our potassium-to-sodium ratio in line. Read food labels carefully. Lower the amount of salt used in cooking. Stop eating heavily salted foods like potato chips, pretzels, cheese, pickled foods, and cured meats.

But the best strategy with salt, as with so many habit changes, is not a defensive one. The best strategy is an offensive, or proactive, one. Let your taste buds awaken from their dull, salty numbness. Get to know the unsalted flavor of foods. Try expanding your culinary herb selection. If you want a salt-like flavor, experiment with some of the natural, flavorful salt substitutes available.

Dosage   To bring the potassium-to-salt ratio into line, make sure you are regularly eating legumes, bananas, and citrus fruits. These are potassium-rich foods. If your body's potassium requirements are not met through diet, supplementation is essential. Athletes and the elderly must pay particular attention to their potassium intake. These habits will help bring your potassium-to-salt ratio into its protective, positive ratio.

The RDA for potassium has been set at 1.9 to 5.9 grams. Physicians who prescribe potassium commonly do so in the form of potassium salts. The amount will range from 1.9 to 3 grams daily.

Unfortunately, potassium in this form can cause a number of side effects, from nausea, vomiting, and diarrhea to ulcers.

In an effort to limit such consequences, some manufacturers of potassium supplements have taken a hint from nature. Because side effects are not seen when potassium is increased through food sources alone, manufacturers are now making natural food-based potassium products.

Most people can handle any excess of potassium. Yet for some groups too much can be extremely harmful. Excessive potassium is of particular concern to individuals with kidney disease. In these people, potassium toxicity can cause heart disturbances and other problematic symptoms. These individuals must pay close attention to the dietary instructions of their doctors.

There are a number of high-quality, food-based potassium supplements on the market. Enzymatic Therapy distributes a product in pill form called Bio-K+, which provides food-grade potassium. This formula includes concentrates from oranges, bananas, and sugar cane juice, along with potassium citrate and chloride. The sugar has been removed from the cane juice. One tablet with meals can help boost potassium levels considerably.

Another good potassium supplement is E-mergen-C from Alacer. This product is a mixture of vitamin C, potassium, other minerals, and B vitamins in the form of a powder. The powder is contained in a packet that can be emptied into a glass and then filled up with about six ounces of water. Two packets a day provides 2,000 milligrams of vitamin C and 400 milligrams of potassium. The potassium is complexed with citrate, ascorbate (vitamin C), tartrate, and aspartate.

Increasing potassium intake can often help leg cramps and sciatica. In talking with my friend and colleague Dr. Michael Murray, he reported a case of a gentleman (John H.) who had sciatica for over 23 years. The patient was very educated about the role of potassium in nerve function. Careful dietary assessment indicated that he was already consuming about 5,000 milligrams of potassium per day. Dr. Murray felt this was still not adequate and recommended the consumption of 24 to 32 ounces of fresh vegetable juice daily, along with three tablets of Bio-K+ three times daily to boost his potassium intake to over 8,000 milligrams each day. Within two weeks of following this recommendation, John's sciatica pain completely disappeared—and has remained so.

Step 6: Take an Omega-3 Oil Supplement

A diet high in fat has been strongly linked to heart disease, stroke, cancer, and other diseases. However, upon closer examination of the data, it becomes clear that the culprit is not fat in general, but saturated fat. Saturated fats are typically animal fats that are semi-solid to solid at room temperature. Vegetable fats are liquid at room temperature and are referred to as unsaturated fats, or oils.

A diet low in saturated fat, but high in unsaturated fat, has actually been shown to exert a protective effect against the above-mentioned diseases. Another way of stating this is that when the amount of animal foods in the diet is low and the amount of plant foods rich in polyunsaturated fats is high, the rate of these diseases is low. Good dietary sources of polyunsaturated fats include vegetable oils, seeds, nuts, and some legumes.

Essential Fatty Acids

The human body cannot function properly without two polyunsaturated fats. These are linoleic and alpha-linolenic acid. These fatty acids are referred to as essential fatty acids because they truly are essential to normal cell structure and body function. Many of the beneficial effects of a diet rich in plant foods are a result of the low levels of saturated fat and the relatively higher levels of essential fatty acids.

Both linoleic acid and alpha-linolenic acid function as components of nerve cells, cell membranes, and hormone-like substances known as prostaglandins. But they have some basic differences, which researchers are increasingly finding valuable. Although both are 18-carbon-length fatty acids, alpha-linolenic acid has three unsaturated bonds, while linoleic acid has only two. The differing location of the first unsaturated bond gives them the more common names by which they are frequently called. Alpha-linolenic acid's first unsaturated bond occurs at the third carbon. It is known as an omega-3 oil. Linoleic acid's first double bond is at the sixth carbon and is an omega-6 oil.

Because of these differences, linoleic acid and alpha-linolenic acid form entirely different prostaglandins. Researchers and physicians are finding that by manipulating the type of dietary oils, body function can sometimes be dramatically altered. In some cases, disease can be treated by this manipulation. The omega-3 oils are showing the greatest promise in this regard.

SOME CONDITIONS IMPROVED BY OMEGA-3 OILS[14]

High cholesterol levels
Stroke and heart attack
Angina
High blood pressure
Rheumatoid arthritis

Multiple sclerosis
Psoriasis and eczema
Cancer (prevention and treatment)

Medicinal Oils

Several plant-derived oils, as well as fish oils, are being used for medicinal purposes. Evening primrose, black currant, and borage oil all contain gamma-linolenic acid (GLA). This is an omega-6 fatty acid that eventually acts as a precursor to some favorable prostaglandins. Although these agents are quite popular as supplements, the research on GLA products is not as strong as the research on omega-3 oils. Because GLA can be formed from linoleic acid, it is difficult to determine to what extent the effects are due to GLA vs. linoleic acid. A further complication of the issue is that most sources of GLA are much richer in linoleic acid than in GLA. For example, evening primrose oil contains only 9 percent GLA, but 72 percent linoleic acid.

In most instances, high linoleic acid-containing oils, like safflower and soy oil, may provide nearly as much benefit as GLA products. And they do this at a fraction of the cost. The only exceptions to this generalization may be in individuals with diabetes and people who cannot form GLA from linoleic acid. GLA supplementation in diabetics has been shown to improve nerve function and prevent diabetic nerve disease.[15]

However, rather than simply relying on common vegetable oils, it appears that most individuals would be better off supplementing their diet with omega-3 oils. According to Harvard's Alexander Leaf, M.D., and other medical experts, our hunter-gatherer ancestors had a ratio of omega-6 to omega-3 fatty acids of five or six to one.[16] This ratio appears to be optimal for our bodies. The ratio of omega-6 to omega-3 fatty acids in the average American's diet is about 24 to 1. By increasing your intake of omega-3 fatty acids (by taking fish oil or flax oil supplements), you can achieve a more favorable ratio. Reversing this ratio can have long-lasting, positive effects on many illnesses, including heart disease, arthritis, stroke, migraine headaches, and other serious and even fatal maladies.

Although most of the research on omega-3 oils have featured fish oils rich in eicosapentaenoic acid (EPA), EPA is manufactured in the body from alpha-linolenic acid. This is the primary essential fatty acid in flax oil. Compared to fish oil, flax oil contains more than twice the amount of omega-3 oil. It is a good source for linoleic acid as well.

Lignans   Flax oil may offer other benefits over fish oil and GLA products. Flaxseeds are the most abundant source of lignans, special compounds that are demonstrating some impressive health benefits: relief of menopausal hot flashes, as well as anticancer, antibacterial, anti-fungal, and antiviral activity.[17]

Perhaps the most significant action of lignans is their anticancer effect. A substantial amount of research has shown that flaxseed lignans are changed by the bacteria in the human intestine to compounds that are extremely protective against cancer, particularly breast cancer.

Specially processed flax oils rich in lignans may be the best kind of flax oil for women in menopause or at risk for breast cancer.

Affordability   Flax oil is the best choice for an oil supplement because it provides the greatest nutritional benefits. And flax oil also has a special benefit: it is inexpensive. EPA (fish oils) and GLA supplements have been shown to be very beneficial in the treatment of many health conditions, but the dosages required to produce the desired health effect are quite high. And that means additional supplements and therefore more money.

In the treatment of rheumatoid arthritis, studies have shown positive results with EPA and GLA supplements at a dosage of 1.8 grams and 1.4 grams, respectively.[18] Most fish oil supplements provide 180 milligrams of EPA per 1,000-milligram capsule. Most GLA supplements provide about 100 milligrams per 1,000-milligram capsule. This means you may need to take as many as ten capsules daily. Taking less than the effective dosage is not likely to produce benefits. In order to achieve the high levels of EPA and GLA required, a person would have to spend $70 to $135 per month.

In contrast to the high price of EPA and GLA products, flax oil costs less than $12 a month (see Table 2.2). A daily dosage of one tablespoon provides about 6 grams of alpha-linolenic acid and 2 grams of linoleic acid.

Table 2.2 Cost Comparison of EFA Products

Source	Daily Dosage*	Average Cost per month
Omega-6 Oils		
Evening Primrose Oil (9% GLA)	1.4 g GLA	$90
Black Currant Seed Oil (17% GLA)	1.4 g GLA	90
Borage Oil (capsules) (22 % GLA)	1.4 g GLA	75
Borage Oil (liquid) (22% GLA)	1.4 g GLA	60
Omega-3 Oils		
EPA (fish oils) (180 mg EPA/1,000 mg)	1.8 g EPA	70
Flaxseed Oil (capsules) (55% alpha-LA)	5.0 g alpha-LA	18
Flaxseed Oil (liquid) (55% alpha-LA)	5.0 g alpha-LA	12

*Estimated therapeutic dosage based on clinical data

Flax Oil   Not all flax oil is created equal. Like other oils, there is tremendous variation in quality and purity as a result of differences in how the oil is expressed. Most flax oils are produced by mechanically pressing the oil through an expeller. During this process, a tremendous amount of pressure and heat can be generated. The higher the heat, the better the yield of oil. Temperatures generally reach 200° F. Interestingly, flax oil processed in this manner can still be referred to as cold-pressed because no external source of heat was added.

Although high temperatures, as well as supercritical fluid extraction, will provide a greater quantity of oil, they produce a lower quality oil. Many manufacturers willingly sacrifice quality for quantity.

However, consumers must be aware that because flax oil is a highly polyunsaturated oil, it is extremely susceptible to damage by heat, light, and oxygen. Once damaged, the oil is a rich source of toxic molecules known as lipid peroxides. These molecules can actually do the body harm and should not be ingested. Lipid peroxides are associated with an extremely bitter taste and rancidity. One of the best ways to measure the quality of a flax oil is by taste. The degree of bitterness is a close approximation of the level of lipid peroxides.

Barlean's Flax Oil   In my opinion, the highest quality flax oil available is Barlean's. The Barleans take great care in making sure their flax oil provides the benefits that Mother Nature intended. They do this by using 100 percent certified organic flaxseed. They then expel the oil through a special procedure called the bio-electron process, which allows the oil to be expressed at a temperature below 96° F. This protects the oil from the damaging effects of heat, light, and oxygen. You can actually taste the difference in quality between Barlean's and other flax oils.

Barlean's flax oil is available at most health food stores. Because of this care in processing, it is recommended exclusively by some of the leading experts in health and nutrition, such as Dr. Michael Murray, coauthor of the *Encyclopedia of Natural Medicine;* Dr. Johanna Budwig, the world-renowned Nobel Prize nominee and top authority on fats and oils; and Ann Louise Gittelman, best-selling author of *Beyond Pritikin.*

The Best Way to Use Flax Oil   Homemade salad dressings are the perfect opportunity to use flax oil. Here is a sample recipe. Simply combine all the ingredients in a blender and mix thoroughly.

BASIL DRESSING

Makes 6 servings (2 tablespoons per serving)

> 1/4 cup flax oil
> 1/4 cup water
> 3 tablespoons fresh lemon juice
> 2 tablespoons fresh basil (or 2 teaspoons dried basil)
> 1 teaspoon finely chopped garlic
> black pepper to taste

If you would like other recipes, or ideas on how to use flax oil, write or call:

> Barlean's Organic Oils
> 4936 Lake Terrell Road
> Ferndale, WA 98248
> 1-800-445-FLAX (3529)

Step 7: Eat a Lowfat, High-Complex-Carbohydrate Diet

I've saved my basic dietary recommendations for last. I do this although I consider my dietary recommendations the most important step of all.

By focusing first on specific nutrients that are critical for good health, the case for my prescription in this section is basically already made. It doesn't matter whether we are looking at antioxidants and cancer, potassium and heart disease, or oils and stroke. When trying to increase your intake of specific nutrients, the first step toward getting on the right track is to eat a lowfat, high-complex-carbohydrate diet. Sadly, the typical American diet acts as a hindrance to good health.[19]

Many people find basic dietary changes to be the toughest part of my seven-step wellness program. People seem to find it easier to start new habits than to change old ones. For instance, many find that adding nutritional supplements as a regular part of their life is easier than making dietary changes.

The key to making the change come easier is to realize just how many delicious, good-for-you foods and food combinations there are out there. Nature produces an amazing and diverse bounty. Food is one of the most wonderful explorations available to us. Yet many of us remain habituated to a stationary treadmill of limited food choices. When talking about changes, many focus on having to "give up" the foods they normally eat. Instead, I invite you to focus on embracing the great and tasty exploration that your new, healthful diet will provide.

Recognize that any difficulty in making any kind of change is largely a matter of perception. Consider both the types of food you eat and the amounts. When eating with their health in mind, many people are amazed at how much food they can eat and still lose weight.

Over the last twenty years, I have found that a very lowfat, high-complex-carbohydrate diet is the most powerful tool in health care. It is useful in preventing disease, and it is useful in treating disease. My experience is the basis of my recommendations. But this is so important that I want to share with you some other evidence supporting it. Then I will give some helpful hints on how to change your dietary habits as painlessly as possible.

What We Are Made to Eat

One way to determine the optimal diet for human health is to compare the human anatomy with the anatomies of other animals. The eating habits of creatures with similar physical characteristics might cast light on our optimal dietary habits. For instance, our jaws and teeth are useful indicators. Human molars are perfect for crushing and grinding plant foods, and front incisors are well suited for biting into fruits and vegetables. Together, these account for twenty-eight of our teeth. The remaining four canine teeth are designed for eating meat. The structure of the jaw allows both vertical and lateral movement, to tear and crush; carnivore jaws only swing vertically.

The other end of the digestive process in humans also supports the herbivore in us. Carnivores typically have a short bowel. Herbivores have a longer bowel length, which is proportionally comparable to humans. This alone provides an interesting perspective on the role of excessive animal products in the growing incidence of colon cancer. While the human gastrointestinal tract is capable of digesting both animal and plant foods, evidence suggests that its design specifications were developed largely to support plant foods.[20]

An appropriate human diet could also be determined by looking at the diets of the animals closest in development to humans, the primates. Researchers who have studied the eating habits of chimpanzees, monkeys, and gorillas provide interesting insights. In general, studies have shown that these primates favor plant foods. Researchers describe them as "herbivores and opportunistic carnivores." By this they mean that from time to time, a meat dinner sounds about right. Primates may on rare occasion eat lizards, eggs, or small animals. But meat is not a staple of most primate meals. Fruits and vegetables are the more likely fare.

The research distinguishing eating habits of different groups of primates also supports the herbivore in the human. Smaller primates get more of their food from animal sources, while orangutans and gorillas, the primates closest to humans in size, rely on animal sources for only 2 percent and 1 percent of their total calories, respectively. The rest of their diet is plant foods.

The average human weight falls between that of orangutans and gorillas. For this reason, some researchers have postulated that perhaps the optimal level of animal foods in the human diet would be 1.5 percent. It's a sobering perspective: Most Americans derive well over 50 percent of their calories from animal foods.

Human Health and Animal Foods

Another productive viewpoint on human dietary choices comes from the field of epidemiology, where we are looking at general health characteristics of a population rather than at specific biomedical data. The adoption of the current American diet by various population groups gives us a tremendous supply of unwitting guinea pigs in what is the largest health experiment of the century. Disease rates are measured over time and against changing dietary habits in various populations. The shift toward a "Western" diet by the Japanese following World War II provided a classic "experiment." Other populations that have been studied are ethnic groups who immigrated here and subsequently adopted the customary American diet.

The evidence is resoundingly clear. A tremendous array of chronic diseases, which were previously virtually unknown, began to be seen when the usual diets of these populations had been largely vegetarian: heart disease, cancer, stroke, diabetes, and arthritis. Their deviation from a predominantly plant-based diet appeared to be a major factor in the increased incidence of these diseases.

By the 1960s and early 1970s, many forward-thinking doctors began to respect this epidemiological information. We began to make the links and prescribe treatment plans based in part on this evidence. Medically, this was a relatively easy step for many of us to take. All it took was a little common sense. Yet those of us who valued this epidemiological data were, in those relatively dark ages of public policy, loudly and publicly dismissed as "quacks."

Yet change has come, if slowly. Finally, in the 1980s, a number of studies began to appear which took a look at the changing health of another population group: United States citizens. Epidemiologists knew that our country had seen a tremendous upswing in killer diseases. Infectious diseases were no longer dominating the list; now we were seeing an array of chronic diseases as the leading killers.

In 1984, the National Research Council's Food and Nutrition Board undertook a comprehensive analysis of diet and the major chronic diseases. This group, which is also responsible for the RDAs, established the Committee on Diet and Health. The U.S. Surgeon

General at the time, C. Everett Koop, M.D., filed his "Report on Nutrition and Health" in 1988. Major medical and health foundations began looking at diet and health. The American Heart Association, the National Cancer Institute, and the American Diabetes Association stepped into the picture.

Finally, after many years of nutrition-oriented physicians calling out in the wilderness for more attention to the relationship between diet and health, light began to dawn.

The findings were convincing. Links were finally established between the typical American diet and many diseases. The diet that is the culprit is the one that our gastrointestinal tract is not built to assimilate. It is the diet that our cousin primates are not choosing. It is the diet through which, by adopting it, our Japanese brothers and sisters are spreading disease amongst themselves. It is a diet low in plant foods, and high in animal foods and refined sugars.

DISEASES ASSOCIATED WITH A DIET LOW IN PLANT FOODS

Metabolic   obesity, gout, diabetes, kidney stones, gallstones

Cardiovascular   hypertension, cerebrovascular disease, stroke, angina, heart attack, varicose veins, deep vein thrombosis, pulmonary embolism

Colonic   constipation, appendicitis, diverticulitis, diverticulosis, hemorrhoids, colon cancer, irritable bowel syndrome, ulcerative colitis, Crohn's disease

Other   dental caries, autoimmune disorders, pernicious anemia, multiple sclerosis, thyrotoxicosis, dermatological conditions

As study after study began to emerge, a remarkably consistent pattern of recommendations emerged.

1. Reduce total fat intake to 30 percent or less of calories. (Many experts say 20 percent or less is optimal.) Reduce saturated fatty acid intake to less than 10 percent of calories. Reduce intake of cholesterol to less than 300 milligrams daily.

2. Eat five or more servings per day of a combination of vegetables and fruits, especially green and yellow vegetables and citrus fruits.

3. Increase the intake of fiber and complex carbohydrates by eating six or more servings per day of a combination of whole-grain breads, cereals, and legumes.

4. Maintain protein intake at moderate levels.

5. Balance food intake and physical activity to maintain appropriate body weight.

6. Limit the intake of alcohol, refined carbohydrates (sugar), and salt (sodium chloride).

Some Practical Tips

You already know that you need to decrease the amount of fat and protein in your diet. You know you need to limit the amount of animal foods you consume. You also know that you need to consume more highly nutritious foods: vegetables, fruits, whole grains, and legumes. But how do you go about making these changes?

I have discovered some mealtime strategies that are useful if you think this transition will be tough. If you always have meat, try having just one lowfat animal food meal a day. Consider eating a meal that is all "side dishes," such as vegetables, rice, potatoes, beans, or fruit. Leave the animal products out. Once you get used to this, try leaving animal products out of your diet two days a week. Eat only grains, vegetables, and fruits for these two days.

Here are five additional easy ways to increase the level of plant foods in your diet.

1. When grocery shopping, stock up first on potatoes, yams, squash, onions, carrots, garlic, a host of salad vegetables, and fruits.

2. Go to the rice, soup, and beans section. Pick up a variety of pre-packaged (not canned) bean soups. Most stores have a good selection of mixes where all you have to do is follow some easy directions, cut up some vegetables, and simply add the spice packet that comes with the mix or add your own spices. If the recipe calls for meat, use only a quarter of what the recipe recommends. Or leave it out all together.

3. Have a piece of fresh fruit or vegetables with every meal.

4. Buy a juicer and try to drink at least twelve ounces of fresh fruit or vegetable juice each day.

5. Invest in some good vegetarian or lowfat cookbooks to help you add spice and variety to your diet.

These changes will seem strange in the beginning. That's in the nature of change. But if you succeed and follow through, you will be surprised at times by how different you feel. You will have new sensations. Consider them your body's way of thanking you. Listen to these sensations. Be thankful that you have this little advertising campaign for healthful living inside you.

If I were to recommend only one therapeutic agent for improving health, it would be this lowfat, high-complex-carbohydrate diet.

Chapter Summary

The Whitaker Wellness Program involves seven steps:

1. Adopt a healthy lifestyle.

2. Become more active.
3. Take a multiple vitamin-mineral formula.
4. Take extra antioxidant nutrients.
5. Take extra magnesium and potassium.
6. Take an omega-3 oil supplement.
7. Eat a lowfat, high-complex-carbohydrate diet.

Take any of these steps and you will improve your level of wellness. Take all of them and you will have a strong foundation upon which to build lifelong health. More power to you!

The Whitaker Wellness Program will improve your overall health by serving as the foundation for enhancing specific body functions and addressing specific health conditions. The rest of the book addresses these specifics, and will work wonders when used in conjunction with the recommendations in this chapter.

PART II

Building Optimal Health

Our goal is to focus on health. Often, it is only a specific body function that is not functioning up to par. There is no disease present, only a slight dysfunction or insufficiency. Part II focuses on promoting overall health by enhancing the function of specific body activities. Practicing the seven steps of the Whitaker Wellness Program will take you a long way, but often certain body systems or organs need additional support.

A Note on Product Recommendations

Most herbs, vitamins, minerals, and nutritional supplements are, as of this writing, still classified as foods by the U.S. Food and Drug Administration (FDA). Many of these substances can produce more direct, focused, medicinal effects than do foods (and many drugs). But manufacturers of these healthful products, for the most part, are prohibited by the FDA from making claims to their health and medical value.

As new information becomes available, the FDA's position fluctuates. All natural products are fraudulent, at best placebos, so they claim one day. Or should the FDA regulate these natural products as a drug, and force manufacturers to undergo the same process regarding safety as prescription and over-the-counter medications?

Until recently, the natural products industry didn't embrace the challenge of self-regulation posed by the FDA. Today, the Natural Products Quality Assurance Council and the National Natural Foods Association are organizing the various trade associations in the natural food industry to help them create their own, industry-wide quality-control standards. Clearly the pressure of FDA threats is one thing that moved the industry to hasten self-regulatory efforts.

For the practitioner of natural medicine, and for the consumer, a great deal of uncertainty still exists about various products and product lines. Every manufacturer claims their product is superior and that their quality-control measures are the strictest. Unfortunately, there are numerous examples where what was claimed on the label did not match up with the chemical analysis of the product. A company might claim to be using an especially effective (more expensive) form of a vitamin or mineral; upon analysis it is discovered that a less expensive, less effective form was actually used. A claim of a certain level of potency is made, but upon analysis each tablet or capsule is found to contain less than the label amount. Or, an herbal product may be made from a part of the plant that has no therapeutic benefit, because the manufacturer can buy this part of the plant cheaply and undercut the price of an honest, effective product.

For all of these reasons, it is critical that you develop relationships with people (doctors specializing in natural medicine or competent health food store personnel) and companies that you can trust. As a physician who prescribes these products, I have a special responsibility. I know what the scientific literature says will help produce the desired effect. It is my responsibility to make sure that the products I give my patients have the power and the potency that the clinical studies suggest is appropriate. For example, if I want to produce the benefits of saw palmetto extract in the treatment of benign prostate enlargement, I had better make sure I prescribe the fat-soluble extract standardized to contain 85 to 95 percent fatty acids and sterols at a dosage of 160 milligrams twice daily.

As I have developed my clinical practice and use of natural products, I have gained reliable confidence in certain products and certain companies. The company I have the deepest level of respect for is Enzymatic Therapy. This Green Bay, Wisconsin, firm has been a leader in bringing top-quality science to its formulations; the list of industry firsts for this company is impressive. Here are just a few of the important natural products Enzymatic Therapy introduced to the United States:

> Saw palmetto extract (85 to 95 percent fatty acids and sterols)
> Ginkgo biloba extract (24 percent ginkgoflavonglycosides)
> DGL (deglycyrrhizinated licorice)
> Glucosamine sulfate
> Enteric-coated peppermint oil
> Predigested-soluble glandular extracts
> Silymarin
> Bilberry extract (25 percent anthocyanosides)

What you are looking for from a manufacturer is to be convinced that what they say on the label regarding ingredients and potency is true. Enzymatic Therapy is not the only company whose products I recommend. Many other products and companies have my utmost respect, based on my own experiences and knowledge.

3

Enhancing Digestion and Elimination

Most of us have finally learned that what we eat is perhaps the single most important influence on our health. Those good foods will be of limited value, however, if our system for digesting, assimilating, and eliminating foods is not functioning properly. The best food in the world is wasted if our bodies are not processing it effectively.

Health concerns, discomfort after we eat, and our body's inability to properly digest food have created a huge market for over-the-counter preparations in this country. Antacids, in particular, are pumped into people's stomachs by the tens of thousands daily. Most people who buy and take antacids do so to relieve the symptoms of indigestion. Some speak of "heartburn." Others feel a bloating or gaseous sensation. Whatever the complaint, there are many better solutions than resorting to antacids.

A properly functioning digestive system is truly remarkable in its ability to efficiently cull from our foods only the useful and necessary nutrients. Chapter 3 studies the digestive system, the kinds of problems that can arise, and some smart choices we can make to assist our digestive processes.

The entire digestive system extends from the mouth through the anus. It includes the gastrointestinal tract, along with a number of organs appended to it. These are the salivary glands, liver, gall bladder, and pancreas. At various steps along the way, glands secrete an array of digestive juices. The compounds in these juices that are most active in digestion are primarily enzymes.[1]

While the formal digestive work begins with the mouth, a more instructive view is to consider that the process actually begins with our brains, and our ideas about what we are going to eat. This extends to the arms and hands that bring it to our mouths. Healthy digestion gets off to a good start depending on what these organs and appendages do. I am talking about our dietary choices.

Some of the digestive processes, such as those involving enzymes, are chemical. Others are mechanical. Chewing is a little of both. Thoroughly chewing food physically breaks it down into more digestible chunks. It also gives your teeth and salivary glands a chance to work together. Salivary glands, by secreting the enzyme salivary amylase, help break down starch molecules into smaller sugars. Meantime, chewing sends signals to the rest of the digestive system: "Get ready, I'm sending food your way."

Hydrochloric Acid

Food passes from the mouth through the esophagus into the stomach. The stomach aids digestion by acting both as a muscle, churning and gyrating, and as a gland, secreting various agents to mix with the food. Until the food gains a semi-liquid consistency, it sits in the stomach. When the food material leaves, it is called "chyme."

Key stomach secretions for digestion are hydrochloric acid and pepsin. Both are required for the absorption of minerals and digestion of proteins. Without proper protein digestion, a cascade of unfortunate health effects can ensue. An immediate sign of something not being quite right is the comment: "I've got indigestion." Another is the quiet, frequently habitual reach for antacids.

Common as this occurrence is, the activity may well be based, for many people, on a mistaken assumption. If asked, most would probably say that their indigestion is caused by having too high a level of acid in their stomach. The stomach, in this scenario, would be over-secreting.

A very strong case can be made that the opposite is more often true. The digestive problems of many people are related to a deficiency in the production of hydrochloric acid. One study concluded that over 40 percent of adults have insufficient levels of this essential digestive agent.[1] This condition is called *hypochlorhydria*. The problem occurs particularly in the elderly. We know that the ability of the stomach to secrete hydrochloric acid decreases with age. One study found over half of people over 60 years of age had hypochlorhydria. At the extreme, when complete lack of gastric acid secretions is found, the condition is termed *achlorhydria*. See Table 3.1.

A couple of sound techniques are available for diagnosing the level of hydrochloric acid in the stomach. One is a laboratory test which provides detailed gastric acid analysis.[2] The other is a good, low-tech "challenge" method developed by nutrition-oriented medical doctor Jonathan Wright.[3]

Heidelberg Gastric Analysis

An electronic capsule attached to a string is swallowed and kept in the stomach. This simple little device measures the pH (acidity level) of

Table 3.1 Common Symptoms, Signs, and Diseases Associated with Low Hydrochloric Acid Secretion[4]

Symptoms	Signs	Diseases
Bloating, belching, burning, and flatulence immediately after meals	Itching around the rectum	Addison's disease
	Weak, peeling, and cracked fingernails	Asthma
		Celiac disease
	Dilated blood vessels in the cheeks and nose	Dermatitis herpetiformis
A sense of "fullness" after eating		Diabetes mellitus
		Eczema
	Acne	Gallbladder disease
Indigestion, diarrhea, or constipation	Iron deficiency	Graves disease
	Chronic intestinal parasites or abnormal flora	Chronic autoimmune disorders
Multiple food allergies		Hepatitis
	Undigested food in stool	Chronic hives
Nausea after taking supplements	Chronic candida infections	Lupus erythematosis
	Upper digestive tract gas	Myasthenia gravis
		Osteoporosis
		Pernicious anemia
		Psoriasis
		Rheumatoid arthritis
		Rosacea
		Sjogren's syndrome
		Thyrotoxicosis
		Hyper- and hypothyroidism
		Vertigo

the stomach. It then sends a radio message back to a receiver which records the findings. After the test, the string is used to pull the capsule back up from the stomach. This is the best test of the ability of the stomach to secrete acids.

Challenge Protocol for Hydrochloric Acid Supplements

Many symptoms and signs can suggest impaired hydrochloric acid secretion. In addition, a number of specific diseases have been found to be associated with insufficient hydrochloric acid output. Either the symptoms or the disease can suggest low stomach acid output.

Not everyone needs detailed gastric acid analysis to determine whether gastric acid supplementation would be beneficial. For many, a simple practical method can be just as useful. It will determine whether you need hydrochloric acid, as well as how much your body needs for proper digestion.

The following challenge method is modified from one developed by Jonathan Wright, M.D. This challenge supports your stomach's ability to produce the levels of acids you need.

1. Begin by taking one tablet or capsule containing 10 grains (600 milligrams) of hydrochloric acid with your next large meal. The hydrochloric acid should be bound to betaine or glutamic acid. The formulation should also include at least 150 milligrams of pepsin. Pay attention to any side effects you may feel. Do you have gas, a burning sensation, or pain?

2. If this does not aggravate your symptoms or produce side effects, begin increasing your dose. At every meal of the same size after that, increase your dose by one more tablet or capsule. For instance, increase by one at the next meal, two at the meal after that, then three at the next meal.

3. Continue to increase the dose until you feel a warmth in your stomach, or other side effects. Do not increase the dose above seven tablets. A feeling of warmth in the stomach means that you have taken too many tablets for that meal. If you have this sensation, take one less tablet for the next meal of that size. It is a good idea to try the larger dose again at another meal to make sure that it was the HCl that caused the warmth and not something else.

4. Once you have found the largest dose that you can take at your large meals without feeling any warmth, maintain that dose at all meals of similar size. (You will need to take less at smaller meals.)

5. When taking a number of tablets or capsules, it is best to take them throughout the meal.

6. With this supplementation, your stomach will begin to regain the ability to produce the amount of HCl you need to properly digest your food. The signs of this quiet healing will be the warm feeling in your stomach again. When you feel this, cut down the dose level. Continue to step the dose down as your stomach begins to produce the gastric acids you need.

A number of companies manufacture hydrochloric acid-pepsin products. The decisive factor in choosing a product is that it should contain sufficient levels of hydrochloric acid and pepsin. Products in capsule form may produce slightly better results than products in tablet form.

Preventing "Heartburn"

Hypochlorhydria is one cause of indigestion; overly acidic stomachs are also a source for many people who are regular users of antacids.

The causes of indigestion are not as simple as the advertising for over-the-counter medications would have you believe.

A further insight into the complexity of factors and symptoms which people try to relieve by taking antacids was provided in 1983 by a leading medical journal, the *American Journal of Gastroenterology*. Authors of the article asked why otherwise healthy people took antacids. The conclusion was that people took them for what they called *heartburn*.[5]

In medical terms, the name for this problem is *reflux esophagitis*. The process is what the name suggests: gastric juices flow out of the stomach back up the esophagus. It's a wrong-way train on the gastrointestinal tract.

Overeating is almost always the cause of this acidic back-eddy. Consumption of fried foods, carbonated soft drinks, chocolate, cigarette smoking, alcohol, and coffee can also be causes. Not surprisingly, with this list, obesity is also linked to reflux esophagitis.

These factors act on digestion in one of two ways. They may increase pressure within the stomach, forcing the contents back upward. Or they may interfere with the activity of the sphincter, the muscle between the stomach and the esophagus which normally prevents emission of fluids. When the emitted gastric juices hit the esophagus, a burning discomfort is produced that radiates upward.

A couch potato's favored response to overeating does not help. Lying down makes heartburn worse. The pain would be better alleviated by helping with the dishes.

Before we talk about treatment, consider a precautionary note on chronic heartburn. This sensation might be a sign that the stomach is pouching out above the diaphragm, a condition known as *hiatal hernia*. This is not likely, however. Only about one in twenty people with hiatal hernias experience reflux esophagitis as a result.

The first step in treating heartburn involves the organ and the appendages previously mentioned: the brain and the arms. Try eating different foods. Or at least tell your arms not to lift so much of it to your mouth. This is prevention at its most direct and basic: reducing or eliminating the most common causative factor. If you have chronic heartburn, experiment first with this brain-arm remedy.

People with heartburn believe that their stomach juices have too much acid. They announce this as if it were the "cause" of the problem, which an antacid will "cure." But note that "over-acidic stomach" is not a cause of heartburn. Nor is an antacid a cure. The former is a sign that something has gone haywire. The latter is a means of suppressing symptoms.

Symptoms of heartburn or indigestion should be viewed as a sign of a significant imbalance during the initial stage of digestion. This imbalance can either be due to poor food selection or impaired digestion.

Reaching immediately for an antacid may not be the best choice because it may not address the real cause. Just remember that heartburn and reliance on antacids is not a natural or healthy condition.

Over-acidity and Precautions on Antacids

A chemical scale called the pH is used to measure acid levels. The scale is used for diverse purposes, such as the evaluation of lake water where acid rain may be a problem, but this scale is also used to measure stomach acidity. Using the pH scale, a neutral substance has a pH of 7. A reading above 7 is alkaline; below 7 it is acid. The optimal pH range of the stomach is between 1.5 and 2.5. The primary acid in the stomach's mix is hydrochloric acid.

Antacids are the chief method people use for neutralizing a stomach that is overly acidic. These pills work by binding free acid, which raises the pH of the stomach. These "neutralizing" antacids don't actually take the pH above absolute "neutral", or 7, on the pH scale. But typically, antacids will raise the pH out of the optimal range for digestion, to a point above 3.5. In doing so, the action of an enzyme called pepsin, which can be irritating to the stomach, is inhibited. Heartburn's warming fire is dimmed or extinguished.

In considering the stomach's role in digestion, remember that hydrochloric acid and pepsin are the two main substances the stomach secretes. Both are necessary for proper digestion. Pepsin helps assist with protein digestion.

This should raise a red flag of concern for antacid users. Like many agents commonly used to ease symptoms, antacids interfere with necessary physiological activity in a healthy body. So while antacids can help provide relief, they must be used wisely and sparingly.

I recommend two first steps for heartburn. The first may be the most effective treatment for chronic reflux esophagitis, though it is not always practical. Consider placing four-inch blocks under the bedposts or frame at the head of the bed. For many chronic heartburn cases, gravity is the best medicine.

The very best products for the problems of over-acidity and heartburn will provide relief for the problem of over-acidity and any related heartburn. Gastro-Soothe from Enzymatic Therapy is an all-natural antacid and contains a special licorice extract known as DGL. DGL helps counter the effects of heartburn. (DGL is discussed further on page 349 as a treatment for peptic ulcer.)

The typical American diet is clearly highly beneficial to the makers of antacids. And consumers have a host of choices. When used occasionally, all antacids are relatively safe, but users should take some precautions.

Antacids Containing Aluminum   Aluminum is linked to impaired mental function and to a number of diseases of the nervous system, among them Alzheimer's disease, Parkinson's disease, Lou Gehrig's disease, and dialysis dementia.[6]

Most of the best-known antacids contain aluminum: Maalox, Rolaids, Digel, Mylanta, Riopan, Wingel, Amphogel, and AlernaGel. These products are potent in neutralizing acid. Manufacturers of these products and the FDA tell us "not to worry" about the aluminum, that aluminum is not absorbed by the body.

Studies, even of low doses of antacids containing aluminum, prove otherwise.[7] Bodies do absorb aluminum. We also know that absorption of aluminum is higher under some very common circumstances, such as after consuming a meal containing citrus fruit, orange juice, soda pop, or other citric acid source. How often are these foods consumed while overeating, which is the single greatest cause of the problem for which people take these aluminum-containing products? Probably pretty often. Aluminum uptake is likely to be highest in the people most likely to use antacids. Impaired kidney function and active Alzheimer's disease also create conditions which promote absorption of aluminum. It is clear to me that significant long-term safety concerns argue against taking antacids with aluminum.

If the FDA banned all aluminum-containing products, it would not remove all possible antacid options. And antacids are not the best remedy for heartburn anyway. Taking preventive measures against the onset of heartburn is the ideal cure.

Baking Soda   Common baking soda (sodium bicarbonate), changed into its effervescent form, is better known to television watchers and heartburn sufferers as Alka-Seltzer. Sodium bicarbonate can be useful for indigestion in short-term therapy.

However, I advise against prolonged use of sodium bicarbonate for chronic indigestion, as it can cause sodium overload. The bicarbonate ion is rapidly absorbed and the pH of the whole body can be altered. This is known medically as *systemic alkalosis*. Nausea, vomiting, headache, mental confusion, and the formation of kidney stones are all associated with systemic alkalosis.

Calcium Carbonate Antacids   When the body is given medicinal agents that counter its processes, the body doesn't usually just lie there and take it. Calcium carbonate antacids (like Tums) have been shown to cause the body to come back strong. This is called a "rebound effect." The stomach attempts to overcompensate for the neutralization of its own secretions. After all, the stomach secretes acids and pepsin for a reason. So three or four hours after calcium carbonate antacids are administered, the stomach begins secreting even more acids. This rebound effect does not appear to significantly hinder the treatment of indigestion. Yet rebound secretions associated with this form of antacid may delay the healing of ulcers.

Calcium in the carbonate form is an effective form of antacid. Yet its strong alkaline nature can be problematic. The risk of kidney stones increases. If milk products are a regular part of the diet, the risk of this side effect increases further.

Many physicians actually recommend using Tums as a calcium supplement. In fact, the carbonate form is the most widely used form of calcium supplement, whether it is taken as an antacid or merely as a calcium supplement. But in fact, there are better forms of calcium for supplementation, which are described in my prescriptions for osteoporosis on page 314.

Calcium Citrate   Ironically, there is a product that is not marketed as an antacid, which may be the best option for treating indigestion. The product is a form of calcium known as citrate.[8] Calcium citrate is showing impressive results in patients with kidney disease. There are signs that, unlike the potential harm from carbonate products, citrate may actually prevent formation of kidney stones.[9] The body's tolerance of calcium citrate is higher than its tolerance for the aluminum-containing antacids.[10]

This form of calcium is also proving to be the best way to take supplemental calcium. While I am not aware of any company marketing calcium citrate as an antacid, you can find calcium citrate products in health food stores as calcium supplements.

One final precaution: Calcium supplementation of any kind may serve to decrease the absorption of other minerals. If a calcium product is being used for its antacid effect, the best recommendation may be to simply take a multi-mineral formula that includes calcium. This way you will replace lost minerals. Base your dosage on the calcium content of the multi-mineral. For an antacid effect, it should be in the 500- to 1,000-milligrams range. In addition, check to see that the chelating agent for the calcium is citrate or another Krebs cycle intermediate. Numerous formulas in health food stores meet this criterion.

The Small Intestine and Digestion

The small intestine is twenty-one feet long. It secretes a variety of protective and digestive substances, and also acts as a mixing bowl for the valuable secretions of the pancreas, liver, and gallbladder. There is hardly an aspect of digestion, absorption, and transportation of food and other ingested materials with which the small intestine is not involved.

The length of this organ is divided into three sections. Each has its particular functions. The first section, ten to twelve inches in length, is the *duodenum*. Its specialty is mineral absorption. The next is the *jejunum*. Roughly eight feet long, the jejunum is the primary place where absorption of protein, water-soluble vitamins, and carbohydrates occurs. The last and longest section is called the *ileum*. Here fat-soluble vitamins, fat, cholesterol, and bile salts are absorbed.

If it is true that we are what we eat, then it's fair to say that we don't exist until it is all absorbed. If the small intestine is not functioning properly, all the good nutrients in an excellent diet can go for naught.

In medicine, problems of the small intestine are called *malabsorption syndromes*. They are characterized by multiple nutrient deficiencies. Examples include celiac disease (gluten intolerance), food allergy or food intolerance, intestinal infections, and Crohn's disease.

Pancreatic Enzymes and Digestion

The importance of the pancreas for digestion cannot be overstated. Each day this little organ pumps nearly a half gallon of pancreatic juice into the small intestine. This juice includes a rich blend of enzymes that are necessary for us to digest and absorb our food.

Amylases   The salivary glands and the pancreas both secrete this enzyme which breaks starch molecules into smaller sugars.

Lipases   Fat cannot be properly digested without lipases, a pancreatic enzyme, and bile. Fats and fat-soluble vitamins are malabsorbed with lipase deficiency.

Proteases   Protein molecules must be broken down into single amino acids to be digested. If protein is not properly broken down, a host of problems can ensue. We see allergic reactions. Toxic substances can be produced if bacteria, rather than enzymes, break down the protein. This process is known as *putrefaction*. Proteases help prevent putrefaction through proper breakdown of proteins.

The value of proteases does not end there. These enzymes are necessary for warding off a growing health problem in our population: parasites. These include bacteria, yeast, protozoa, and intestinal worms. Proteases have the leading role in keeping the small intestine free of these microscopic critters.[11] Intestinal infections, including chronic candida infections of the gastrointestinal tract, are also much more common in individuals lacking protease and other digestive secretions.[12]

The list of known benefits from this multifaceted enzyme goes on. Proteases are important in depositing immune complexes in body tissues. They help prevent tissue damage during inflammation. We need them to form fibrin clots.

The Health of Your Pancreas

Our bodies provide us with a complex array of signs when we are having problems with the function of the pancreas. If you frequently have gas, indigestion, or abdominal bloating and discomfort, the pancreas may not be doing its job. Another less obvious sign is the passing of undigested food in the stool.

Nutrition-oriented physicians gather information about such signs and symptoms to help us assess pancreatic function. We will often then do something that many conventional doctors rarely do. Perhaps because most doctors are not trained to look at diet and nutrition, most doctors won't consider looking at the other end of the nutrition equation: our stools. To gain a clearer and more specific reading on the health of the pancreas, a nutrition-smart doctor may choose a comprehensive stool and digestive analysis. (These are available to physicians from Meridian Valley Laboratory, 1-800-234-6825, or Great Smokies Diagnostic Laboratory, 1-800-522-4762.)

Laboratory analysis will evaluate the level of excess fat and nitrogen in the stool. The test will show whether or not there are other partially or incompletely undigested food elements. It will also measure the health of the bacterial flora. These assessments help indicate the general health of the pancreas and the specific level of pancreatic enzymes being dumped into the intestines.

Pancreatic Insufficiency

Cystic fibrosis, a rare, inherited disorder, is the most severe example of pancreatic insufficiency, but mild insufficiency of the pancreas is thought to be quite common, particularly among the elderly.

Pancreatic enzymes are the most effective treatment for pancreatic insufficiency and the malabsorption, impaired digestion, nutrient deficiencies, and abdominal discomfort that may be associated with it. Fresh hog pancreas (pancreatin) is the source for most commercial preparations.

Sometimes manufacturers make choices that appear to be in our best interests, but later don't prove to be. This is the case for some pancreatin products. Most enzyme products are coated with a substance to keep them from being digested in the stomach. This is so they can reach the small intestine intact. At first this process, called "enteric coating," seemed to be a good idea. But we now know, from numerous studies, that enzyme preparations that are non–enteric-coated out-perform enteric-coated enzymes. If used for digestive purposes, the non–enteric-coated products must simply be taken prior to a meal. If you are using them for their anti-inflammatory effects, studies show they should be taken on an empty stomach.

The United States Pharmacopoeia (USP) has established strict definitions for the activity levels in pancreatic enzymes. This determines specific levels of the key enzymes. A 1X pancreatic enzyme product (pancreatin) must have in each milligram at least 25 USP units each of amylase and protease activity, and at least 2 USP units of lipase activity.

Manufacturers may make a stronger product. If so, it is given a whole number multiple of 1X to indicate its strength. A full-strength, undiluted product with 10 times the USP standard would be 10X. Full-strength products are preferable to lower-potency pancreatin products, because those with lower potency are often diluted with salt, lactose, or galactose to achieve the desired strength (4X or 1X). For a 10X USP pancreatic enzyme product, the dosage would be 500 to 1,000 milligrams three times a day. The timing would depend on whether you are taking them for digestion (take immediately before meals) or anti-inflammatory effects (take on an empty stomach).

One of the best pancreatic enzyme preparations has a couple of additional helpful factors. The product is Mega-Zyme, from Enzymatic Therapy. This product includes two natural agents from the pineapple and papaya, the digestive agents bromelain and papain. Some people choose to use these enzymes alone as a vegetarian substitute for treating pancreatic insufficiency.[13] In Mega-Zyme, these products are combined with pancreatin and ox bile, providing the best results.

Sometimes a therapeutic trial is extremely effective in determining whether supplementing digestive enzymes can help with digestion. One dramatic case in which I utilized digestive enzymes comes to mind. The patient was a five-year-old girl who had experienced diarrhea almost from the moment she was born. She had been in and out of hospitals for extensive tests and close evaluation. Despite the best that conventional medicine had to offer, no diagnosis could be made. As a result of both her diarrhea and medical treatment with drugs attempting to slow down the activity of the bowel, she was virtually entirely debilitated. I suggested she take some digestive enzymes, including betaine hydrochloride and pancreatin. When I saw the patient one month later, her parents reported that the problem had stopped almost immediately after the first dose of the digestive enzymes. The child began gaining weight and experienced dramatic increases in her energy and activity levels.

I was as surprised as the parents were and was equally surprised that no conventional medical doctor had thought to simply support the child's digestive process with enzymes. Obviously, poor digestion was the cause.

Food Allergies, Proteases, and Pancreatin

A half-century ago, studies were performed which showed how effective pancreatic enzymes can be in preventing food allergies.[14] Proper protein digestion is not possible without these enzymes. Food allergies are just one of the problems that can result from incomplete digestion of proteins. If a person doesn't secrete enough proteases, multiple food allergies will often result.

The Liver, Bile, and Digestion

Each day the liver secretes about a quart of bile into the small intestine or the gallbladder. Almost all of it, 99 percent in fact, is then reabsorbed.

This bile plays a number of important roles in proper digestion. It works inside the ileum, the third and longest section of the small intestine, to assist in absorbing oils, fats, and fat-soluble vitamins. Like the pancreatic enzymes, bile helps free the small intestine of potentially harmful microorganisms.

Bile also has a role in the functioning of our bowels. This liver secretion assists in keeping the stool soft by aiding in the incorporation of water. Many commercial digestive aids contain bile, usually ox bile, for this reason. These ingested agents have a mild laxative effect by helping soften the stool. Constipation is the result if not enough bile is available and the stool becomes too hard.

The amino acids choline and methionine can also be helpful in increasing the output of bile. A number of nutritional products to assist digestion include these agents. (See Chapter 5, for more information about these formulas which support healthy function of the gallbladder and liver.)

The Large Intestine and Digestion

The last few years have seen increased awareness of the role of the colon, or large intestine, in health. This organ, which is about five feet long, has some important features that have not been spotlighted. It functions in absorbing water and, in a more limited way, in absorbing the final products of digestion. The large intestine also helps to absorb electrolytes (salts).

The focus on the colon has rightfully been on ensuring that it functions properly in its capacity as a holding tank for waste products, and in elimination. One concern about colon malfunction is bacteria. If wastes do not move through the colon in a timely fashion, the colon becomes a very hospitable medium for growing harmful bacteria.

The choices people make about the foods they eat are clearly linked to most colon problems. Chronic constipation usually reflects a low-fiber diet. Colon cancer, diverticulitis, hemorrhoids, and irritable bowel syndrome are among the other bowel problems associated with the typical American diet.

Making choices that create a healthy colon are simple, though habit changes may be difficult. Increasing dietary fiber is the key. With this change, transit time of stools is quicker. So is the frequency and quantity of bowel movements. Toxins have less time to be absorbed from the stool into the body. The painful and even deadly major diseases of the colon can often be prevented.

A therapeutic approach to the colon must begin with complying with a diet which, as noted throughout this book, also makes us healthier in dozens of other ways. Eating more whole grains, legumes, nuts, seeds, and fruits is the most effective way to raise the fiber content of our diets, and assure the proper working of the digestive system.

Chapter Summary

Eating well is the best way to ensure good digestion. Many of the health problems that arise in the passage of food through the gastrointestinal tract will decrease or disappear when you make the right food choices.

Yet, simply eating well does not alone mean that your body is going to get the full benefit of your healthy dietary habits. If the digestive tract is not functioning properly, many important nutrients may not be properly absorbed.

For some individuals, achieving optimal digestion will include not only proper diet, but the use of supplements which will assist with digestion. These may include pancreatic enzymes (taken just before meals), and hydrochloric acid and pepsin (taken with or just after meals).

A number of types of antacids are available. Each has different properties. Some have potentially severe side effects. Use them only rarely and wisely.

Consulting a nutrition-oriented physician may be the best start in determining your optimal road to digestive health. The physician may use special diagnostic procedures to pinpoint your problem areas. One may be the Heidelberg gastric analysis, which assesses the level of hydrochloric acid secreted by the stomach. Many people are surprised to learn that they suffer from a lack of acidity, not over-acidity. Another test a nutrition-oriented physician may order is a comprehensive stool and digestive analysis.

4

Enhancing Detoxification

During the last twenty-five years, environmental activists have made a point that few will deny: we live in a polluted environment. Toxins are virtually inescapable. The water we drink, the food we eat, the air we breathe, the medicines we take, even the bacteria in our intestines: all can add to the pollution of our bodily systems. Many people respond to the multitude of polluting sources in our environment with a shrug. They accept these pollutants as a fact of modern life. Others choose to become engaged in some activity to help clean up our environment.

Whether or not a person decides to become politically active, clear steps can be taken to personally limit the effect of these toxic environmental substances on our health. The steps are called detoxification.

In medical school, we all learned that the liver is the most important organ in removing and eliminating toxic chemicals from the blood. We learned about liver disease. The diagnostic sciences are a strength of biomedicine. But we learned next to nothing about how to sustain or improve the natural health of the liver. Most Western medical education does not teach physicians to treat the whole person; we were not taught to spend time with our patients and ask the questions that would elicit critical information about the toxins they might be encountering in their environments. Nor were we encouraged to help patients to see that they have an active role to play in their own health.

The liver was not designed to deal with the pollutants that have become a part of modern life in the last 100 years. Now, more than ever, we must take an active role in understanding the ways in which pollutants may be affecting our personal health. We must personally ensure that we provide our systems with the best opportunity to dump these toxic loads. Our health is directly tied to our ability to "detoxify."

There are many ways to enhance this process. Let's first look at some possible sources of toxins and some of the symptoms that may be signs of toxicity. Physicians may use diagnostic tests to gain a clearer picture of the role toxic substances may be having on your health, and these will be examined briefly.

Sources of Toxins

Heavy Metals

Environmental contamination due to industry is the primary source of the extremely toxic compounds known as heavy metals. Included are lead, mercury, cadmium, arsenic, nickel, and aluminum. Over a billion pounds of lead alone are dumped into the atmosphere each year by industrial sources and leaded gasoline. Some of this lead is inhaled. Some of it drifts onto our crop lands or into our watersheds. It is ingested as we eat and drink.

Other sources of heavy metals are diverse, and even surprising. Mercury is in cosmetics, contaminated fish, and dental fillings. Lead is in cooking utensils, pipes that carry water, solder on tin cans and pesticide sprays. Cigarette smoke contains lead and cadmium. Most commercial antacids can leave aluminum residues in the body, as can cookware.

Toxic Chemicals, Drugs, Alcohol, Solvents, Pesticides, Herbicides, and Food Additives

We are all exposed to an endless supply of inescapable substances that can stress the liver. Pesticides and herbicides are now closely linked to production of the food most Americans consume. They also get into the ground water we all drink. Each year, an additional 600,000 tons of these toxic chemicals are pumped into our environment. Customary American habits also put stress on the liver. Consuming substantial amounts of alcohol is one. Food additives and some medicines are others.

Symptoms and Known Health Effects of Toxins

Research into what is called environmental medicine, or the health effects of toxic substances on humans, is a growing field. But pollutants have already left their marks on human health. The major industrial interests creating these toxins must consider how their everyday activities are associated with environmental health problems and, like the rest of us, begin changing their destructive habits into constructive ones.

In time, additional research will certainly expand and deepen our knowledge of the many ways modern life has been saturated by this sea of poisons. A great deal is known already, as the field of environmental medicine has grown. Until all the results are in, common sense is our best guide.

Individuals working in certain professions or trades are more likely than others to have high exposure to industrial toxins: gasoline station attendants, roofers, printers, miners, solderers, battery makers, dental workers, and jewelers. For environmentally aware physicians, any one of these occupations will send up a red flag.

Conservative estimates suggest that nearly 25 percent of the people in the United States suffer to some extent from heavy metal poisoning. The heavy metals tend to accumulate in the brain, kidneys, and the immune system.[1] They can disrupt normal function. Increased exposure to toxins of many kinds are linked to diverse health problems, including an increased risk for cancer. And as noted, the full, long-term health effects of chronic exposure to even very low levels of toxic compounds have not been fully determined.

Heavy metal poisoning and poisoning by other kinds of toxins all create an overloaded liver. Symptoms include fatigue, headache, muscle pains, digestive disturbances, and constipation. Other symptoms may include anemia, pallor, dizziness, and poor coordination.[1] Because toxic chemicals, like heavy metals, have an affinity to nervous tissue, another cluster of psychological and neurological symptoms may appear. Examples are abnormal nerve reflexes, depression, mental confusion, and tingling in the extremities.[4]

Children show an additional, awful effect. Numerous studies link learning disabilities to the stores of heavy metals in children's bodies. Lead is the major culprit.[2] The negative effects do not stop there. The heavy metals are also associated with other disorders, including criminal behavior. Luckily, we are finding that "getting the lead out" can reverse some of these problems.[3]

Diagnosing Toxic Conditions

To fully appreciate the complex functioning of the body, I sometimes tell my patients to give a human or anthropomorphic shape to specific organs. Picture yourself as the human liver. Your job is to detoxify the blood. You do a good job of it. The toxins hit your desk, you work them over, and pass clean blood through. A job well done.

Now imagine an incredible onslaught of toxins. Work piles up. You crank up your speed to get it done, hoping that it's a one-time event. Unfortunately, the onslaught doesn't stop. The toxins keep piling up. Your energy drains. You know you'll never get ahead of the game. You're tired. You want to quit your job.

Table 4.1 Causes of Cholestasis

Presence of gallstones	Certain chemicals or drugs:
Alcohol	Aminosalicylic acid
Endotoxins and other gut-derived bacterial toxins	Chlorothiazide
	Erythromycin estolate
Hereditary disorders, such as Gilbert's syndrome	Mepazine
	Phenylbutazone
Pregnancy	Sulphadiazine
Natural and synthetic steroidal hormones:	Thiouracil
	Hyperthyroidism or thyroxine supplementation
Anabolic steroids	Viral hepatitis
Estrogens	
Oral contraceptives	

Many naturopathic and nutrition-oriented physicians have a word for the overworked and overtired condition that results. They call it "sluggish liver" or "congested liver." Exposure to toxic chemicals causes great stress on the liver. Bile flow diminishes. The liver simply doesn't do as good a job of detoxifying any longer.

One test which is a good screen for heavy metal toxicity is a hair-mineral analysis. Sometimes the test is inconclusive. A more sensitive test uses the chelating agent EDTA (edetate calcium disodium). It's called the eight-hour mobilization test and must be performed by a licensed physician. For a period of eight hours after injection of the EDTA, the level of lead excreted in the urine is measured.

The medical name for the impairment of bile flow in the liver is *cholestasis*. Cholestasis can be caused by a variety of agents and conditions. These are listed in Table 4.1.

Many of the conditions listed in Table 4.1 are marked by changes in laboratory tests of liver function. Examples of these markers are serum bilirubin, alkaline phosphatase, SGOT, LDH, and GGTP. These tests, however, are somewhat crude. The liver needs to be significantly damaged before these tests will record changes. An individual may have symptoms related to liver malfunction, but maybe they are not yet severe enough to alter laboratory values.

Often this is the case with the condition that nutrition-oriented doctors refer to as "sluggish liver." These doctors may order additional, more sensitive tests, such as the serum bile acid assay and various clearance tests.

Clinical judgment based on medical history remains the major diagnostic tool for sluggish liver. Generally the physician, and patient, will find that the interview of the patient leads to evidence of exposure to toxic chemicals, alcohol, drugs (especially birth control pills), or hepatitis.

A Well-Rounded Detoxification Plan

A smart plan to assist in detoxifying an overstressed liver begins with the Whitaker Wellness Program (see Chapter 2). Some special alterations to my general prescription will specifically assist your detoxification process.

Adopt a Healthy Lifestyle

Plan to enjoy regular physical activity. Exercise assists the digestive and detoxification process.

Diet

A lowfat, high-complex-carbohydrate diet will remove a number of the most routine stresses on the liver. For successful detoxification, it is helpful to be a bit more strict with the diet than usual. Don't allow quite so many breaks from optimal food choices. Eliminate all alcohol, sugar, saturated fats, drugs, and any other substances that you suspect may be toxic to the liver.

Then focus your food choices on some special foods rich in nutrients that assist liver function and combat heavy metal poisoning. One group consists of foods that are sources of water-soluble fibers: pears, apples, legumes, and oat bran. Another are the cruciferous vegetables (broccoli, cabbage, Brussels sprouts). Herbs and spices like cinnamon, licorice, and garlic are helpful, as are beets, carrots, dandelion, and artichokes. Very important are foods high in sulfur: onions, garlic, and legumes. In general, keep to fresh fruits and vegetables, whole grains, legumes, seeds, and nuts.

High-Potency Multiple Vitamins

Detoxification will help put these nutrients to work. Give special attention to taking them regularly and vitamins will provide a strong basic grounding for a detoxification program.[5]

Special Supplements and Fasting

I recommend two additional important components for a successful, well-rounded detoxification plan. One is the use of special nutritional and herbal supplements, which are very helpful in boosting the functioning of the liver. (These supplements and their detoxifying actions are described in detail beginning on page 82.)

The second is a time-honored means of cleansing and detoxification which dates back centuries. It is used as a means to enhance physical health and has also been a sacred part of religious practices in many areas and eras of our world. The practice is fasting. I recommend that individuals wishing to detoxify and stay clean complete a fast of three days in length at the change of each season.

The special nutritional supplements alone can help the liver gain strength. Fasting alone can also help. Combining a good regimen of supplements with a seasonal fasting program is optimal.

If we once again give an anthropomorphic shape to the stressed liver, and imagine ourselves as that overworked, tired, sluggish organ, the idea of a minor vacation from regular duties seems very attractive.

Fasting

A system-wide side effect of the drug-oriented medical culture is that many time-honored, valuable therapies have become neglected. Today's medical doctors receive few classroom hours and virtually no clinical training in nutrition. Rarely are therapeutic strategies involving proper foods and nutritional supplements recommended. Even more rare is a doctor who will think to recommend abstention from food for a limited period: Fasting.

Existing medical literature holds substantial evidence that fasting can be extremely beneficial. Growing awareness of the problem of industrial pollution provoked one of the most important of these studies in 1984. The *Journal of Industrial Medicine* published a report involving individuals who had unwittingly ingested PCBs (polychlorinated-biphenyls) through eating contaminated rice oil.[6] The subjects underwent controlled fasts of a week to ten days in duration. Some observed "dramatic" relief of symptoms and all reported some relief. The report confirmed other studies of the value of therapeutic fasting for PCB-poisoned patients.

The medical literature supporting fasting suggests a multitude of diverse applications. Leg ulcers, irritable bowel syndrome, chemical poisoning, allergies, impaired appetite, obesity, depression, bronchial asthma, neurosis, rheumatoid arthritis, eczema, schizophrenia, and psoriasis are among the health problems for which fasting has been recommended.[6]

This therapeutic tool is probably one of the oldest therapies known to humankind. Fasting is classically defined as abstinence from all food and drink, except water, for a specific period of time.

A form of fasting that is more prevalent than total abstinence is a juice fast. Typically, it will last three to five days. This way, the fasting individual does not totally abstain from taking in nutrients. Instead, three or four 8- to 12-ounce juice "meals" are taken each day. A benefit of incorporating juice in a fast is that some of the side effects that may accompany a strict water fast are diminished—headaches, tiredness or

Two very important liver substances, SAM (S-adenosylmethionine) and glutathione, and supplements that can assist the liver in producing and utilizing these critical detoxification substances are the key to the healthy liver. A compound of the milk thistle called silymarin is one of the most potent liver medicines known.

SAM (S-adenosylmethionine)   This substance is made in the liver from the essential amino acid methionine. Steroid hormones like estrogens are detoxified in the liver and then assisted in their excretion by SAM.

Estrogens are known to promote cholestasis. These hormones can be particularly problematic in pregnant women and in women taking birth control pills. In addition, the membrane fluidity in the liver can be decreased by estrogens. This harms bile activity.

Understanding of SAM has been enhanced by its study in Europe, where SAM is available as a drug.[8] This study has shown that estrogen-related liver damage can be prevented by SAM. Bile activity can also be restored through SAM's positive effects on membrane fluidity.

Lipotropic Factors   While SAM is not currently available in the United States, various agents known to increase the levels of SAM are available. These agents are referred to as "lipotropic agents," and help to lift the liver's sluggishness by helping it decongest. They promote the flow of fat and bile to and from the liver, thus enhancing both liver function and fat metabolism. Among the lipotropic agents are methionine, betaine, choline, and folic acid.[9]

Glutathione   This substance is perhaps the most important compound, and is required for virtually all liver detoxification processes. Glutathione performs a critical physiological alchemy.

Heavy metals and many toxins are fat-soluble. Excretion through bile is the only way that fat-soluble compounds can be effectively eliminated from the liver. But virtually all (99 percent) of fat-soluble compounds are reabsorbed after they are excreted. This is how liver bile is replenished. This replenishment would be a deadly cycle, if it weren't for glutathione. While glutathione doesn't turn straw into gold, its alchemy is as valuable. The substance converts fat-soluble toxins into a water-soluble form. They are then more efficiently excreted via the kidneys.

Like SAM, levels of glutathione are also determined, and can be enhanced, by lipotropic factors. Glutathione can be protected by methionine and cysteine, into which methionine is converted, when the load of toxins in the liver are high.[10] Elimination of heavy metals like lead and mercury is dependent on glutathione and therefore on the agents which are necessary for glutathione synthesis.[11]

Supplements for Detoxification

In Chapter 2, in my prescription for wellness, I include a basic supplement for detoxification. I recommend it in my foundation plan because the modern world exposes all of us to literally countless toxins. This is the high-potency vitamin-mineral formula. Vitamins C and E and beta-carotene are potent antioxidants. Simple nutrients like B vitamins and trace minerals also help eliminate toxins.[5] Of great use in detoxification are formulas which contain lipotropic factors. Examples are Liv-A-Tox from Enzymatic Therapy and Lipotropic Complex from Nature's Life. Nutrition-oriented physicians use these formulas effectively for a number of liver problems, including serious conditions such as hepatitis, chemically-induced disease, and cirrhosis.

While all of us sharing this modern world have increased exposure to potentially liver-damaging pollutants, those who know they are steadily exposed to toxins can additionally benefit from supplemental methionine and cysteine. To get more of these compounds into your liver, take either Chem-Ex from Enzymatic Therapy (three capsules daily) or N-acetylcysteine (500 milligrams daily). Several other suppliers have N-acetylcysteine, including TwinLabs. Its product name is NAC.

Silymarin   Some people still refuse to acknowledge that plants can have potent medical effects. I find the place to start opening them up to this reality is to mention the druggy effects of the coffee bean, the tobacco leaf, and the coca leaf. That gets them thinking. With this opening, I often tell them about the milk thistle and its known value for the liver, and point out that digitalis, morphine, and aspirin are all plant-based drugs.

After mentioning the potentially liver-damaging effects of coffee, cigarettes, and coke, I find it fitting to focus on a plant that is a great friend to the liver.

The milk thistle produces a group of flavonoid compounds called silymarin. Silymarin's activity in the liver includes antioxidant protection against free radicals. In general, silymarin inhibits various factors which damage the liver.[12] Silymarin also is known to stimulate the generation of new liver cells. It is one of the most potent liver medicines known.[13]

The effect of these flavonoid compounds of milk thistle on the alchemy of fat-soluble into water-soluble compounds of glutathione is impressive. Silymarin has been shown to increase glutathione levels by as much as 35 percent. Detoxification reactions may increase accordingly.[14]

In focused studies, silymarin has been shown to prevent glutathione depletion due to toxins and alcohol, by limiting fatty infiltration of the liver caused by these substances. A range of liver diseases have been found to be helped by silymarin. Examples are cirrhosis, gallbladder inflammation, and hepatitis.[11] (Milk thistle and its silymarin compounds are also discussed in the section on hepatitis.)

Most of the major supplement companies market a silymarin product, including Milk Thistle X from Enzymatic Therapy, Thisyln from Nature's Way, and Milk Thistle Powder from Nature's Herbs. Recommended dosage varies, but is generally between 70 to 120 milligrams three times a day.

Lethal Toxicity

If you have been exposed to near-lethal doses of toxic chemicals, a more comprehensive medically-supervised detoxification program is indicated. For example, many Vietnam war veterans were exposed to high levels of Agent Orange. This deadly pesticide contains the toxic chemical dioxin.

Here is a story of a Vietnam vet named Mark who was exposed to high levels of toxic solvents and rodent control chemicals, as well as Agent Orange, during the war. In 1968, his boat in the Mekong Delta of Vietnam was sprayed twice with Agent Orange. He remembers a deep, choking, gagging cough that he never had before. He also developed a skin condition called *chloracne.*

Back in the United States, Mark noted persistent lung congestion, extreme fatigue, short-term memory disturbances, and sexual problems. Following several months of exposure to oil-based paint fumes at work, Mark became totally dysfunctional. He had numbness and tingling in his hands and feet, loss of eye-hand coordination, and severe, unpredictable swings of mood and temperature. He could not drive a car. He would routinely pass out if exposed to the common fumes of modern life. He actually had to carry an oxygen bottle around with him.

When he began detoxification, Mark was on complete disability and had spent tens of thousands of dollars on visits to conventional physicians. Since they could not find a specific cause, they kept insisting that it was in his head. They were right. Mark was suffering from toxic overload, his brain was loaded with these toxic agents.

Remember, most toxic chemicals, particularly the pesticides, herbicides, and solvents, are stored in the fat tissues. The organs that contain the most fatty substances, and therefore are the greatest storage depots for toxins, are the brains and kidneys.

Fortunately, Mark had heard of the Northwest Healing Arts Center in Bellevue, Washington. It is run by naturopathic physician, Walter Crinnion, N.D., who has been attacking built-up toxicity with a multipronged approach for the last ten years.

Removal of toxic substances from the body is called *depuration.* To stimulate the body to eliminate stored toxins, Dr. Crinnion uses a seven-point program. It includes:

1. A diet containing lots of fresh, pesticide-free vegetables and vegetable juices, beets, radishes, artichokes, and dandelions which, according to Dr. Crinnion, increase the flow of bile from the liver. Meats, concentrated oils, and high-calorie, refined foods are avoided. These add to the strain on the liver.

2. Nutritional supplements, particularly vitamin C, up to 12,000 milligrams daily; beta-carotene, 200,000 IU daily; L-cysteine, 500 to 2,000 milligrams daily; and silymarin, 360 milligrams daily.

3. Constitutional hydrotherapy that consists of alternating hot and cold towels on the abdomen and back. (This therapy has been used for centuries in Europe.

4. Frequent supervised colonic irrigations.

5. Various homeopathic remedies.

6. Body therapies such as manipulation, acupressure, trigger point therapy, and others.

7. Psychoneuroimmunotherapy, a complicated word for techniques to identify and eliminate various emotional stresses and disturbances.

To further support the elimination of stored toxins, Dr. Crinnion places patients on an exercise and sauna program. Exercise tends to mobilize the fat tissues. The sauna is used to increase the elimination of toxins by promotion of sweating.

Mark required seven weeks of this intensive detoxification program. Now he no longer carries his oxygen bottle. His mood swings have dramatically lessened. His energy is returning. And his brain is functioning again.

In a similarly toxic patient, Dr. Crinnion found nine toxic chemicals in his blood. Included was DDE, the breakdown product of DDT, which measured 8.0 micrograms per liter. Eighteen days later, eight of the toxic chemicals were gone and the DDE had dropped to 3.9 micrograms per liter.

If you have been exposed to toxic chemicals, you might want to call Dr. Crinnion's office for information about their program (206-747-9200). Also, the American Academy of Environmental Medicine (303-622-9755) offers a referral service for physicians who specialize in chemical sensitivity and toxicology.

Chapter Summary

Detoxification of harmful substances is an ongoing process in the body. Modern life has substantially increased the "toxic load" on our systems. Toxins such as heavy metals, solvents, pesticides, and microbial toxins are known to cause significant health problems. The ability to detoxify is a major factor in determining an individual's health status.

A rational approach to aiding the body's detoxification mechanisms can include the use of periodic short fasts (3 to 5 days) or longer, medically supervised fasts. To truly support the body's detoxification processes, I recommend a long-term detoxification program. This involves adopting a healthy diet and lifestyle, and using nutritional and herbal products to support the detoxification functions of the liver. Short, three day juice fasts (as described) at the change of seasons are a good way to help prevent the accumulation of toxic substances in the body.

People who have been severely poisoned by toxic chemicals should consult the American Academy of Environmental Medicine and ask for a referral to a physician who specializes in this field.

5

Enhancing Brain Power

Alzheimer's. Our fear of losing our mental function is now stronger than the fear of cancer and any other disease. The reason for this fear is obvious: To participate in society in a normal way you have to have normal mental function.

Sadly, this fear of memory loss or mental deterioration, if not of Alzheimer's itself, is reasonable, from a strictly statistical perspective. The problem, called "senile dementia" in the elderly, is quite common. Estimates suggest that three out of every twenty of our elderly suffer from this condition in some form. Two-thirds of the elderly in nursing homes have some mental deterioration.

Individuals with dementia begin to feel moodiness and irritability. Childish behavior is often seen, and the self-centeredness that goes along with it. From a physiological perspective, in the case of Alzheimer's, nerve cells in key areas of the brain are found to be destroyed. A transmitting agent in the brain called *acetylcholine* is in decreased supply. Levels of other neurotransmitters are down. Connections don't get made. Irritability seems to be a very reasonable response to such a condition.

While, for many of us, our terror of the "A-word" makes it unmentionable, the growing menace that is Alzheimer's disease has stimulated more research into brain and memory function. These studies of mental activity cast light on all kinds of dementia. We are discovering that we are not helpless. The normal aging process does not have to mean progressive loss of mental function. In fact, we can enhance our brain power by following some basic steps.

Brain Function, Atherosclerosis, and Food

Much of the health research in the United States has been undertaken in the last half-century. The typical subject of this research has been the adult male, so we know that this typical American has been eating a very high-fat, low-fiber diet. Over 50 percent of his calories come from meat. He isn't a very healthy specimen. He probably has arteries as hard as lead pipes.

What would the outcomes have been if the subjects had all followed the Whitaker Wellness Program (outlined in Chapter 2), and exercised good sense in their health habits? Most of the information we have is general to this particular, unhealthy population group, who are not following any wellness plan.

The total number suffering severe dementia alone is over 1.5 million. Most of the people analyzed quite likely had lifelong, unhealthy diets. Given the nature of average nursing home cooking, most of the individuals were probably eating poorly when the study was undertaken. Many were, to a greater or lesser extent, atherosclerotic.

Atherosclerosis is linked to diminished brain function, because brain function is dependent upon oxygen. Roughly 20 percent of the body's total oxygen supply is used by this little three-pound organ, the brain. In addition, the brain is so metabolically active, that virtually every known nutrient, vitamin, and mineral is required for it to function properly. How do these nutrients and oxygen get to the brain? Through the blood. What does atherosclerosis do? It pinches off the flow of blood to the brain. It slows the supply of oxygen and nutrients to the brain.

In short, the high incidence of dementia in our elderly may be caused in large part by the poor diet of the average American.

The brain is highly dependent on a constant supply of blood, oxygen, and nutrients. Increased mental activity raises the brain's needs. Dimished blood flow to the brain or "cerebral vascular insufficiency" is extremely common in the United States. The chief reason is the high rate of atherosclerosis in our population. The flow of blood to the brain can be severely blocked by atherosclerotic plaque.

How does this cerebral vascular insufficiency appear as symptoms? Short-term memory loss, ringing in the ears, dizziness, headaches, depression, and impaired mental performance are all associated with this condition. Such symptoms especially hound the elderly. In fact, this cluster of symptoms is so common in our elderly population that they are often referred to by a phrase which implies that they are unavoidable: "symptoms of aging."

The best long-term measure that an individual can take to prevent progressive loss of mental function is to eat a healthy diet, such as the one described in Chapter 2. This is especially important for the elderly. Studies have shown that the major determining factor in mental function of people over the age of sixty is nutritional status.[1]

Brain Function and Specific Nutrients

Impaired mental function can be caused by a deficiency of virtually any individual nutrient. Some are necessary for the manufacture of critical brain compounds. Others are vital in the brain's exacting chemistry. Many common nutrients assist in transmitting messages from one nerve cell to another.

The breadth of the effects of deficiencies of even a single nutrient are pointed out in a key reference book for nutrition-oriented doctors, *Nutritional Influences on Mental Illness: A Sourcebook of Clinical Research.* The author, Melvyn Werbach, M.D., who is on the faculty of the UCLA School of Medicine, writes: "It is clear that nutrition can powerfully influence cognition, emotion, and behavior. It is also clear that the effects of classical nutritional deficiency diseases upon mental function constitute only a small part of a rapidly expanding list of interfaces between nutrition and the mind."[2]

Dr. Werbach makes a fascinating point regarding the use of nutritional supplements. Mainstream medicine will accept that correcting nutritional deficiencies discovered through laboratory analysis can restore normal mental function. But are there deficiencies which conventional laboratory tests don't discover? Werbach reports what I have experienced repeatedly in my clinical practice. He writes: "Even in the absence of laboratory validation of nutritional deficiencies, numerous studies using rigorous scientific designs have demonstrated the benefits from nutritional supplementation."

We are dealing here in the realm known as "subclinical," with symptoms such as depression, fatigue, and mental disorders. These are the symptoms that mainstream medicine will likely dismiss as "in the mind" of the patient, when, in my experience, they are actually "in the brain." Studies have shown that, even when there are no demonstrated nutrient deficiencies, improved mental functioning can be gained through supplementing the diet with minerals and vitamins.

A telling recent study of children provides one example of the value of nutritional supplements in assisting mental function. Published in *The Lancet,* a respected British medical journal, the study showed that supplements increased intelligence in children who were not previously malnourished. The supplement was a simple multivitamin-mineral formula.[3]

Mainstream medicine has so far been reluctant to embrace the value of supplementation, particularly for this cluster of symptoms. With the information that is available, however, I believe it is safe to make one simple claim: The potential value of supplements in supporting brain activity is, at the very least, a strong argument for Step 3 of the Whitaker Wellness Program—take a multiple vitamin-mineral formula.

Another important point to consider is that the group of symptoms associated with nutrient deficiency and dementia can also occur if the brain is not getting enough glucose, or blood sugar. Paying attention to the relationship between meals and these symptoms is a good way to get a reading on whether low glucose levels are behind such symptoms. (This is discussed in more detail in the section on hypoglycemia, page 277.)

Zinc

Research provoked by Alzheimer's has cast some light on the role of zinc in nutrient-brain relationships. Postmortem analyses of the brains and cerebral spinal fluids of individuals with Alzheimer's have found marked decreases in zinc levels. Zinc deficiency has been suggested as a key contributor to the progression of Alzheimer's disease.[4]

One study found that eight of ten patients showed improvement with supplemental zinc. Each day, 27 milligrams were administered. Medical staff and family members called the response of one 79-year-old patient "unbelievable." Improvements in other patients included better communication, understanding, social contact, and memory. Other studies in Europe have confirmed these results.[5]

Zinc deficiency is one of the most common nutrient deficiencies in the elderly. One requirement for proper zinc uptake heightens the likelihood of zinc deficiency with this population. The absorption of zinc into the bloodstream, and from there to the brain, is facilitated by picolinic acid. This substance binds to zinc in the intestines and helps move it on its way to where it is needed. The catch is that picolinic acid is secreted by the pancreas, and most elderly people have some pancreatic insufficiency.[6]

Some manufacturers of zinc products, aware of this possible deficiency, provide this mineral already bound to picolinic acid. I recommend this form of zinc for supplementation. The study (noted above) which showed the value of zinc supplementation in individuals with Alzheimer's might have shown even higher positive responses had zinc picolinate been used, instead of zinc aspartate.

Enzymes of all kinds require zinc more than any other trace mineral. Zinc is required by many antioxidant enzymes and enzymes responsible for tending to DNA, the genetic blueprint of all body cells. All cellular processes are impaired with zinc deficiency.

One interesting perspective on the importance of zinc in dementia is offered by DNA experts. If DNA is ineffectively handled by the nerve cell enzymes which require zinc, formation of neurofibrillary tangles and plaques could ensue. Nerve cells could be destroyed. In this view, zinc deficiency, even pancreatic insufficiency which restricts zinc uptake, could set off a domino effect. Zinc-deficient enzymes may lead to error-prone handling of DNA and eventually to the symptom cluster known as dementia.

The relative lack of research that is being done on zinc's importance is unfortunate. But zinc, like other natural products, cannot be patented, and manufacturers would rather pursue marketing a drug that they can patent. The government is the only other possibility for funding the major research that this evidence recommends. But such a progressive governmental stance has not been forthcoming.

Meantime, many people, our elderly in particular, may needlessly be buffeted by mental deterioration. They may be unnecessarily irritable and irritating to those closest to them. Nutrient-deficiency dementia may needlessly be filling nursing home beds. Over $10 billion of the $21 billion spent annually on nursing home care represents money spent on those said to have some level of dementia. The escalating social costs associated with this serious health condition should, one hopes, eventually lead to more research and support for a natural approach to healing.

Iron

In the elderly, difficulty in maintaining a conversation and decreased attention span can be related to deficiencies in iron. In children, in whom iron deficiency is the most common nutrient deficiency, the symptoms too often get tagged as "learning disability."

In the United States, low iron is the most common mineral deficiency. Studies have shown that iron deficiency is especially high in certain portions of the population, like children and the elderly. Iron deficiencies have been found in 30 to 50 percent of the individuals of some groups studied.[7] Pregnant women and teenage girls are also particularly prone to low levels of this essential mineral.

Studies in which iron is supplemented to levels required by the body have shown that normal mental function returns with supplementation. This points out a fascinating characteristic of nutrition-oriented medicine. "Senile dementia" and "childhood learning disabilities" would seem to be unrelated. Each diagnosis has spawned its own, distinct, mainstream medical protocols. Yet here, influencing both of these diseases, is a common nutrient deficiency: iron. Studies have shown that other common nutritional factors are also involved in both conditions.

What would happen to all the vast categories of diseases if everybody was simply well-nourished? In addition to zinc and iron, B12 and folic acid are often found to be deficient in individuals suffering impaired mental function.

Folic Acid, B12, and Other B Vitamins

Folic acid and B12 work together in nerve cell replacement and in manufacturing a number of nerve transmitters. Two-thirds of geriatric patients in one study were found to be deficient in folic acid. Nearly one out of every three psychiatric patients have folic acid deficiencies, according to other studies.[1] Deficiencies are associated with various mental symptoms, including dementia. In the United States, folic acid deficiency is the most common vitamin deficiency.

What happens with supplementation? With psychiatric patients, studies have shown a decrease in the length of hospital stays after folic acid levels are increased. In many individuals, complete resolution of a range of mental symptoms has resulted from folate supplementation.

Deficiencies of folic acid and vitamin B12 are often missed. This is due to a prevailing belief that an individual must first show signs of anemia. Yet problematic changes in other tissues, related to deficiencies in vitamin B12 and folic acid, can occur long before the blood shows as anemic.[8] Vitamin B12 deficiency, in particular, is significant in Alzheimer's patients.[9]

Supplementation has resulted in complete reversal of the resultant mental symptoms in some, though not the majority, of cases. One hypothesis suggests that prolonged low levels of these nutrients may lead to irreversible changes that cannot respond to supplementation. It is unfortunate, however, that since some individuals do respond to supplementation, serum B12 and folate levels are often not measured if no signs of changes in the blood are evident.

A look at other B vitamins reveals a similar pattern of support for the value of good diet and supplementation in improving mental function. Low levels of Vitamin B1 or niacin are often found in newly admitted psychiatric patients. Significant energy metabolism decreases and altered brain chemistry are typical outcomes of niacin deficiency. Nerve-transmitting substances require Vitamin B6, or pyridoxine. Again, low levels are found in depressed patients. In addition, vitamin B6 deficiencies are particularly associated with depression in women taking birth control pills, a condition which usually responds to supplementation.[4]

Heavy Metals and Alzheimer's

Chapter 4 discussed the affinity that aluminum, lead, mercury, cadmium, and other heavy metals have for brain tissue. If mental functions are impaired, a good screening test for heavy metals is the hair-mineral analysis. Normal brain chemistry can be severely disrupted by these metals. Dementia can be produced by high levels of heavy metals, which are known to alter neurological activity and are associated with creating psychological disturbances.[10]

One of these metals, aluminum, has gained special attention in Alzheimer's research. This metal can enter the body in a variety of surprising ways. Many underarm deodorants include aluminum. Most of the most popular antacids have aluminum in them. Other sources are cooking pans, drinking water, wrappings, foils, and many processed foods.

The role of aluminum in Alzheimer's is hotly debated. The debate commenced when the senile plaque and neurofibrillary tangles of deceased Alzheimer's patients were found to have elevated aluminum levels.[11]

Whenever an agent that is common and marketed profitably is associated with disease, hot debate will ensue. What if aluminum were conclusively accepted as a causative agent in Alzheimer's? Whose bottom line might suffer as a result?

Often, when profit is at stake, interested parties get together with government-sponsored research to create "objective" research. Research questions might be framed in a way that will support the answer that the interested business want to hear, so the studies are presented to the public as contradictory to original findings. Evidence is found to be "inconclusive." Claims will be made that there is "no significant scientific consensus," so government will not be able to act. Harmful practices continue, positive practices do not gain support.

In the case of the controversy over aluminum and Alzheimer's, it is fair to say that aluminum's role is still not definitive. But we know enough already to make a decision based on common sense.[2] I recommend that your aluminum exposure be kept as low as possible. There are so many polluting forces in our lives over which we have little personal control, why not cut our losses on those we can control?

Creating the proper environment for healthy mental functioning can occur, first, by having the foundation of a good diet. Second, make sure that certain key nutrients such as zinc and iron are available and work to prevent accumulation of the heavy metals that may harm brain activity. Two other agents may also have particularly valuable roles in enhancing mental activity. They do so by supporting brain metabolism.

Ginkgo biloba

As mentioned, one of the primary causes of mental deficiencies is poor blood flow in the brain or "cerebral vascular insufficiency." An answer to this problem may come from a plant which has been used for medicinal purposes since 2800 B.C. It is found in the oldest Chinese books on herbal medicine, known as *materia medicas*. The plant may provide the most important medicinal plant extract available as we enter a new millennium—nearly 5000 years later. The plant is *Ginkgo biloba*.

Ginkgo works in a number of important ways to assist the brain.[12] The effect of the plant on cerebral vascular insufficiency has been widely studied. An analysis of forty of the scientific articles reporting on this subject noted ginkgo's clear value in treating the "symptoms of aging" in the elderly. The studies looked at an extract of ginkgo which was standardized for the level of Ginkgo flavonglycosides (heterosides).[13]

Any skepticism about the quality of this research was also answered in the study. The ginkgo research methods were found to be at the same level as those employed to study an FDA-approved drug, Hydergine (ergoloid mesylates). The FDA approves the use of this drug for dementia, including Alzheimer's.

Ginkgo does not only assist the brain by increasing its supply of blood and oxygen. This plant has been shown to increase the ability of brain cells to make use of glucose. Energy production is improved. Nerve signal transmissions are improved. Brain wave tracings are improved.

Diverse population groupings have been shown to benefit from administration of ginkgo. The memory of college students as well as the elderly have shown improvement. Ginkgo facilitates short-term memory by increasing the speed of nerve impulses.[14]

This fascinating plant is sometimes called the "oldest living fossil." The Permian period, 200 million years ago, has shown evidence of Ginkgo's existence then. The Ice Age destroyed its habitat throughout most of North America and Europe, but it continues to grow in China, where it is honored as a sacred tree and is cultivated for its medicine.

In recent years, this plant has reached a highly valued status in Europe. In France, 1.5 percent of all prescription sales are for ginkgo leaf extract. The figure is 1 percent in Germany. In both of these countries, the extracts of the ginkgo leaf are among the leading prescription medicines. Worldwide, some 10 million prescriptions for the extract of this plant leaf were written in 1989; roughly 100,000 physicians prescribe ginkgo as a regular part of their practices.

Given the wide range of values of extract of Ginkgo leaf, it is not surprising that studies in Alzheimer's patients are promising. At this time, extracts from this ancient tree appear to delay and possibly reverse some mental deterioration in the early stages of the disease. Sufferers may be able to maintain normal lives for a longer period.

While the ginkgo appears to have only marginal value in well-developed Alzheimer's, it may be very useful to a significant number of individuals who may be being misdiagnosed with this disease.

Alzheimer's cannot be conclusively established except through a post-mortem biopsy. An "Alzheimer's patient" who is suffering from severe mental deterioration tied to cerebral vascular insufficiency could clearly benefit from ginkgo.

I strongly urge individuals looking for a good ginkgo product to find the quality which matches the extract used in the gingko studies in Europe. Look for the level of ginkgo flavonglycosides advertised on the label. Find one which is standardized for 24 percent for these important agents. A number of American suppliers offer an extract which is similar to the form of the plant used in European studies. The recommended dose for the 24 percent extract is usually 40 milligrams each day.

The way that ginkgo begins to produce positive results points out an important characteristic of many natural therapies. Many natural agents take time. Drug medicine teaches us to expect "fast, fast, fast relief." But think for a minute how long it has taken for your diet to create atherosclerosis, and for atherosclerosis to effect the efficiency of your cerebral vascular system. Does it make sense that positive, long-term benefits be expected overnight?

With ginkgo, the effectiveness may not be felt for twelve weeks. While most people note some improvement in just two to three weeks, others take longer to respond. Studies have shown that the length of time a person uses this plant leaf is very important. One review looked at twenty carefully conducted studies. Over 750 patients were involved. They had been administered ginkgo for varying periods of time, ranging from two weeks to a year. The average was four months. The conclusion: "It seems that the longer the treatment is continued, the more obvious and lasting the result. Even at the end of a year, it was found that improvement was continuing and adherence to the treatment was good. At least eight days are necessary for the clinical effects to be felt."[15]

Ginkgo is clearly a powerful natural product, yet it is extremely safe. No significant adverse reactions to ginkgo have been reported. On a rare occasion, however, ginkgo can cause a mild headache or dizziness. If this occurs, try to work through it, as more than likely these symptoms will disappear with a little time.

Phosphatidylcholine

Sometimes the logic of known chemical pathways leads researchers on chases which do not prove to be very productive. At this time, this seems to be the case, for most individuals, with a component of soy lecithin called *phosphatidylcholine*.

The logic is simple. Levels of the neurotransmitter, *acetylcholine*, are decreased in Alzheimer's patients. Acetylcholine is formed when the enzyme acetylcholine transferase combines choline with an acetyl molecule. Couldn't phosphatidylcholine supplements provide the enzymes with the choline they need?

At this time, the research has been disappointing.[16] Where some positive effects have been discovered, the levels of phosphatidylcholine necessary do not appear to be practical, either therapeutically or economically. In general, studies have shown inconsistent effects in both normal and Alzheimer's patients.[17] Very high doses, on the order of 20 to 25 grams per day, have been required to produce a benefit. But high consumption of lecithin is also associated with a number of side effects, including diarrhea, gastrointestinal pain, nausea, bloating, and even anorexia.

If this agent is used for a patient with poor memory or moderate dementia, I recommend that a preparation containing 90 percent phosphatidylcholine be used. Most commercial lecithin has only 10 to 20 percent phosphatidylcholine and even the "phosphatidylcholine" supplements generally have only 35 percent. The high-percentage preparation is necessary due to the dosage required for an effect. It also helps cut the likelihood of side effects. The patient should start with just 2,000 milligrams per day, three times each day with meals. If the desired effect is not achieved, the program should be canceled after a month. The benefits are simply outweighed by the costs.

DHEA

One of the most powerful tools for the improvement and maintenance of brain function is DHEA (dehydroepiandrosterone). DHEA is a steroid-like hormone which is the most abundant hormone in the bloodstream. It is found in extremely high concentrations in the brain. As DHEA levels decline dramatically with aging, low levels of DHEA in the blood and brain are thought to contribute to many symptoms associated with aging, including senility.[18]

Although DHEA itself has no known function, it does serve as the source for all other steroid hormones in the body, including sex hormones and corticosteroids. Therefore, the function of DHEA seems to be in supplying the body with what it needs to maintain optimum levels and balance of all the steroid hormones that regulate the body's activities.

Over the last decade, studies have demonstrated that declining levels of DHEA are linked to such conditions as diabetes, obesity, elevated cholesterol levels, heart disease, arthritis, and other age-related diseases.[18] In addition, DHEA shows promise in enhancing memory and improving cognitive function.

Dr. Eugene Roberts, a distinguished neurobiologist at the City of Hope in Duarte, California, has been working with DHEA and related hormones for years. How DHEA improves memory is unknown, but Dr. Roberts feels, as do others, that DHEA improves the overall communication between nerve cells.[19]

One study looked at a 47-year-old woman with a lifelong learning and memory disturbance who had received all kinds of therapy for her problem. None had worked. Blood levels of DHEA were found to be abnormally low in this patient. Supplements of DHEA produced marked improvement. Now on a maintenance level of DHEA, she has started and has maintained a business, an activity she had never done before.[18]

In another study, Alzheimer's patients had blood levels of DHEA that were lowering, by 48 percent, the body's ability to respond normally to stimuli.[10] In essence, DHEA seems to rejuvenate the systems required for optimal functioning of the human body. It helps protect the body from the malfunctions associated with age. The exciting part of the action of DHEA is that it may reverse many of the aspects of aging previously thought to be irreversible.[18]

The level of DHEA necessary to improve brain power appears to be 25 to 100 milligrams per day. All of the human and animal studies on DHEA have found that it is exceptionally safe. The only side effect that has been mentioned with doses greater than 90 milligrams per day is infrequent and mild masculinization of women. This appears as facial hair or a drop in the voice timbre. These side effects go away with cessation or reduction in dosage of DHEA.

DHEA is a prescription item, and many physicians are unaware of it, because it cannot be patented. The drug companies do not promote it. If you or your physician would like more information on DHEA, including more references and where to get it, send a self-addressed stamped envelope for information to:

The Whitaker Wellness Institute
4321 Burch Street, Suite 100
Newport Beach, CA 92660

Chapter Summary

Normal brain function requires adequate nutrient, glucose, and oxygen levels. One factor in mental deficiency is the high degree of atherosclerosis in the United States, which hinders the ability of the brain to take up oxygen and nutrients.

To enhance mental function, the goal is not just to provide adequate levels of these factors; the goal is to provide optimum levels.

This can be done though following a healthy diet and lifestyle, exercising, and using specific nutritional supplements. Nutrients especially critical to proper brain function include iron, zinc, folic acid, vitamin B12, and other B vitamins.

The extract of *Ginkgo biloba* leaves is demonstrating great promise in improving mental function, especially in the elderly. It accomplishes this by improving the supply of oxygen and nutrients to the brain as well as by improving the rate of the transmission of the nerve impulse. Phosphatidylcholine preparations are worth a try in individuals with impaired memory and mental function. And research on DHEA is indicating that it may be one of the most promising methods to improve brain power.

6
Enhancing Adrenal Function

An image has stuck with me from a research study which I will describe later in this chapter. The researchers were testing a substance by watching how well mice responded to it. They wanted to see its effect on energy and exhaustion. So the researchers forced the mice up on a vertical rope. Because the rope was revolving downward on a pulley, the mice were climbing what seemed to them to be an endless rope.

"Climbing an endless rope"—what a picture. Life can feel like that sometimes. Somehow we've ended up on this endless rope, which some unseen hand is revolving.

A familiar myth tells a related story. In the myth of Sisyphus, he is forced to roll a boulder up a hill all day, only to have it roll back down. The next day it's the same. Up the hill. Down the hill. Up the hill.

Both of these stories actually understate the difficulties and pressures that modern life presents. Our challenges are not quite so well-defined and clear-cut. They're multiple. They come from all sides: Family. Work. Finances. Environment. Health. Expectations. Demands. Even vacation and holidays can feel like they belong in the "stress" column. No wonder two of the most familiar phrases in our daily slang are "stressed out" and "burned out."

These are good phrases to describe the kind of stress going on inside us. And what exactly is going on in our bodies when we are under stress? What can we do about it?

Stress and Burnout

The Body Responds: General Adaptation Syndrome   Technically speaking, a number of different factors can trigger the biological changes that are called "the stress response."[1] Physical or emotional trauma, toxins produced by microorganisms, heat or cold, and toxins from the environment are all among the triggers.

The stress response is part of what is called the General Adaptation Syndrome. The adrenal glands are the power center for this process. This control system for the body is equipped to handle everyday stresses and the rare major trauma. Unfortunately, the system can get maxed out.

The three stages of the General Adaptation Syndrome are alarm, resistance, and exhaustion.

Under Fire: The Alarm Stage   Some truly amazing things can happen when the adrenal glands are kicked into action by fright or challenge. These two little glands above the kidneys send a surge of adrenaline into the system. It is this power surge which gives us the true stories of people lifting seemingly impossible loads, a car off a family member, or a treasured piano from a fire.

This response is kind of like the science fiction android character Data on *Star Trek.* Maximum brain. Maximum muscle. In short, maximum protection.

In fact, during the first alarm phase, blood is shunted away from the skin and most internal organs. Digestive secretions are halted, since they are not critical. The heart and lungs get continued and increased blood, because these organs are needed for maximum response. The rate of the heart and the force of its contraction both increase under the stimulation of adrenaline's messages. Breathing rate increases. To reduce body temperature and eliminate toxins, the body sweats. The liver dumps stored glucose into the bloodstream. Blood, carrying its fuel of glucose and oxygen, is rushed to the brain and muscles. Alert!

This process is also called the body's "fight-or-flight" response. Reactions in the brain to the stressors set off this response. The alert stage of the general adaptation syndrome is usually a short-lived phase.

Stress: The Resistance Stage   After the initial alert, the body hunkers down into its longer-term response strategy. The body uses the "resistance reaction" for fighting infection, meeting an emotional crisis, performing strenuous tasks, or dealing with other stressors.

It's a siege state. Different hormones kick in. At the top of the list are the corticosteroids, secreted by the adrenal cortex. These hormones help ensure that the body has a large supply of energy long after glucose stores are depleted. The corticosteroids do this by stimulating the conversion of protein to energy. And they help to keep blood pressure elevated by retaining sodium.

A prolonged siege which keeps the resistance reaction running can bring great damage. Cancer, high blood pressure, and heart disease are all associated with extended stress. Like a war of attrition, supplies are depleted. The organs weaken. The last stage of the adaptation response kicks in.

Burned Out: The Exhaustion Stage   "Burned out" is beautifully descriptive. In this third stage of the general adaptation syndrome, organs are weakened. Most at risk are those most used in the first two stages: the heart, the blood vessels, and the adrenals. Glucocorticosteroid stores, our ammo dumps, get depleted. Insufficient amounts of glucose and other nutrients are taken up into the body. Hypoglycemia results.

Less obvious, but just as problematic, is the toll taken on the other organ systems from prolonged stress. The digestive system can get out of whack. Impaired adrenal function leads to fatigue and low immune function. The organs which are lower priority during stress response are depleted, while other organs are overextended.

Under continued stress, the adrenal glands actually shrink. This adrenal exhaustion allows acute infections to become chronic. The body can't fight them off as well. Fatigue, too, can become chronic. It's the feeling of "not being able to get that energy back." Hypoglycemia and allergies are also promoted if we don't tend to the health of our adrenals. Compared to the many stresses over which we have no control, working to create optimal adrenal function is an achievable best goal.

A note of caution: Individuals who have taken cortisone have a special concern. A side effect of this drug is the shrinking or atrophy of the adrenal gland.

Coping with Stress

One of the best ways to support the adrenal glands is to learn to deal with stress effectively. Everyone has their own pattern for coping with stress. Not all patterns are positive. A good place to start is to take a look at your own coping patterns. Here are some types of stress response that can be harmful:

> Dependence on chemicals
> Overeating
> Smoking
> Too much television
> Emotional outbursts
> Feelings of helplessness
> Overspending
> Alcohol
> Excessive behavior

The challenge is to discover how to move away from these negative coping strategies. These negative strategies tend to be called "taking the edge off," an edge off of the tension of stress. Some use the relaxant of alcohol. Some attempt to "blow off steam" through anger, and often get steamed up further. Others just try to forget the pressure through some excessive, escapist behavior.

Once these patterns are recognized, the trick is to work to replace them with new behavior patterns, which I call "positive coping strategies." These new behaviors help to counter the depletions of the General Adaptation Syndrome. We need to give our adrenal systems a chance to recover and heal. To do this, it's best to find pleasures that can become new habits. These are habits which, instead of "taking off the edge," actually help replenish our depleted organs.

Top on the list is a habit that is vastly important but often overlooked. That's getting enough sleep. Try turning off that 10:00 P.M. show and going to bed earlier for a week. See how it feels. Take naps. Learn to take short cat-naps. Taking walks and sinking into a good book are also excellent ways to relax. With both activities, it is likely that far more than your adrenals will feel the benefits. Regular exercise and appropriate relaxation are critical for adrenal health.

The "Relaxation Response"

I was told a story once about a short walk a friend took down a pathway over the ridge and into the Grand Canyon. He was accompanied by a friend from Queens, New York, who had almost never left that city, or its pace, in his whole life. To this New York visitor, the vast quiet of the Grand Canyon seemed very strange, even frightening. He didn't know what to make of it. So he did what was his custom: He talked. He talked to ward off the quiet.

This vignette exemplifies a literally dis-quieting fact of many modern lives. Quite a number of people have never been completely relaxed and many fight relaxation or calmness as if "it" were bad or dangerous. Their familiar stress levels remain perpetually high.

People who can't relax, who have time pressures, or specific health concerns, have provoked increasing interest in learning more quick, sure-fire ways of relaxing. Some are turning to age-old techniques, like meditation and prayer. Self-hypnosis, biofeedback, and progressive relaxation are other methods. A common denominator of most of these techniques is a simple reminder to breathe in a more relaxed manner.

The effect of these techniques on the body is called the "relaxation response."[2] This response counters the drains put on the system by the stress response. What technique you choose depends only on what is most agreeable to you. The important thing is to set aside each day at least 5 or 10 minutes of time for conscious relaxation.

The method that I use and teach at the clinic is a meditation technique that utilizes a mantra. A *mantra* is any word that you simply repeat over and over in your mind. It is done while you are sitting or lying quietly with no distractions, and you repeat the word to yourself as a way to to sweep out all other stimuli. For instance, when you hear a car's horn blow or someone talking in the next room, simply focus on your mantra and allow it to overwhelm all bodily sensations and external stimuli. Studies on this form of meditation have shown that it produces a deep state of relaxation. Other forms of relaxation can accomplish the same thing, but the mantra form is easy to master and easy to do.

Self-Management in Time

"Fighting the clock"—how much of our lives seem to be in a losing race with the digital ticking away of time? It's a tough race to win. Beating the clock is something that one does, if ever, only by a hair. Getting an errand done before picking up a child at daycare. Sealing an overnight mail package just as the Federal Express pick-up arrives. I would say this is not beating the clock. This is a draw. Meantime, we are being beaten down by this feeling of time pressure.

The crush of our lives has created a great interest in what is called *time management.* The name is misleading. No one manages time. It goes on its ticking way, whatever brilliant delusions we may have about managing it. Only one basic idea should be kept in mind when you are thinking about managing time: what you are doing is managing yourself—in the context of time.

Tip 1. Set priorities. You can only accomplish so much in a day. Decide what is important. Limit your efforts to taking steps to achieve that goal.

Tip 2. Organize your day. There are always interruptions and unplanned demands on your time. Create a definite plan for the day, based on your priorities. Avoid the pitfall of always letting "immediate demands" control your life.

Tip 3. Delegate authority. Delegate as much authority and work as you can. You can't do everything yourself. Learn to train and depend on others.

Tip 4. Tackle tough jobs first. Handle the most important tasks while your energy levels are high. Leave the busywork or running around for later in the day.

Tip 5. Minimize meeting time. Schedule meetings to bump up against the lunch hour or quitting time. That way they can't last forever.

Tip 6. Avoid putting things off. Work done under pressure of an unreasonable deadline often has to be redone. That creates more stress than if it had been done right the first time. Plan ahead.

Tip 7. Don't be a perfectionist. You can never really achieve perfection. Do your best in a reasonable amount of time, then move on to other tasks. If you find you have the time later, come back and polish the work some more.

This "self-management" perspective on time management reflects a central perspective in the field of natural health care. "Managing time" is as impossible as managing the body with drugs. The drug cortisone is a classic example. It can be an effective drug. It acts, like many drugs, by supplanting the body's natural process. But chronic use will shrink the adrenal gland, harming the system it was meant to manage. As the side effects worsen, the idea of managing the body with cortisone proves to be an illusion. The body tends to rebel against being "managed" this way.

Both time and the body's processes are, for all that we do know, fundamentally mysterious. A nutrition-oriented physician seeks to understand and support these mysteries rather than supplant the body's own mysterious and complicated processes.

When it comes to adrenal stress, learning to relax is an important technique for assisting the body's recuperative abilities. A good diet and some specific supplements offer additional ways to assist the adrenal system in stressful times.

Adrenal Health

Times of stress are times to make sure that the body has some important basic nutrients. A key concern is to guarantee that the body has the building blocks the adrenal glands need to manufacture hormones. Among these are vitamin C, vitamin B6, magnesium, zinc, and pantothenic acid.[3] Supplementing these at mere RDA levels will not provide the optimal support. This is another time when a high-potency multiple vitamin-mineral complex may be appropriate.

Of special importance are the body's potassium levels. Loss of potassium ions ranks with depletion of adrenal hormones as the top biochemical change associated with exhaustion. When cells lose potassium, they become less effective. Eventually they die. You can redress this by making certain that your diet has a high potassium-to-salt ratio. (In Chapter 3, the importance of this ratio is described in detail, including specific ways to create this ratio. If the goal is to support the adrenals, I recommend at least 3 to 5 grams of potassium daily.)

Oral Adrenal Extracts

One way to support adrenal function is to give it additional adrenal agents, using preparations made from the adrenal glands of animals. Their value is indicated in cases marked by persistent fatigue, reduced resistance, and inability to cope with stress.

These extracts have been used in medicine for over half a century.[4] Two types are available. One is made only from the adrenal cortex. These contain small amounts of corticosteroids. For this reason, they may be used as a "natural" cortisone in severe cases of allergy. They may also be used in cases of inflammation such as rheumatoid arthritis, psoriasis, eczema, and asthma.

The other form is extract made from the whole adrenal. Often these are presented in formulations that include various essential nutrients important for adrenal activity. One of the best supplements I have found is Raw Adrenal (Enzymatic Therapy). It uses a bovine (beef) adrenal in a predigested, soluble, concentrate form. It also includes most of the nutrients that are particularly helpful for low adrenals, such as vitamin C, pantothenic acid, vitamin B6, and betaine.

Dosage will depend on two factors. First, the product or formulation used. Second, the individual will need to gauge the level of stimulation he or she desires from the product. In the case of Raw Adrenal, I usually suggest one to two capsules with meals.

Ginseng

In the late 1950s and early 1960s, a famous Russian pharmacologist, I.I. Brekhman, performed a series of fascinating studies on the energy-enhancing activity of ginseng.[5] In one, radio operators were given a ginseng extract. They were found to transmit with fewer mistakes and more rapidly than those given a placebo. In another, Soviet soldiers were administered the extract. They were tested after a stressful physical exertion, a three-kilometer race. Once again, those taking ginseng outperformed those on placebos. Ginseng was shown to enhance the ability of the body to cope with both physical and mental stresses.

These studies prompted some animal research.[6] Remember the unlucky mice on the endless rope? The researchers, also using a placebo group, set up two tests to evaluate the performance of mice before becoming exhausted. One group was set to swimming in cold water. The other climbed the endless rope. In both cases, exhaustion came later with the group taking ginseng. A clear, dose-dependent relationship to the time before exhaustion was established. The higher the dose, the longer the mice could carry on their activity. The studies established the value of the ginseng root as an anti-fatigue agent.

The term *adaptogen* is used to explain the activity through which ginseng helps create these positive results. In a more common phrase, the herb is considered a *general tonic*. The term implies that the herb is good for the overall tone of the body. Ginseng is also referred to specifically as an *adrenal tonic*. The root, particularly that of a type of ginseng known as Panax ginseng, promotes the pituitary gland to release the adrenocorticotrophic hormone (ACTH). ACTH is useful for people who have taken corticosteroids such as prednisone, or who have been under severe stress.

The modern term adaptogen is a more descriptive term used to describe the general tonic effects of Siberian and Panax ginseng. An adaptogen is defined as a substance that (1) must be innocuous and cause minimal disorders in the physiological functions of an organism; (2) must have a nonspecific action (it should increase resistance to adverse influences by a wide range of physical, chemical, and biochemical factors); and (3) usually has a normalizing action regardless of the direction of the pathologic state. According to tradition and scientific evidence, both Siberian and Panax ginseng possess this kind of equilibrating, tonic, antistress action.

Siberian ginseng, also known as *Eleutherococcus senticosis*, and Panax ginseng, also known as Chinese or Korean ginseng, are the two most popular species of the plant. They are recommended for many reasons, all of which are backed up by good clinical research. They can restore vitality in debilitated individuals, increase feelings of energy, and promote better physical and mental performance. They are also often used to enhance liver function, offset some of the negative effects of cortisone, and protect against radiation damage.

Studies have shown that both Panax and Siberian ginseng can also help offset some of the negative effects of stress.[7] The antistress action is presumed to be mediated biochemically by mechanisms that control the adrenal glands. In particular, ginseng delays the onset of the alarm phase and reduces the severity of the general adaptation response.

The type of effect you desire is the best guide in deciding which ginseng you should take. Siberian ginseng is generally regarded as less potent than Panax ginseng. Therefore it may be the best choice for low or mild stress. Long-standing problems, however, or the negative effects of chronic use of prednisone or other corticosteroids, may be better assisted by the stronger Panax ginseng.

Ginseng shares with adrenal extract the characteristic that the amount an individual wants to take varies greatly. The Russians provide us one model for administering ginseng: they suggest a cyclical use. That is, take it for a two- to three-week period. Then discontinue it for two weeks. Follow this pattern cyclically. Each individual's response will be unique. Too much ginseng, for some people, can cause unpleasant side effects: nervousness, anxiety, irritability, insomnia, and hypertension. Two additional side effects have been noted by women: breast pain and menstrual changes. If you have any disagreeable side effects, lower the dose or discontinue using ginseng.

Consumers in the United States have a difficult decision to make in selecting a ginseng product. If you buy ginseng and don't feel any effect from the product, consider that you may have purchased a product that is inferior to the ginseng that was administered to the Soviet soldiers, the radio operators, and the mice that were studied.

A good ginseng product is relatively expensive to grow and produce. Its strength depends on a number of factors, including which parts of the root are used and the source and the soils in which it is grown. The age of the root is critical. A mature ginseng plant will take years to grow. Methods of preparation can also affect its strength.

For these reasons, many of the ginseng products in the U.S. marketplace are inferior. Ginseng is often found blended with adulterants or diluted with excipients. Sometimes it is found to be without any of the active agents.

In looking for a good ginseng product, check for one that shows a standardized amount of an active ingredient. For Panax ginseng, the ingredients are called *ginsenosides*. Ginsana, Herbal Choice, and Enzymatic Therapy are among the companies selling reliable Panax products.

Appropriate dosage (as I have said) varies greatly from individual to individual. For people using Panax ginseng for adrenal support, for instance, a typical dose should contain a ginsenoside content of at least 15 milligrams, one to three times daily. The Ginsana product, for instance, is a 7 percent ginsenoside extract; the proper dose would be 200 milligrams, one to three times each day. Lower doses can be used for general tonic purposes.

Good suppliers of Siberian ginseng are Enzymatic Therapy, Sibergin, Nature's Herbs, and Herbal Choice. The ingredient for which this ginseng is typically standardized is its *eleutheroside E* content. Look for it standardized at greater than 1 percent. An initial dosage to begin evaluating the benefit of Siberian ginseng standardized at this level would be 100 milligrams, three times each day.

Chapter Summary

The adrenal glands control many body functions and play a critical role in our resistance to stress. If an individual has experienced a great deal of stress, or has taken corticosteroids for a long period of time, the adrenal glands will shrink and not perform properly. The individual will be susceptible to chronic fatigue, reduced resistance, and allergies.

We can support our adrenal glands by learning how to deal effectively with stress through the regular use of relaxation techniques and exercise. In addition, the adrenal glands can be supported by eating a high-potassium diet, along with taking nutritional supplements, adrenal extracts, and ginseng.

7

Enhancing Immune Function

Very often people announce a sickness by saying they have a "cold bug", or a "flu bug." These infectious critters are a familiar part of our conversations around the workplace and home. Almost everyone accepts the power of these "bugs" at face value. Having a "bug" can serve as full and complete explanation for a person's low energy, sickness, absence, or even as the cause of major chronic problems.

This view of disease encapsulates perhaps the core bias in conventional medicine. A germ or pathogen deemed responsible for causing a disease must first be discovered. The job of a physician is to kill it. The weapon of choice is a drug.

We are all constantly exposed to viruses and other organisms, but we don't always get sick. And not all of us gets sick even when "a bug is going around." Why?

Some light is cast on this question by other statements we sometimes hear from people who get sick. A person might say: "I wasn't taking good care of myself," or, "I wore myself down from working too hard," or, "I've been stressed out lately." These people seem to think that their susceptibility or resistance to disease is the key to why they got sick.

This latter perspective focuses not on the germ, but on the health of what is called "the immune system." This system is responsible for protecting us from infection, allergy, and even cancer. Most conventional medical doctors either undervalue or overlook altogether the importance of a susceptibility or "host." If host susceptibility is acknowledged, it tends to be as an afterthought. Many doctors don't think to focus their treatments on this important component of the disease picture.

A great way to think about this approach to a healthy immunity is to consider what it takes to be a lousy host of a party. How could you make sure someone would have a bad time and not want to return? First, get to know what your guests like, then serve what they dislike. If they love their burgers, serve them tofu. If they love hard rock, give them Mozart. If they think all natural health care is quackery, go on forever about the value of vitamins! If it's the end of the party and people aren't leaving, make some big changes: Change the environment. Remove the darkness. Turn on the lights. Remove the pleasure. Stop the music. Glare at them. Guests are not going to want to hang around.

Make your body into a very inhospitable environment for "flu bugs," "cold bugs," and other diseases. This chapter focuses on some specific steps an individual can take to limit "host susceptibility" to disease.

Pasteur, the Germ, and the Host

Most people have heard of Louis Pasteur, the nineteenth-century physician and researcher who discovered the antibiotic effects of penicillin. Pasteur played a major role in the development of the germ theory. This theory holds that different diseases are caused by different infectious organisms. Much of Pasteur's life was dedicated to finding substances that would kill the infecting organisms. Pasteur and others since him who pioneered effective treatments of infectious diseases have given us a great deal for which we all should be thankful.

During the same era in which Pasteur lived, another French scientist, Claude Bernard, also made major contributions to medical understanding. Only Bernard had a different view of health and disease. Bernard believed that the state of a person's internal environment or *milieu interieur* was more important in determining disease than the organism or pathogen itself. In other words, Bernard believed that the internal "terrain," or host susceptibility, to infection was more important than the germ. Physicians, he believed, should focus more of their attention on making this internal terrain a very inhospitable place for disease to flourish.

Bernard's theory led to some rather interesting studies. In fact, a firm advocate of the germ theory would find some of these studies crazy. One of the most interesting was conducted by a Russian scientist named Elie Metchnikoff, who discovered white blood cells. He and his research associates consumed cultures containing millions of cholera bacteria, yet none of them developed cholera. The reason: Their immune systems were not compromised. Metchnikoff believed, like Bernard, that the best way to deal with infectious disease was to focus on enhancing the body's own defenses.

During the last part of their lives, Pasteur and Bernard engaged in scientific discussions on the virtues of the germ theory and Bernard's perspective on the internal terrain. On his deathbed, Pasteur said: "Bernard was right. The pathogen is nothing. The terrain is everything."

Unfortunately, modern medicine hasn't grasped Pasteur's final insight, as though they went to court and got Pasteur's last testament thrown out. Pasteur's germ legacy was all that was inherited by them, and so they focus almost entirely on the pathogen. Modern medicine has largely forgotten the importance of keeping the "terrain" healthy and strong and inhospitable to disease-causing germs.

The Whitaker Wellness Program is based upon the thinking of Bernard, which Pasteur eventually embraced. In modern terms, "enhancing the terrain" means enhancing the immune system. The basic steps of the wellness program outlined in Chapter 2 are all steps that strengthen the immune system. They enhance resistance. Taking those steps now is like turning on the lights, turning off the dissonant music, and saying: "Okay, disease, your party is over. Get out of here."

The best way to stimulate immune function is to take a comprehensive approach. Stress, pollution, and poor diet are all tied to lowered immunity. A complete strategy involves appropriate changes in your lifestyle, exercise habits, attitude, and diet, in addition to nutritional supplementation, glandular therapy, and herbs.

Magic Laughter, Stress, and Susceptibility

Picture this. You learn from your doctor that your aches and tiredness are indeed indicators of a serious disease. As part of your therapy, the doctor sends you down to a special "pharmacist": your local video store. The doctor has prescribed Marx brothers movies, and old *Candid Camera* reruns. Instead of (or together with) "magic bullets," the doctor has prescribed "magic laughter." The doctor's perspective is that having a good laugh can actually help the body heal.

Does this sound a little unusual? Twenty years ago it would have been considered utterly foolish. This began to change in 1979. A former editor of the *Saturday Review,* Norman Cousins, wrote a book called *Anatomy of an Illness.* In this autobiographical story of his response to a serious illness, he "prescribes" himself humorous reading and movies. He attributes his success in regaining his health to the positive emotional state he was able to create in himself.[1]

Cousin's story is now supported by a growing body of scientific evidence.[2] Both sides of the coin are proving to be true. Positive mental states support the immune system. Grief, anger, fear, and other negative states have been shown to be a drag on immune response.[3]

The person on the street who has a little common sense may well have been able to provide us this insight. But a benefit of the research now available is that we have some more specific understanding of what is taking place on the biochemical level. And that has helped us develop a comprehensive plan for assisting the immune system.

A major player is stress.[4] The relationship is so clear that the level of immune suppression in a person is usually proportional to his or her level of stress. Biochemically, stress increases secretion of hormones by the adrenals. Chief among these are the corticosteroids and adrenaline. The body's energy goes into "fight or flight." Energy withdraws from such mundane needs as digestion and healing. White blood cell activity is inhibited. The thymus gland, the master gland of the immune system, actually shrinks. Immune function is dramatically inhibited.

It is as though, with a "bad" or "stressed" attitude, the host loses the ability to confront the partying disease agents. It hasn't the will to turn on the lights or turn off the music. Grousing from the next room about the unruly behavior of a few malingering guests in the living room just allows the behavior to go on. The disease says: "I guess they don't mind. They seem to have just gone to sleep. Let's party!"

For healthy immunity, it is important to develop a plan to limit and manage stress.

Lifestyle, Diet, and Resistance

Following the Whitaker Wellness Program provides the foundation for giving your immune system the best shot at protecting you. People who follow those seven steps just don't get sick as often or for such long duration.[5] Some practices are known to be particularly important. In general, it helps to "get regular."

Regular exercise
Regular meals
Regular sleep (at least seven hours per night)

Food intake should focus on more green vegetables. A primarily vegetarian diet is optimal. Maintaining proper body weight is also important. And smoking is known to be a major encumbrance to healthy immune performance.

Studies show that dietary habits can affect immune activity, whether undernourishment or overeating is the defining character. Involved in both of these scenarios is an agent called *sugar*.

Sugar "Supplementation"

Imagine the food industry taking the following proposal to Congress: "We have a plan to create a national diet which will guarantee that, on average, each and every American will eat at least 150 grams of sugar each day."

The Congressperson responds: "Now, is this sugar that comes with our food or will people be needing supplements? You're talking about a person taking 150 capsules of 1,000 milligrams each. That's even more than Dr. Pauling recommends for vitamin C, isn't it?"

The food industry spokesperson is reassuring: "Oh no, we're not talking about people adding supplements to their diets. No, instead, our plan laces sugar into just about everything, from ketchup to cured meat. Those who want to, are free to add additional spoonfuls when they drink or eat. We maintain an individual's freedom to choose."

Now picture a representative of the FDA at the hearing. Such a representative, working in the public interest, might use research on sugar and immunity to speak against the food industry's proposal: "Members of Congress, allowing this dietary proposal will damage the immunity of Americans. The ingestion of 100 grams, just two-thirds of the amount of the sugar proposed by the food industry, is known to significantly harm white blood cell activity. These important cells, called neutrophils, won't be as able to engulf and destroy bacteria. Within 30 minutes of ingesting this sugar, white blood cell activity will slow. It won't recover for five hours. The food industry is proposing that people consume 150 grams each day, day in and day out, through the year. To support this proposal for sugar supplementation, you will create an America full of people with chronically depressed immune systems."[6]

Actually, over 150 grams of sugar, per person, each day, are consumed, when nonsucrose sources are also included. The immunity of Americans, particularly those with infections or chronic problems, including chronic fatigue, is unnecessarily compromised by the amount of sugar added by the food industry to our foods.

Overconsumption

White blood cells optimally have great freedom to search and destroy. They migrate to the areas of infection or cancer and go to work. Studies have shown that this migratory ability is hindered when the bloodstream has higher levels of fatty acids, bile acids, cholesterol, and triglycerides. These blood conditions are linked to many chronic problems, such as hypertension, atherosclerosis, diabetes mellitus, and joint disorders. Meantime, basic immune response is also compromised. The overconsumption of fats, sugars, and calories typical of the diets of the obese, all greatly reduce immune activity.[7] The problem is complicated further because these diets often don't have enough positive nutrients to support immunity. It's a one-two punch to the immune system.

Undernutrition

In Chapter 5, I looked at the way many of the so-called "symptoms of aging," such as forgetfulness and irritability, may actually be due to poor nutrient intake. The relationship between the immune system and diet adds a dimension to this understanding. It appears that the so-called "age-related" depressions of immune function may be similarly nutritionally based.

A number of studies have shown that immune function in the elderly is enhanced following regular administration of a vitamin and mineral formula.[8] Levels of infections went down in the elderly who were taking the supplement, compared to a group taking a placebo.[8] Major studies have concluded that between 20 percent and 66 percent of the elderly consume substantially less than the RDA for many nutrients.[9]

In fact, undernutrition is considered the most common cause of immunodeficiency in the world. The value of the insurance policy of a good vitamin-mineral formula is evident again.

The Master Gland of the Immune System

Just below the thyroid gland and above the heart is a soft bib-like gland with two pinkish lobes. Right after birth, the gland develops rapidly. In the elderly, it often shrinks. This master gland of the immune system is extremely susceptible to the free radical and oxidative damage caused by stress, infection, chronic illness, and radiation. When stressed, it shrinks or becomes, in medical terms, *involuted*. This important gland is the thymus gland.

The thymus releases hormones which regulate many immune functions. Low levels of these hormones, such as thymosin, thymopoetin, and serum thymic factor, raise susceptibility to infection. The elderly and people with chronic conditions, including AIDS, tend to be low in these hormones.

The AIDS epidemic has brought to public attention a type of white blood cell for which the thymus also plays a critical activity. These are the T lymphocytes or T-cells. One measure of the development of AIDS is lowered T-cell levels.

The thymus is involved in producing T-cells. I consider them the Special Forces of the immune system. The medical term for their work is *cell-mediated immunity.* T-cells assist the immune system without need for antibodies.

The list of harmful conditions against which host resistance is maintained by these cells is long and diverse. The growth of bacteria, fungi, parasites, and yeast, including candida albicans, is mediated by these cells. The production of T-cells by the thymus creates resistance to many viruses, including herpes simplex, Epstein-Barr, and viruses involved with hepatitis. The relationship is so strong that often merely having these problems is a sign that T-cell production is not what it should be.

Altered thymus function is found in a number of additional conditions, including migraine headaches, rheumatoid arthritis, hayfever, and allergies.

Nutrition-oriented physicians who are working with patients to increase the health of the immune system focus on enhancing thymus activity. The critical components are: (1) diet and nutrient intake, particularly zinc; (2) antioxidant status; and (3) supplementation with thymus extracts.

Diet and Nutrition

Virtually every single vitamin and mineral is critical to good health, but certain nutrient factors are associated specifically with mental deficiencies and immune deficiencies.[10] A review of available studies particularly shows the dual value of zinc in the elderly population.[11]

Let's look at one study of forty-four patients. All were institutionalized, which allowed for good control in the study. This was a placebo-controlled, crossover trial of sixteen weeks. In short, a tightly controlled study. The results were impressive. In those supplementing zinc, food intake actually increased, and basic nutrition improved. Levels of serum albumin were restored and serum thymulin, a thymus hormone, was increased.[12]

Zinc is an important cofactor in the manufacture, secretion, and function of the thymic hormones. When zinc levels are low, T-cell numbers go down. White blood cells become inefficient for a range of activities. Zinc also has antioxidant activity, which is important in maintaining thymic integrity. Supplementation has shown these effects to be reversible, as was found in the study of the elderly.

One health claim for supplements that has been turned down by the FDA is the role of zinc in improving elderly immune function. Considering that reasonable supplementation is neither costly nor risky, the FDA's position does not make sense.

In Chapter 5, I described the known connection of zinc to the mental health of our elderly. Recall that perhaps 15 percent of our elderly are estimated to have some level of senile dementia. In general, zinc deficiency is one of the most prevalent nutrient deficiencies among the elderly. Most elderly people would probably appreciate a supplement that is likely to help their mental and physical health. The FDA could allow a health claim that states: "For the elderly, zinc supplementation is likely to assist with mental health, immune status, or both."

Zinc's value doesn't end here; there are numerous other important roles for this essential mineral in our health.

High-dose zinc supplementation, however, does have some risk associated with it. With 45 milligrams a day, copper levels can be depressed, which in turn could negatively effect the LDL to HDL cholesterol ratio. This ratio shift has not yet been found. But conservative supplementation suggests that low-dose zinc is the way to go.

Other nutrients besides zinc are important cofactors in thymic activity. Supplementation of vitamin B6 and vitamin C have also been shown to increase cell-mediated immunity and thymic hormone function.

Antioxidants and Thymic Activity

Vitamin C, vitamin E, beta-carotene, and selenium, as well as zinc, have an additional important value in maintaining a healthy thymus. As antioxidants, they can help enhance the immune system by preventing the thymic involution brought about by the stress of free radicals. One view of chronic fatigue syndrome is that individuals with this condition have an "oxidative imbalance." This means that their systems have too high a level of prooxidants compared to antioxidants in their systems. Activity of the thymus is disturbed. Achieving oxidative balance may be a promising strategy for individuals with chronic fatigue, and other conditions associated with impaired immune function.

Optimally, the diet of an individual should be rich in these antioxidants. Supplementation can also help guarantee that these important nutrients are available to protect the thymus from free radical assault.

Thymus Extracts

One of the fascinating characteristics of thymus extracts in immune enhancement is its balancing role. Thymus extract is associated with enhancing T-cell production in AIDS patients, where production of these Special Forces agents is low. It acts similarly with cancer and chronic infections. In other conditions, T-cell activity is too high. This happens in autoimmune diseases and in problems like allergies and migraines. The Special Forces get out of control. Here, thymus extract helps diminish T-cell production, thereby normalizing it. We refer to this as "broad-spectrum immune enhancement." It's a balancing role.

This balancing is one of the general concepts of therapy with all glandular extracts. The activity of the corresponding human gland is improved. The biochemical activity produced by the extract depends on what the system needs. Unlike most drugs, these extracts don't supplant the body's natural abilities. They assist them.

A great deal of specific data shows the value of oral administration of thymus for diverse conditions. Among them are hepatitis B, asthma, and hayfever. At a biochemical level, T-cell defects in AIDS have been corrected. The depression in the numbers of peripheral leukocytes due to cancer chemotherapy has also been turned around.[13]

The extract is also proving to be an excellent therapeutic agent for a number of problems that children face, including early food allergies. Recurring childhood respiratory illnesses have been helped. Double-blind studies showed that respiratory tract infections in children could not only be eliminated, but that treatment over the course of a year improved other immune parameters. This value in chronic problems suggest that thymic extracts may be an answer to a range of chronic infections, including chronic fatigue.[14]

Quality thymic extracts are made from predigested calf thymus. Extracts rich in thymus-derived polypeptides were used in the studies noted above. Unfortunately, the consumer can face a problem in finding a good thymus product. At this time, manufacturers have a great deal of leeway in their manufacturing practices. So dosage varies depending on the strength of the product.

I feel the best thymus extract currently on the market in the United States is found in two products from Enzymatic Therapy, ThymuPlex and Thymulus. The Thymulus product contains the very same thymus extract used in ThymuPlex, but is without other ingredients. It does, however, contain an extract of the immune-potentiating Chinese medicinal plant known as *Astragalus membranaceous.*

Each tablet of ThymuPlex contains 375 milligrams of active polypeptide fractions from calf thymus. ThymuPlex is a great nutritional formula for general immune enhancement. My usual recommendation to people needing immune system support is two tablets, twice daily, with meals. The product also includes nutrients essential to immune and thymus functions, such as L-lysine. It also includes herbal extracts from goldenseal, blue flag and echinacea. The last of these remarkable immune-enhancing plants, echinacea, deserves special mention.

Echinacea and the Immune System

During 1992 and 1993, the value of certain herbs began to get favorable airtime in the mainstream media. One of the first to gain serious exposure was *echinacea.*

For the indigenous people of North American, echinacea had more uses than any other plant. It had both internal and external applications. Insect bites, wounds, burns, and abscesses were treated topically. For various infections, joint pains, and toothache, echinacea was taken orally. The plant was also used as an antidote for snakebite. Generally, the part of the plant used was the root.

The results are compelling. Like the thymus extract, echinacea has a broad spectrum of effects on immune function. The activity is nonspecific and is due to a wide range of active plant components. Echinacea increases white blood cell activity, particularly the activity of those cells known as macrophages. These are large white cells found in the spleen, the liver, and the lymph nodes. Macrophages filter the lymphatic fluid and blood, and destroy bacteria, cellular debris, and other foreign particles. Macrophages are the "Pac-Man" blood cells. They engulf harmful particulate matter, a process called *phagocytosis.*[15]

When echinacea was sold as a kind of panacea in the late nineteenth century, its main promoter, H. C. H. Meyer, called it Meyer's Blood Purifier. In 1909, the AMA dismissed echinacea as "unworthy of further scrutiny until more reliable evidence is presented in its behalf." Yet, seventy-five years later, here we are finding that, by stimulating macrophage activity, echinacea can quite reasonably be called a blood purifier.

Recent clinical studies have further supported at least some of the early claims made for echinacea. The range of effects is impressive. Macrophages stimulated by echinacea produced increased amounts of various immune-enhancing compounds, such as interleukins, interferon, and tumor necrosis factor. Colds and flus have responded well. Respiratory and urinary tract infections, vaginal infections, chronic vaginitis, and other infectious conditions have all been treated positively with echinacea.[15]

A recent double-blind study in Germany looked at preventive treatment against viral infections using echinacea (4 milliliters twice daily of the fresh juice of the above-ground portion of *Echinacea purpurea*). Results showed a decreased frequency of infection in patients susceptible to the common cold.[16] The number of patients remaining healthy in the echinacea-treated group was 35.2 percent, compared to 25.9 percent in the placebo group. In addition, the length of time between infections was much longer in the echinacea group (40 days) compared to the placebo (25 days). When infections did occur in the group receiving echinacea, they were less severe and tended to resolve quicker. Patients showing evidence of a weakened immune system (T4 to T8 ratio less than 1.5) benefited the most.

The most thoroughly researched echinacea products are produced from the fresh-pressed juice of *Echinacea purpurea*. EchinaGuard from Nature's Way and EchinaFresh from Enzymatic Therapy are two excellent products to choose from. Other forms of echinacea may be just as beneficial. Some other companies marketing good sources of echinacea include: HerbPharm, Gaia, Eclectic Institute, and McZand. As a general immune enhancer, echinacea can be given in any of the following forms three times daily:

Dried root (or as tea)	0.5–1 gram
EchinaGuard or EchinaFresh	4 ml (2 teaspoons)
Tincture (1:5)	2–4 ml (1–2 teaspoons)
Fluid extract (1:1)	1–2 ml (0.5–1 teaspoons)
Solid (dry-powdered) extract	
(6.5:1 or 3.5% echinacoside)	100–250 mg

When used at the recommended dosages, there is no danger of toxicity with echinacea.

A final comment on this remarkable herb. Its growing popularity in warding off colds and infections has given it a reputation as a "natural antibiotic." Echinacea will, in fact, work in many situations where a conventional medical doctor might prescribe an antibiotic. But to give the herb the name *antibiotic* misses an important point. Echinacea does not attack the infecting pathogen like an antibiotic does. Instead, in diverse ways, echinacea stimulates the ability of our bodies, at a cellular level, to get the job done the way that our bodies like to get it done. The science is there to support this assertion. As a physician, I look for that. Yet my instinct as a human also raises its hand in salute of this herb's activity. Isn't a supportive relationship with the body's own healing processes a great relationship for a healing agent to have?

Chapter Summary

Most natural therapeutic approaches work to stimulate the body's healing processes. The heart of this strategy is to enhance the functioning of the immune system and its master organ, the thymus.

The best foundation for a healthy immune system is a diet, lifestyle, and dietary supplement program such as the Whitaker Wellness Program (see Chapter 2). Limiting stress and developing and maintaining a positive attitude assists immunity. Closer adherence to certain dietary guidelines is particularly recommended for those who are working to recover from or throw off chronic problems. Sugar and fats are particularly problematic and should be avoided.

Some nutrients, such as zinc and the other antioxidants, are especially important for a healthy immune system. In addition, preparations containing calf thymus tissue and echinacea can be extremely helpful in restoring healthy immune system function.

8
Enhancing Weight Loss

"I am going to lose weight!" Many of us have made this pledge at one time or another. All of us have certainly heard it. For me, it always evokes an image of a forced march. Gritted teeth. Clenched jaw. Single-mindedness of purpose. And not much fun. I picture a little creature on the pledging person's shoulder taunting them for what will happen if they don't lose weight. How does one respond upon hearing this pledge from a friend or associate? Isn't it usually with stories of diets one has tried and most likely failed?

I often find myself responding to such a resolution with an internal shrug. I expect that the person's resolve will give out, and that the taunting creature on the person's shoulder will take up residence in the person's brain, whispering: "I told you so. I knew you couldn't do it."

Weight loss is big business in the United States. The business is big for same reason that "disease management" is such a big business (as described in Chapter 1). In the case of medicine practiced as disease management, patients keep coming back for medical care because all that was addressed the first time were the symptoms, not the cause, of the problem. Similarly, many diets and weight-loss programs don't work over the long run. Weight goes down and goes back up again, like a yo-yo. In fact, the "yo-yo effect," as it is known, refers to a more serious phenomenon. Weight is often not just regained after a diet program. People actually become heavier, and desire increases to try a new dieting program. The yo-yo goes up and down.

Now make a different kind of pledge: "I plan to be healthier." Another vista unfolds. A person can make many choices on the road to health. This resolution is a positive one, affirming life. As noted in Chapter 7 on immune function, a positive approach already assists in bolstering a person's health. When I hear a resolution to become healthier, it usually invites a conversation about what it means to be healthy. It stimulates gathering and sharing of our own favorite healthy habits and techniques. Thus, more positive energy circles around the person embarking on a healthier life.

The optimal weight-loss program is not, at its core, a weight-loss program. It's a program for health whose basic features, with some individual variation, are the foundation I present in the Whitaker Wellness Program (see Chapter 2): healthy diet, adequate exercise, and a positive mental attitude.

The Oprah Winfrey Example

In the past five years, through the medium of television, many Americans were made aware, at least peripherally, of a weight-loss story exemplifying both of these approaches. In 1988, Oprah Winfrey lost 67 pounds, by following a 400-calorie-a-day liquid protein diet. Just after her much-publicized success, I predicted that she would gain back the weight, and it took her very little time to balloon back up to an all-time high.

I don't claim to be a prophet. But I do understand the mechanisms that produce obesity. I know what's wrong with the way most Americans, including Oprah, used to try to lose weight.

The old method of dieting was to starve yourself thin. This method simply does not work in the long run. Low-calorie dieting disrupts the body's metabolism. The body thinks famine has struck. It dramatically slows down metabolism to avoid starvation. When you do start eating again, even at normal calorie intakes for your weight, the depressed metabolic rate ensures rapid weight gain. That is what happened with Oprah. Her quick weight loss on a low-calorie diet was followed immediately by rapid weight gain.

In 1993, Oprah began a new attempt to achieve permanent weight loss. This time I predict she will make it. By the beginning of 1994, her noticeably thinner figure was once again being featured on the cover of tabloids. Her method of weight loss was nothing fancy. What Oprah did was make a total commitment to achieving health rather than losing weight. She decided she would learn what she needed to do in order to be healthy. She ate highly nutritious, lowfat meals and began exercising twice daily.

Will Oprah keep the weight off this time? I believe she will.

The Whitaker Prescription for Weight Loss Through Health

Over the past 15 years, I have used a weight-loss program successfully in my clinical practice. I prescribe this program not only to help people lose weight, but also to lower their blood pressure and improve blood glucose control. My program is a straightforward, rational approach to successful, permanent weight loss. It is designed to help your body stop storing fat, and start burning it. It's designed to help you become healthy.

I now employ seven steps in my program. All of these steps directly reflect my basic Prescription for Wellness. Four are mandatory. The other three are optional. These are additional natural therapies that specifically assist the chronically overweight in regaining health.

MANDATORY HEALTH MEASURES

1. Eat. Don't starve yourself.
2. Choose carbohydrates and proteins over dietary fat.
3. Eat more dietary fiber.
4. Exercise at least five times a week.

OPTIONAL ADDITIONAL ASSISTANCE TOWARD HEALTH

5. Use special nutritional substances.
6. Use thermogenic formulas to burn fat.
7. Use *Malabar tamarind* as a lipogenic inhibitor.

Step 1: Eat. Don't starve yourself.

I believe that one of the most important dietary recommendations for people trying to lose weight is to eat more. That's right, *eat more*. The biggest mistake people make when trying to lose weight is trying to starve themselves thin.

If the body is not fed, it feels that it is starving. The body is no fool. It wants to hold on to its food sources as long as possible. The result: metabolism will slow down. This means less fat will be burned.

So, eat to lose weight! But choose high-fiber, lowfat foods. These foods can help you achieve long-term, permanent results.

The tips below really seem to work. Focus first on what you need to do. Make affirmative decisions. You will benefit from each decision. At the same time, begin to create the positive mental attitude that will help keep your immune system healthy and your plan for health on *Go*.

ENHANCE YOUR HEALTH

1. Eat regular, planned meals. Eat slowly. Enjoy your meals. Allow your body time to realize it has been fed.
2. Drink a glass of fresh fruit juice 30 to 45 minutes before your main meal. The fructose (fruit sugar) in the fresh juice will dampen your appetite, resulting in less mealtime calories.

3. Eat large quantities of fresh vegetables and salads at all your meals. Fill yourself up with these foods.
4. Eat high-fiber, whole grain breads and cereals.
5. Take advantage of the amazing array of fresh fruits available when you select your dessert.
6. Drink a glass of fresh vegetable juice if you want a snack. Or eat a piece of fruit, or a salad.
7. Choose restaurants that offer healthy food choices when you eat out.

PROTECT YOUR HEALTH

1. Reduce intake of fatty foods, spreads, salad dressings, butter, and other sources of fats. Keep fat intake to a minimum.
2. Cut down on white bread and refined cereals.
3. Eliminate high-calorie desserts and sweets.
4. Avoid alcohol and soft drinks.
5. Avoid fast-food restaurants.
6. Avoid snacking.
7. Avoid eating late at night. Calories tend to be stored rather than burned for energy.

The choices available to you by pursuing weight loss through health opens up a whole world of exploration. These proven tips can help guide you into this new place.

Step 2: Choose proteins and carbohydrates over dietary fats.

A common view of obesity reduces the problem to caloric intake. This reductive perspective leads to a simplistic prescription: Eat fewer calories. This unfortunately promotes the yo-yo effect of starvation diets.

An approach to weight loss through health appreciates that the body is actually more complicated than that. And more interesting. Working with this understanding of the body actually offers pleasures in the process of weight loss.

Excess calories are not the problem. The issue is excess calories from fat. Even if an individual takes calories from carbohydrates and protein in excess, they are seldom converted and stored as fat.

The way the body treats protein calories is quite different than either fats or carbohydrates. It is true that, if taken in excess, many problems can ensue from too much protein. The liver and kidneys become stressed, for instance. But protein calories don't lead to obesity. This is because proteins are metabolized and utilized rapidly. By-products are quickly excreted. The body doesn't have an efficient metabolic pathway by which protein can be turned into fat.

Let's look at carbohydrate calories. The body's metabolic pathways for these are "expensive" to the body. I call them "high-overhead." The body burns nearly a quarter of carbohydrate calories simply to store them. By comparison, only 3 percent of fat calories are used to digest, transport, and deposit fat.

If the body's method of dealing with carbohydrate calories were analyzed by a productivity consultant, the consultant's report would probably deem those calories inefficient and wasteful. Weight-loss through health takes advantage of the opportunity in this apparent "waste." In fact, complex carbohydrates taken in excess tend to increase the body's metabolic rate. The body's furnace gears up for what our productivity consultant would call "wasteful" metabolic reactions. Yet if a person is overweight, wasting calories is a good thing.

We generally associate the idea of "burning up calories" with an external physical activity. Yet this process also commences whenever we consume food. A certain portion of what we eat goes into creating heat. It keeps the body's furnaces charged.

This process may also be the best single indicator for determining whether a person is likely to be overweight.[1] In an overweight person, heat production after eating often increases by less than 10 percent. For a lean Jack Spratt, on the other hand, heat production may increase by up to 40 percent following a meal. The overweight person will not "waste" as many calories as the lean person.

In medical terms, this process of converting food to heat is called "diet-induced thermogenesis." Here's where the choice of high-complex-carbohydrate calories becomes particularly important. Thermogenesis actually increases under the influence of carbohydrates. Fats, on the other hand, slow down thermogenesis. So fat calories are doubly harmful. A high percentage are taken up and stored in the body. And the body's burning of wastes slows down.

That a lowfat diet is successful in weight control has been proven beyond any reasonable doubt. Consider the example of the traditional Japanese diet, which consists primarily of rice, vegetables, soy foods, and fish. While the typical American diet gets 40 percent of its calories from fat, the traditional Japanese diet typically contains less than half this amount. The rate of obesity is much lower in Japanese people who consume this traditional diet. But when Japanese individuals start eating the standard American diet, the rate of obesity, as well as the risk for heart disease and cancer, increases dramatically.[2] The rate of obesity for Japanese people living in the United States is seven times higher than in Japan.

A Menu for Losing Weight through Gaining Health

Here is a one-week sample menu to help you design a lowfat diet. By substituting similar foods here and there, this menu can serve you indefinitely. You will lose weight without dieting.

MONDAY

Breakfast
Oatmeal
Ripe banana for sweetener (cook with oatmeal)
Nonfat milk

Mid-morning snack
Fresh apple, pear, or grapefruit (these fruits are high in pectin, a "slimming" type of fiber)

Lunch
Mixed salad (sprouts, tomatoes, parsley, lettuce, cabbage, carrots, celery, and other fresh vegetables) with low-calorie salad dressing or MCTs (discussed on page 133)
1 rye crispbread cracker (Wasa and Ryvita are good brands)

Mid-afternoon snack
Carrot sticks, celery, and other fresh vegetables
1 rye crispbread cracker

Dinner
Mixed salad
Whole grain spaghetti or pasta (without egg)
Marinara sauce (make your own or choose brands low in salt and fat)
Fresh fruit dessert

TUESDAY

Breakfast
Buckwheat pancakes (use egg whites only for eggs in batter; add no butter or margarine. Spray skillet with Pam or other no-calorie vegetable oil spray)
Unsweetened fruit spread for topping
Herb tea or coffee substitute

Mid-morning snack
Fresh apple, pear, or grapefruit

Lunch

Mixed salad

Lentil soup (fresh lentils, soaked and cooked with onions, carrots, herbs, and seasonings to taste, with no salt or oil. Use a thermos to carry to work.)

Mid-afternoon snack

Carrot sticks, celery, and other fresh vegetables

1 rye crispbread cracker

Dinner

Mixed salad

Stuffed bell pepper (cooked bell peppers stuffed with steamed brown rice, tomatoes, fresh kernel corn, pimento. Season with hot spices or stone-ground fresh mustard.)

Fresh fruit for dessert

WEDNESDAY

Breakfast

Seven-grain hot cereal

Banana, apricot, or raisins (cooked with cereal for sweetener)

Nonfat milk

Herb tea or coffee substitute

Mid-morning snack

Fresh apple, pear, or grapefruit

Lunch

Pita surprise (whole grain pita or pocket bread, stuffed with sprouts, onions, tomatoes, parsley, cucumbers, seasoned with mustard—if you use enough stone-ground mustard, this healthy vegetable sandwich will taste like a hot dog!)

Mid-afternoon snack

Carrot sticks, celery, and other fresh vegetables

1 rye crispbread cracker

Dinner

Mixed salad

Steamed vegetables (broccoli, carrots, snow peas, and celery) served over steamed brown rice

Fresh fruit for dessert

THURSDAY

Breakfast
Belgian waffles (1 cup whole wheat flour, 1 cup nonfat milk, 3 beaten egg whites; grease waffle iron with Pam)
Unsweetened fruit spread for topping
Herb tea or coffee substitute

Mid-morning snack
Fresh apple, pear, or grapefruit

Lunch
Mixed salad
Vegetable soup (simmer vegetables with spices and herbs; no salt or oil)

Mid-afternoon snack
Carrot sticks, celery, and other fresh vegetables
1 rye crispbread cracker

Dinner
Mixed salad
Baked potato with nonfat sour cream
Corn

FRIDAY

Breakfast
High-fiber cereal
Fresh strawberries
Nonfat milk
Herb tea or coffee substitute

Mid-morning snack
Fresh apple, pear, or grapefruit

Lunch
Garbanzo inroad (cooked garbanzo beans with onions and raw bell peppers. Mash until smooth; stuff into pocket bread with lettuce and tomato.)

Mid-afternoon snack
Carrot sticks, celery, and other fresh vegetables
1 rye crispbread cracker

Dinner

Mixed salad

Chinese revelation (steamed brown rice with Chinese vegetables—beans, sprouts, water chestnuts)

Season with tamari sauce (diluted half and half with water)

Fresh fruit for dessert

SATURDAY

Breakfast

½ cantaloupe

Cracked whole wheat cereal (cooked with banana for sweetener)

Nonfat milk

Herb tea or coffee substitute

Mid-morning snack

Fresh apple, pear, or grapefruit

Lunch

Homemade tomato soup (use any cookbook recipe, but omit the oil and salt; season with herbs and spices)

Mixed salad

Mid-afternoon snack

Carrot sticks, celery, and other fresh vegetables

1 rye crispbread cracker

Dinner

Mixed salad

Steamed garden vegetables (carrots, corn, cucumbers, bell peppers, mushrooms—seasoned with herbs and spices)

Whole grain roll

SUNDAY

Breakfast

Scotch oat cereal (cooked with banana for sweetener)

Nonfat milk

Unsweetened applesauce

Herb tea or coffee substitute

Mid-morning snack

Fresh apple, pear, or grapefruit

Lunch

Mixed salad

Black bean soup (use any recipe, without oil and salt)

Season with lemon juice

Mid-afternoon snack

Carrot sticks, celery, and other fresh vegetables

1 rye crispbread cracker

Dinner

Mixed salad

Succotash (lima beans and fresh corn cooked with onions and spices)

Black-eyed peas flavored with onion

Pita bread

Fresh fruit for dessert

Step 3. Eat more dietary fiber.

I have described elsewhere in this book how natural health therapies generally seek to work with the body's own processes. In this chapter, I have mentioned one particular way this is also true when the concern is obesity: how eating more complex carbohydrates stimulates thermogenesis.

"Eating more" is not usually a core recommendation of a diet plan. Yet what we know about the body's processes argues in still another way that eating more is the way to both health and weight loss. Knowledge of the body's process begs people struggling with excess pounds to eat more fiber. A fiber-deficient diet has a well-established connection with obesity.[3]

Here is how this works. You eat more fiber-rich foods, or take fiber supplements. Your body sends you the message of fullness. The feeling of hunger decreases. A number of clinical trials have demonstrated that this communication between an obese person and the body does in fact take place. In one, a daily supplement of 5 grams of fiber led to decreased caloric consumption.[4]

Increasing fiber intake has a number of positive effects. People tend to eat more slowly when eating high-fiber foods. Fiber stimulates the release of cholecystokin and other appetite-suppressing hormones. It assists with intestinal bulking. In addition, fiber helps move more calories through the bowel to be excreted as feces.

Another positive side effect of increasing fiber is that it limits the incidence of colon cancer.

But many researchers believe the prime effect of fiber on obesity is fiber's role in improving glucose metabolism. Blood sugar problems, such as hypoglycemia and diabetes, are closely associated with diets deficient in fiber. Fiber assists in improving glucose tolerance.

A number of clinical trials have looked specifically at supplementing the diet with fiber. Studies have shown positive benefits for blood sugar control. This data suggests that, in addition to eating a high-fiber diet, supplementing the diet with additional fiber may provide additional benefit in obesity. Taking grams of fiber before each meal reduces your appetite.

The best fiber sources to use for weight loss are psyllium, guar gum, glucomannan, gum karaya, and pectin, because they are rich in water-soluble fibers. There are many fiber products from which to choose.

I have a couple of important recommendations for those considering fiber supplements. First, avoid products that add a lot of sugar or other sweeteners to camouflage the taste. Second, be sure to drink adequate amounts of water when taking any fiber supplement. This is especially important if you take fiber in a tablet form. Finally, if you have a disorder of the esophagus, do not take fiber supplements in a pill form. They may expand in the esophagus and lead to obstruction of the intestinal tract. This can be an extremely serious disorder.[5]

Step 4. Exercise at least five times a week.

The importance of lack of exercise in the development of obesity is most evident in studying childhood obesity. Studies have demonstrated that childhood obesity is associated more with inactivity than it is with overeating.[6] Strong evidence suggests that 80 to 86 percent of adult obesity begins in childhood. It could therefore be concluded that lack of physical activity is the major cause of obesity.

These conclusions are quite alarming for the health of Americans. The increasingly sedentary behavior of our technology-surrounded offspring does not bode well for their healthy future.

Physical inactivity is a major reason why so many Americans are overweight. People who tend to be physically active generally have less of a problem with weight loss. Regular exercise is a necessary component of a weight-loss program, due to the following factors:

1. When weight loss is achieved by dieting without exercise, a substantial portion of the total weight loss comes from lean tissue, primarily as water loss.

2. When exercise is included in a weight-loss program, there is usually an improvement in body composition: a gain in lean body weight, an increase in muscle mass, and a decrease in body fat.

3. Exercise helps counter the reduction in basal metabolic rate (BMR) that usually accompanies dieting alone.

4. Exercise increases the BMR for an extended period of time following the exercise session.

5. Moderate to intense exercise may have a suppressing effect on the appetite.

6. Those subjects who exercise during and after weight reduction are better able to maintain the weight loss than those who do not exercise.

Exercise promotes the development of an efficient method to burn fat. Muscle tissue is the primary user of fat calories in the body. The greater your muscle mass, the greater your fat-burning capacity. If you want to be healthy and achieve your ideal body weight, you must exercise.[7] (Please re-read the section on exercise in Chapter 2.)

Step 5: Use special nutritional substances.

Liver function is disturbed in a large percentage of overweight individuals. Nutritional factors that improve the liver's ability to break down and metabolize fat are very important components of a weight-loss plan. As mentioned in Chapter 4, lipotropic agents like choline, methionine, betaine, and folic acid promote the flow of fat and bile to and from the liver. In essence, they produce a "decongesting" effect. They promote improved liver function and fat metabolism.

Formulas containing lipotropic agents, such as Liv-A-Tox from Enzymatic Therapy and Lipotropic Complex from Nature's Life, should be used to facilitate the utilization of fat.

In addition, carnitine and coenzyme Q10 are two other nutrients to consider. Both are essential in the burning of fat and have been shown to help lower body weight. Because carnitine is expensive I would use it as a weight-loss aid only if you have known problems with the liver, such as elevated liver enzymes indicating liver damage, or if cholesterol or triglyceride levels are elevated. The dosage for carnitine is 300 milligrams in such cases, three times daily.

Coenzyme Q10 (CoQ10) may offer better results than carnitine. It is also a little less expensive. CoQ10 deficiency may be a contributing factor to the diet-induced thermogenesis observed in some overweight individuals. In one study, low serum CoQ10 levels were found in 52 percent of overweight subjects tested.[8] Subjects were given 100 milligrams a day of CoQ10, along with a 650 kilocalorie diet, for eight weeks. The average weight loss in the CoQ10-deficient group was thirty pounds. Those with initially normal levels of CoQ10 lost just twelve and three quarters pounds. This study suggests that about 50 percent of overweight individuals may be deficient in CoQ10. For maximum benefit, take 20 to 30 milligrams of CoQ10, three times daily.

Another nutritional factor to help lose weight is medium-chain triglycerides (MCTs). MCTs are saturated fats separated out from coconut oil. They range in length from 6 to 12 carbon chains. In contrast, the long-chain triglycerides (LCTs), are from 18 to 24 carbons long. The LCTs are the most abundant fats found in nature. They are the storage fat for both humans and plants.

This difference in length makes all the difference in how MCTs and LCTs are utilized. Unlike regular fats, MCTs do not cause weight gain. In fact, they promote weight loss.

MCTs increase thermogenesis. The body wastes caloric energy by producing heat and increasing the body's metabolic rate.[9] In contrast, LCTs are usually stored in the fat deposits. Their energy is conserved and the individual's metabolic rate decreases.

LCTs are like heavy, wet logs that you put on a small campfire. Keep adding the logs, and soon you have more logs than fire. MCTs, by comparison, are like rolled-up newspaper soaked in gasoline. They not only burn brightly, they burn up the wet logs as well. In one study, the thermogenic effect of a high-calorie diet containing 40 percent fat as MCTs, was compared to one containing LCTs. The average metabolic rate was determined.[10] The thermic effect (calories wasted 6 hours after meal) of the MCTs was almost twice as high as the LCTs. With MCTs, 120 kilocalories were used as compared to 66 kilocalories over the six hours. Researchers concluded that the excess energy provided by fats in the form of medium-chain triglycerides would not be efficiently stored as fat. Rather, the MCTs would be burned. A followup study demonstrated that MCT oil given over a six-day period can increase diet-induced thermogenesis by 50 percent.

In another study, researchers compared the effects of single meals of 400 calories composed entirely of MCTs or LCTs.[11] The thermic effect of MCTs over six hours was 300 percent higher. Since the MCTs went directly to the liver and were burned, they had no effect on the blood's fat level. The LCTs elevated blood fats 68 percent. Researchers concluded that, "long-term substitution of medium-chain triglycerides for long-chain triglycerides (MCTs for LCTs) would (possibly) produce weight loss if energy intake remained constant."

I recommend that 10 to 20 grams of MCTs be used as a food each day. This is one-third to two-thirds of an ounce, about 3 to 6 teaspoons. The caloric content of this amount is 130 to 260 calories. It could be used as an oil for salad dressing, a bread spread, or simply taken as a supplement.

One patient of mine, Al C., was already healthy, eating a lowfat diet, and exercising regularly. In November of 1992, he weighed 219 pounds. He began using medium-chain triglycerides as a spread on bread and as a salad oil. He also occasionally supplemented his diet with MCTs in capsule form. He continued his exercise and other aspects of his diet. By February of 1992, four months later, he had lost 30 pounds, weighing in at a lean 190.

Sound Nutrition, Inc., has a pure medium-chain triglyceride oil called Thin Oil. This product can be used as a food in salad dressings and pasta. While you can cook with medium-chain triglycerides, I personally recommend adding the oil after cooking. (Their product is available only by phone orders at 1-800-844-6645.) Sound Nutrition also has Thin Oil-Butter Flavor that can be used as a bread spread, on potatoes, and on popcorn.

A note of caution: MCTs can produce ketones. When I use them in my diabetic patients, I instruct patients to be extra careful about their glucose control. Diabetics should not use MCTs unless under a doctor's supervision.

Step 6: Use thermogenic formulas to burn fat.

A number of dieting schemes that have a reputation for stimulating the yo-yo effect feature stimulants. There are excellent reasons for using certain of these agents, but they do not have a history of working well over the long run if used alone.

For this reason I strongly urge all individuals choosing Step 6 to do so in the context of the first four steps, in particular, of this program. Eat, don't starve. Choose carbohydrates and proteins over fatty foods. Eat more fiber. Exercise. These four steps will bring you the best possible results from adding a thermogenic formula to your weight-loss program.

Getting started on a new path is often the toughest part. I recall an image in Jack London's novel, *The Call of the Wild.* The sled dogs were tied up to an extremely heavy sled. It didn't look like the sled could budge. In truth, the runners of the sled were frozen to the snow from sitting there. The sled needed coaxing back and forth before the dogs broke it free of the ice and they set out on their journey.

Starting on any program for changing habits can be like that. We're a little iced-up in our old ways. We can find it hard to budge. Complicating the problem is that most of us have been trained by the popular medical culture and false advertising to expect signs of change rapidly. We can get frustrated if a new program for weight loss, or even for health, does not give us some immediate rewards. Sometimes a little "kick-start" is very helpful.

Thermogenic formulas can be particularly helpful in this start-up period, before the clear vistas from new health habits have been established.

The sympathetic or autonomic nervous systems of many over-weight people no longer function adequately.[12] As a result, they have a slower metabolism. A number of plant stimulants are known to have a positive effect on metabolism.

Two major thermogenic agents are caffeine and ephedrine. In experimental and clinical studies, ephedrine has been shown to promote weight loss.[13] Increased metabolic rates in fat tissue and diminution of appetite seem to be its mechanisms. In other words, thermogenic formulas appear to help you stop storing fat and start burning it. Herbal sources of these thermogenic agents can be used.

Thermogenic formulas should not be used indefinitely. The two classes of people who seem to benefit the most are: (1) those with a history of many low-calorie diets, who have regained any weight lost, or perhaps gained weight as a result of the metabolism slowing down; and (2) those with a long history of obesity. In either case, the use of thermogenic formulas can be likened to the use of kindling to start a fire.

One animal study revealed a substantial benefit from ephedrine alone, measured as 14 percent decrease in weight and 42 percent decrease in body fat. But when the researchers combined ephedrine with caffeine or theophylline, the decreases jumped to 25 percent and 75 percent respectively. Here is the clincher: when caffeine or theophylline alone was administered, no significant loss in body weight was found.[14]

The results of these animal studies have been affirmed by human studies. One showed overall metabolic rates up by nearly 10 percent. Signs were evident that impaired thermogenic response to food in overweight subjects was on the mend. The body's ability to break down fat cells was stimulated. Ephedrine together with caffeine or theophylline was shown to be at least twice as effective as ephedrine alone.[15]

Before choosing to use a thermogenic formula, I recommend that you review the following important considerations:

1. Be sure of the levels of ephedrine and caffeine. I recommend using products that use herbs in amounts standardized for levels of the active compounds. This allows an individual to know clearly what the dosage is, and to modulate it as appropriate. Enzymatic Therapy's product, Escalation, is a well-defined formula. We also use Kal's Diet-Max formula in our clinic; although the level of ephedrine and caffeine are not clearly stated on the label, I trust this company is providing adequate amounts in the dosages they are recommending.

2. Consider the ratio of ephedrine and caffeine. The studies on the synergism between these two components used certain levels of each. Optimally, a formula will reflect these amounts and ratios. For ephedrine, the amount would be 20 to 40 milligrams per day; for caffeine, 80 to 100 milligrams. In the case of Escalation, a dose of 30 milligrams ephedrine and 100 milligrams caffeine would be achieved with one capsule, twice daily. For reference, the level of stimulants compares to two-thirds of a cup of coffee (caffeine) and one dose of over-the-counter nasal decongestant (ephedrine).

3. Eliminate other caffeine sources. Take your formula early in the day. While taking the formula, remove other stimulants such as coffee, black tea, and colas from your diet. This allows you to experience more clearly the effect of the thermogenic formula.

4. Remember that people respond differently to stimulants. Some individuals eliminate ephedrine and caffeine from the body more rapidly than others.[17] Some have greater sensitivity than others. Thermogenic formulas are not for everybody.

5. Watch for possible side effects. Plant stimulants can produce generalized effects in the body. These include dizziness, tremor, anxiety, insomnia, and high blood pressure. Pay attention. Cut back on your dose, or discontinue using the formula if any side effects become problematic.

6. Consult with your physician. Some individuals should not take thermogenic formulas before consulting with a physician: those with high blood pressure, heart disease, or who take antidepressant medication.

The side effects of the stimulatory action of these plants are not a problem in most circumstances. Double-blind studies on overweight individuals showed side effects in less than 10 percent of the subjects.[16] Following eight weeks of use, those receiving the ephedrine plus caffeine formulas had no more side effects than those taking a placebo. In studies where individuals were given higher rates of ephedrine and caffeine than I have recommended, blood pressure, blood glucose, and cholesterol levels showed no significant change. Here, the researchers were using 60 to 150 milligrams of ephedrine and 150 to 600 milligrams of caffeine.

Step 7: Use Malabar tamarind as a lipogenic inhibitor.

Lipo means fat, *genic* means production. *Lipogenic* means fat production. One way to assist weight loss is to inhibit fat production by taking substances that are lipogenic inhibitors. One such agent is a natural component of fruit of the Malabar tamarind (*Garcinia cambogia*). The component is hydroxycitrate.

The Malabar tamarind is a yellowish fruit that is about the size of an orange. It has a thin skin and deep furrows that are similar to an acorn squash. It is native to South India, where it is dried and used extensively in curries. The dried fruit contains about 30 percent hydroxycitric acid.

Hydroxycitrate has been shown to be a powerful inhibitor of fat formation.[18] It also has other effects that promote weight loss. One study showed hydroxycitrate produced a "significant reduction in food intake, and body weight gain" in rats.[19] In other words, hydroxycitrate is not only a powerful inhibitor of fat production, it also suppresses appetite.

On its own, the Malabar tamarind may offer a safe, natural aid for weight loss, when taken at a dosage of 500 milligrams, three times daily. Two commercial sources are Ultra Lean (Schiff) and Citrin (Twinlab). However, by combining it with a thermogenic formula, an even greater effect may be noted. In addition to inhibiting the production of fat, there is also, through the thermogenic formula, an increase in the burning of fats.

Products containing a combination of nutrients, thermogenic aids, and a lipogenic inhibitor like Malabar tamarind may offer the greatest benefit. For example, the formula LipoTherm (available from the Vitamin Shoppe, 1-800-223-1216) provides such a combination. The daily dosage of LipoTherm and similar combination products would be based on the thermogenic compounds. For LipoTherm, a dosage of one or two capsules in the morning and early afternoon would be sufficient for most individuals. Like all stimulant-containing formulas, do not take LipoTherm near bedtime.

Special Note: Thyroid Hormones

Significant obesity is one of the hallmark features of an underactive thyroid (see section on hypothyroidism, page 281). I often use thyroid supplements to help stimulate metabolism in an obese individual who needs to lose weight. However, the use of thyroid hormones as a means to accelerate weight loss in overweight subjects is a hotly debated subject. Numerous studies have demonstrated that thyroid hormone supplementation can effectively accelerate weight loss, and that is also extremely useful in overcoming the adaptive decreased metabolic rate associated with prolonged obesity. However, there is concern for potential side effects.[20] Thyroid hormone medications must be prescribed by your physician. But you may have good results with some of the nutritional thyroid preparations (described on page 282; see hypothyroidism).

Chapter Summary

Successful, permanent weight loss requires a commitment to health. The Whitaker Prescription for Weight Loss through Health is a scientifically sound and clinically proven program to help you achieve your ideal body weight. The foundation of the program is a special application of key steps in the Whitaker Wellness Program. Some special botanical and nutritional agents can additionally assist in strengthening a comprehensive program. This program is designed to help your body stop storing fat and start burning it. Get off the yo-yo and get started on the road to permanent health!

PART III

Specific Health Conditions

P art III features specific recommendations for a number of common health conditions. Before you read on, I want to remind you of some important guidelines.

- Do not self-diagnose. Proper medical care is critical to good health. If you have symptoms suggestive of any illness discussed here, please consult a physician, preferably a holistic medical doctor (M.D.), osteopath (D.O.), naturopath (N.D.), chiropractor (D.C.), or other natural healthcare specialist.
- If you are currently on a prescription medication, you absolutely must work with your doctor before discontinuing any drug.
- If you wish to try the natural approach, discuss it with your physician. Since your physician may be unaware of all the natural alternatives available, you may need to educate him or her. Bring this book along with you to the doctor's office. The natural alternatives being recommended are based upon published studies in medical journals. References are provided if your physician wants additional information.
- Remember, although many natural alternatives, such as nutritional supplements and herbs, are effective on their own, they work even better if they are part of a comprehensive natural treatment plan that focuses on diet and lifestyle factors, such as the Whitaker Wellness Program, described in Chapter 2.

Acne

Dr. Whitaker's Prescription for Acne:

1. Follow the Whitaker Wellness Program.
2. Use Derma-Klear Acne Treatment Program from Enzymatic Therapy:
   a. Take one capsule of Akne-Zyme, twice daily.
   b. Wash face or affected area with Derma-Klear Acne Treatment Cleanser, twice daily.
   c. Apply Derma-Klear Akne Treatment Cream one to three times daily, as directed on label.
3. Eliminate all refined or concentrated sugars from the diet.
4. Do not eat foods containing trans-fatty acids, such as milk, milk products, margarine, shortening and other synthetically hydrogenated vegetable oils, or fried foods.
5. Avoid foods high in iodized salt.
6. Avoid using greasy creams or cosmetics.
7. Wash pillowcases regularly in chemical-free (no added colors or fragrances) detergents.

Description

At puberty, increased levels of the hormone testosterone are found in both girls and boys. Testosterone stimulates glands located beneath hair follicles to enlarge and produce a mixture of oils and waxes. The value of this secretion, called sebum, is in lubricating the skin and preventing water loss. Testosterone also promotes the cells that line the skin pores out of which hair follicles pass to produce more keratin.

Together, sebum and keratin block skin pores, and blackheads (comedones) form. Bacteria overgrow. Enzymes are released which break down sebum. This produces inflammation (papules). Whiteheads (pustules) or "pimples" are the result. Because sebaceous glands are concentrated in the highest levels on the face, shoulders, back, and chest, this is where these little horrors pop up.

The most familiar form of acne is *acne vulgaris.* It affects the hair follicles and the oil-secreting skin glands. Acne vulgaris is known by the skin conditions noted above. *Acne conglobata* is a more severe form. Deep cysts form. Skin can be permanently scarred.

Comments on the Whitaker Prescription for Acne

My approach to acne is a comprehensive natural approach designed to improve the health of the skin. Avoid using harsh prescription drugs or over-the-counter creams and lotions. It is a successful prescription because it addresses the underlying features that contribute to acne.

My treatment plan features the Derma-Klear Acne Treatment Program from Enzymatic Therapy. The program consists of three separate products: a nutritional product, Akne-Zyme; a skin cleanser to remove excess sebum and oil, Derma-Klear Akne Treatment Cleanser; and a natural antibacterial cream, Derma-Klear Akne Treatment Cream.

The nutritional product, Akne-Zyme, is composed of nutrients essential to healthy skin. These include zinc, vitamin A, and vitamin C, in a base of sublimed sulfur, bromelain, and other natural elements that nourish the skin.

Zinc is probably the most important single nutrient in the treatment of acne. Zinc is critical to the utilization of vitamin A by the skin. It is also essential in wound healing, immune system activity, inflammation control, and tissue regeneration, all of which are important in successful treatment of acne. Unfortunately for adolescent boys, serum zinc levels are lower in 13- and 14-year-old males than in any other age group.[1]

Several double-blind studies have shown zinc to produce similar results to tetracycline in treating superficial acne. It actually shows superior results compared to this strong antibiotic in treating deeper forms of acne.[2] Although some people in studies showed dramatic improvement immediately, the majority usually required twelve weeks of supplementation before good results were achieved. Again, natural therapeutics often take time.

Akne-Zyme also provides high levels of vitamin A. This vitamin, like the synthetic vitamin A drug called Accutane, has been shown in many studies to reduce sebum production and other factors which contribute to the formation of pimples.[3] Although many of the studies using vitamin A to treat acne utilized extremely high dosages, I have found that high doses of vitamin A are not necessary. The trick is to introduce other nutritional factors, like zinc, vitamin B6, selenium, and vitamin E in the care program. These nutrients work with vitamin A in promoting healthy skin.[4]

A safe and effective recommendation for acne is to take one capsule of Akne-Zyme twice daily. This dosage will provide 30 milligrams of zinc and 10,000 IU of vitamin A. Because high doses of vitamin A during pregnancy can cause birth defects, women of child-bearing age should use birth control during treatment with Akne-Zyme (or any other high-dose vitamin A product). This is a very cautious approach. The level of vitamin A required to produce birth defects is thought to be at least 25,000 IU. Any risk, however, is simply not worth it.

The Derma-Klear Acne Treatment Cleanser and Cream provide sulfur in a base of herbal extracts. This combination helps remove excess sebum from the skin and assists in preventing overgrowth of bacteria and conditions that lead to closure of skin pores. This helps reduce inflammation and redness.

Age Spots

Dr. Whitaker's Prescription for Age Spots:

1. Follow the Whitaker Wellness Program.
2. Take 50,000 IU of beta-carotene per day.
3. Take 40 milligrams of *Ginkgo biloba* extract (24 percent ginkgo flavonglycosides), three times daily.
4. Use Imedeen, three tablets twice daily.
5. Apply Reviva Labs Brown Spot Cream each night before going to bed.
6. Stay out of the sun.

Description

Certain molecules throughout the body can become partially damaged by free radicals. Like debris in an unkempt yard, this cellular debris collects in our bodies over time. Some of this debris clumps together on the skin to produce brown spots, commonly known as *age spots*. Just as white spots on the fingernails can point to a zinc deficiency, so the number and severity of age spots on the skin can signal the level of oxidative damage throughout the body. This accumulation of cellular debris is known as *lipofuscin*.

Comments on the Whitaker Prescription for Age Spots

It is easier to prevent lipofuscin deposits than it is to reverse them. Foremost in the prevention of age spots is to avoid excessive sun exposure and to use sunblocking creams when you are out in the sun. The second step is making sure your intake of antioxidants, especially beta-carotene, is high. If you are prone to age spots, I recommend 50,000 international units (IU) of beta-carotene per day.

It is also a good idea to take ginkgo (see Chapter 5). Ginkgo helps prevent lipofuscin deposits in the brain, which are thought to play a major role in causing age-related memory loss. When looking for a ginkgo product, make sure the product is standardized to contain 24 percent ginkgo flavonglycosides. Read labels carefully. Most major suppliers of herbal products provide high-quality ginkgo products, including Enzymatic Therapy, Nature's Herbs, Nature's Way, and Kal.

I also recommend a product called Imedeen from Scandinavian Naturals. Imedeen is composed of a special protein and glycosaminol-glycan concentrate from fish. Several clinical studies have shown that Imedeen can significantly improve the health of the skin and help the skin look younger. The oral dose studied is 380 to 500 milligrams daily.[1] Imedeen is especially effective for sun-damaged skin, and is available at most health food stores. If you cannot find it, call The Vitamin Shoppe (1-800-223-1216) or L&H Vitamins (1-800-221-1152).

If you are really bothered by age spots and want to try a more cosmetic approach, you can use creams containing the bleaching agent hydroquinone. It is not known exactly how hydroquinone creams work, but they can reduce the darkness of the spots by about 50 percent. It is even more important to avoid sun exposure or use sunscreen when using bleaching creams. Reviva Brown Spot Cream is a brand that can be found in most health food stores or through the major mail-order houses.

Anemia

Dr. Whitaker's Prescription for Anemia:

Iron-Deficiency Anemia
Take two capsules of Ultimate Iron (Enzymatic Therapy) twice daily.

Folic Acid-Deficiency Anemia
Take 400 micrograms of folic acid, twice daily.

Vitamin B12-Deficiency Anemia
1. Initially, have your doctor inject you with 1,000 micrograms of vitamin B12, once a week for four weeks.
2. Take a 1,000-microgram sublingual vitamin B12 tablet daily.

Description

Anemia refers to a condition in which the blood is deficient in red blood cells, or the hemoglobin (iron-containing) portion of red blood cells. The primary function of the red blood cell (RBC) is to transport oxygen from the lungs to the tissues of the body. There, RBCs exchange the oxygen for carbon dioxide. The symptoms of anemia, such as extreme fatigue, reflect both a lack of oxygen being delivered to tissues and a buildup of carbon dioxide.

There are several different types of anemia. The major categories are:

Anemias due to excessive blood loss
Anemias due to excessive red blood cell destruction
Anemias due to deficient red blood cell production

Most anemia is due to deficient red blood cell production. In most cases, anemia is secondary to blood loss or a nutrient deficiency. Iron deficiency is, by far, the most common nutritional cause of anemia. Deficiencies of folic acid or vitamin B12 can also lead to anemia.

Any case of anemia should be properly diagnosed by a physician to identify the cause. Treatment must be directed at the underlying cause. My recommendations for nutritional deficiency anemias are given below.

Comments on the Whitaker Prescription for Anemia

When I need to prescribe an iron supplement, I usually use Enzymatic Therapy's Ultimate Iron. Each capsule contains 30 milligrams of ferrous succinate and 250 milligrams of liquid liver fractions. Ultimate Iron provides highly absorbable iron and is relatively free from side effects like nausea, constipation, or diarrhea, common to other iron supplements.

Ultimate Iron includes the liver fractions rich in "heme" iron. Of the two forms of dietary iron, "heme" iron and "non-heme" iron, "heme" iron is more efficiently absorbed. It is iron bound to hemoglobin and myoglobin. While heme iron is absorbed intact, non-heme iron is dependent upon ionization and complex transport mechanisms.[1] A breakdown of these mechanisms can harm your body's ability to uptake non-heme iron. In addition, non-heme iron is extremely susceptible to blocking agents, such as fiber, phosphates, calcium, tannates, and preservatives. Heme iron is not affected by these factors.

In addition to iron, Ultimate Iron provides other blood-building factors: vitamin C, folic acid, vitamin B12, and fat-soluble chlorophyll. It is a very good formula for any type of anemia as it provides many factors necessary for the manufacture of red blood cells.

Angina

Dr. Whitaker's Prescription for Angina:

1. For severe angina, take intravenous EDTA chelation therapy.
2. In general, follow Whitaker Wellness Program.
3. Take 500 milligrams of carnitine, twice daily.
4. Take 30 to 100 milligrams of coenzyme Q10, three times daily.

5. Take two tablets Rogenic (Enzymatic Therapy), three times daily with meals.
6. Study *Reversing Heart Disease* (Warner Books, 1985), to learn more.
7. If cholesterol levels are high, follow recommendations on page 193.

Description

Angina describes a squeezing or pressure-like pain in the chest. Angina is caused by an insufficient supply of oxygen to the heart muscle. Since physical exertion and stress cause an increased need for oxygen by the heart, symptoms of angina are often preceded by these factors. The pain may radiate to the left shoulder blade, left arm, or jaw. The pain typically lasts from 1 to 20 minutes.

Angina is almost always due to atherosclerosis. This is the buildup of cholesterol-containing plaque, progressively narrowing (and ultimately blocking) the blood vessels supplying the heart, the coronary arteries. This blockage results in a decreased blood and oxygen supply to the heart tissue. When the flow of oxygen to the heart muscle is substantially reduced, or when there is an increased need by the heart, angina results.

You should be aware that a special type of angina exists that is not related to a buildup of plaque on the coronary arteries. It is known as *Prinzmetal's variant angina* and is caused by the spasm of a coronary artery. This form of angina is more apt to occur when the body is at rest. It may occur at odd times during the day or night, and is more common in women under age fifty. It usually responds to magnesium supplementation.

Comments on the Whitaker Prescription for Angina

Angina is a serious condition that requires strict medical supervision. In the severe case, as well as in the initial stages in the mild to moderate patient, prescription medications may be necessary. Eventually the condition can usually be controlled with the help of natural measures.

If there is significant blockage of the coronary artery, my recommendation is not bypass surgery. I recommend a safer, more effective therapy known as intravenous EDTA chelation. Most modern-day cardiologists place a great deal of trust in the angiogram, an X-ray procedure where dye is injected into the coronary arteries to determine where blockages might be. These blockages can be opened with balloon angioplasty (or another catheterization technique) and coronary artery bypass surgery.

Angiograms

If you have angina, your physician is most likely urging you to get an angiogram. Your physician may be telling you: "Look, you are a walking time bomb. Unless we do this angiogram to find the blockages to your heart and do something about them, you could have a fatal heart attack at any time."

These terrifying words from cardiologists keep heart surgeons very busy. Patients submit to surgical procedures assuming that the search for heart artery blockage is necessary for adequate treatment. I believe this assumption is simply not true.

My book, *Reversing Heart Disease* (Warner Books, 1985), includes a chapter on the angiogram. I believe this procedure is too often misused in order to facilitate the business of bypass surgery and angioplasty. Since 1985, "business" has gotten better. Today, over a million angiograms are performed each year—for a total of over $10 billion.

Not all cardiologists will use this aggressive approach. Dr. Thomas Graboys, a Harvard cardiologist, has published the results from several studies which suggest successful alternatives to the "let's catheterize" approach of some cardiologists.[1] In his most recent study (JAMA, November 11, 1992), 168 patients were told that they needed to have a cardiac catheterization to determine the degree of blockage and consequent need for additional therapy. These patients then came to Dr. Graboys for a second opinion. He used noninvasive, less expensive tests to check out the angiogram recommendation. These tests included an exercise stress test; the echocardiogram, which uses sound waves to assess the function of the heart; and the Holter heart monitor, worn by the patient for 24 hours. Dr. Graboys determined that 134 patients, or 80 percent, did not need the catheterization. For the remaining 20 percent, he recommended a change in medication or treatment and observation for two months. At the end of those two months, he concluded that the majority of these patients did not need catheterization. In all, out of 168 patients, Dr. Graboys recommended that 6 patients, less than 4 percent, required catheterization.

Contrary to the doom-and-gloom proclamations of the original cardiologist, these 168 patients experienced only a 1.1 percent annual fatal heart attack rate over a five-year period. This rate is much lower than the mortality rates associated with either coronary artery bypass surgery (5 to 10 percent) or angioplasty (1 to 2 percent). Dr. Graboys concluded that "in a large fraction of medically stable patients with coronary disease who are urged to undergo coronary angiography (heart catheterization), the procedure can be safely deferred."

Basically, Dr. Graboys demonstrated that you do not need an angiogram to determine if bypass surgery or angioplasty is required. Noninvasive testing to determine the functional state of the heart is far more important in determining the type of therapy that is needed than the invasive search for blocked arteries. Only if the heart is not functioning well is the angiogram needed to see if surgery should be done.

The bottom line is that most aggressive "replumbing" techniques have been found to be irrelevant to the typical course of the disease; blockages found by an angiogram are usually not relevant to the patient's risk of heart attack. The most sophisticated study of bypass surgery—the Coronary Artery Surgery Study (CASS)—demonstrated that healthy-hearted patients with one, two, or all three of the major heart vessels blocked did surprisingly well without surgery.[2] Regardless of the number or severity of the blockages, each group had the same very low fatality rate of 1.6 percent a year; the survival rate was 98.4 percent. That same year, the average fatality rate from bypass surgery was 10.1 percent, about one death per ten operations.

The past decade has seen a proliferation of both bypass surgery and angioplasty, in spite of strong scientific evidence that neither may be helpful in the long run for the overwhelming majority of patients. In general, the only reason for the current 800,000 bypass and angioplasty surgeries performed each year is the high number of working cardiologists and surgeons in the medical community.

If there is no difference in heart attack rate in patients with one vessel blocked, compared to those with all three vessels blocked, the significance of any blockages found on the cardiac catheterization is not much. This possibly unnecessary operation, supposedly to save your life, is about five to ten times more deadly than the disease!

Blockages are not an accurate estimate of the reduction of blood flow in the artery. According to a study in the *New England Journal of Medicine* in 1984, researchers at the University of Iowa measured blood flow in over forty-four blockages demonstrated by the angiogram in thirty-nine patients.[3] Much to their surprise, they found no correlation between blood flow and the severity of the heart artery blockage. In other words, the angiogram was worthless.

The authors concluded that the blockages found on the heart catheterization simply do not correlate with blood flow restriction. They also commented that "the results of these studies should be profoundly disturbing on the coronary arteriogram (heart catheterization)." They added that needed information "cannot be determined accurately by conventional angiographic approaches."

If your physician recommends that you have a coronary angiogram (catheterization), the chances are eight out of ten that you do not need it. The critical factor in determining whether you do need one is how well your left ventricular pump is working. It doesn't have to do with the degree of blockage or the number of arteries affected. It has to do with the ejection fraction, the amount of blood pumped out by the heart with each beat. For example, if the heart is filled with 100 milliliters of blood and pumps out 50 milliliters, the ejection fraction is 50 percent. If it only pumps out 40 milliliters, the ejection fraction is 40 percent. Generally, a healthy heart will have an ejection fraction of 50 percent or greater, but the heart never pumps all of the blood in its chambers.

There are, however, a couple of conditions when bypass is helpful: when the left main coronary artery is blocked; when the patient has severe anginal pain that is unresponsive to all forms of therapy; and when there is evidence of three blockages of the main coronary arteries and the ejection fraction is less than 40 percent. In these cases, surgical patients tend to do better than nonsurgically treated patients.[4]

Using this criteria, it is estimated that greater than 90 percent of all bypass procedures are unnecessary. If this surgery were performed only on appropriate candidates, the heart surgery industry would probably suffer significant financial losses.

Here are ten important points to bear in mind about heart disease, angiograms, angioplasty, and heart bypass operations.

1. Relying on angiograms is an inaccurate method to determine what is going on with the disease.

2. The best that can be said about bypass surgery and balloon angioplasty is that they are irrelevant to the course of the disease, in all but the most serious cases. Patients electing not to have the surgery live just as long or longer than those having surgery.[5]

3. Bypass does not increase blood flow to the heart muscle in most cases. "Successful bypass" may even reduce blood flow.

4. The cardiopulmonary pump used during bypass surgery can causes brain damage in any patient. This damage can lead to memory loss, paralysis, and personality changes after the operation.

5. The number of blood vessels blocked is usually irrelevant to the need for bypass surgery. The main determining factor is how well the left ventricular pump is working.

6. Bypass surgery or angioplasty are not curative; they do not address the reasons why the plaque developed in the first place.

7. Due to changes in blood flow, the section of the artery upstream from the graft has accelerated plaque formation (closure) at a rate ten times higher than the rate in an ungrafted coronary artery. This closure is probably the major reason these patients do so poorly over time.

8. Up to 90 percent of bypass procedures are done when the ejection fraction is greater than 50 percent, which indicates a healthy heart.[2]

9. After a bypass operation, the risk of subsequent heart attack is actually higher than in patients similarly at risk who are treated with drugs.

10. Between 25 percent to 33 percent of patients over 80 years of age die within one year of bypass surgery. This mortality rate is far greater than with nonsurgical therapy.[2]

Get a Second Opinion

If an angiogram is recommended, have a second opinion from a good cardiologist. Follow the steps below:

1. Take the following key reference list to your local library and obtain copies of these articles from the *Journal of the American Medical Association* and the *New England Journal of Medicine*. Most public libraries have these medical journals, and most mainstream physicians respect them.

> Graboys TD, et al.: Results of a second opinion program for coronary artery bypass surgery. JAMA 268:2537–40, 1992.
> Graboys TD, et al.: Results of a second opinion program for coronary artery bypass surgery. JAMA 258:1611–14, 1987.
> Winslow CM, et al.: The appropriateness of performing coronary artery bypass surgery. JAMA 260:505, 1988.
> Hueb W: Two to eight-year survival rates in patients who refused coronary artery bypass grafting. Am J Cardiol 63:155–9, 1989.
> CASS Principle Investigators and their Associates: Myocardial infarction and mortality in the coronary artery surgery study (CASS) randomized trial. New Engl J Med 310:750–8, 1984.

2. Read the articles carefully, with dictionary in hand.
3. Take the articles with you to the physician who will be rendering the second opinion. Request that they follow the protocols outlined by Dr. Graboys for both the angiogram and cardiac bypass operation.
4. If the doctor is unwilling to follow these protocols, seek out another cardiologist.

I strongly recommend, before visiting another cardiologist for a second opinion, that you try to find a qualified chelation specialist immediately. Contact the American College of Advancement in Medicine (ACAM), 23121 Verdugo Drive, Suite 204, Laguna Hills, CA 92653, 1-800-532-3688 (outside California), or 1-800-435-6199 (inside California). Or, if you live in one of the states surrounding the Great Lakes, contact the Great Lakes Association of Clinical Medicine, 70 West Huron St., Chicago, IL 60610, 312-266-6246.

Intravenous EDTA Chelation Therapy

Many cardiologists may tell angina patients: "If you do not have heart surgery, you are going to die. There are no alternatives." In most cases, this is simply not true. For most patients, there is a safer, more effective, less expensive alternative. This is EDTA chelation therapy.

EDTA, or if you prefer its scientific name, ethylene diamine tetraacetic acid, is an amino acid-like molecule. When slowly infused into the bloodstream, it binds with minerals such as calcium, iron, copper, and lead, and carries them to the kidney, where they are excreted. EDTA chelation has been commonly used for lead poisoning. In the late 1950s and early 1960s, however, it was found to help patients with angina, cerebral vascular insufficiency, and occlusive peripheral vascular disease.[6]

Early understanding of EDTA's positive effect was that it opened blocked arteries by chelating out the calcium deposits in the cholesterol plaque, similar to the way in which EDTA chelates out heavy metals such as lead. However, it now appears that the beneficial results are more likely related to chelating out excess iron and copper, minerals that, in the presence of oxygen, stimulate free radical activity. Free radicals damage the cells in the artery and are a primary reason for atherosclerosis.

The initial results with EDTA therapy were remarkable. In a series of 283 patients treated by Dr. Norman Clarke and his colleagues from 1956 to 1960, 87 percent showed improvement in their symptoms. Heart patients got better, and patients with blocked arteries in the legs, particularly those with diabetes, avoided amputation.[6]

Dr. Daniel Steinberg and associates then undertook a review of the process of atherosclerosis. They concluded that it "is dependent on the presence of some metals (copper and iron) and can be completely inhibited by chelating agents such as EDTA."[7]

In spite of its obvious benefits to heart patients, EDTA fell into disfavor in the mid-1960s, for two reasons. First, the surgical approach to heart and vessel disease was more profitable. Second, the patent on EDTA that was held by Abbott Laboratories expired, so there was no longer a financial incentive for drug companies to fund further research. The impact on medical practice was greater than just the lack of support for research. The removal of direct financial support for EDTA also meant that there was no money for getting the word about the effectiveness of this treatment out to patients, physicians, and medical educators.

Fortunately, a small group of practicing physicians, who organized themselves in 1972 as the American College for the Advancement of Medicine, continued to use EDTA chelation therapy. The association was their means to advance this practice.

In the early days, some rather serious problems were still to be worked out. Giving too much of the EDTA, or giving it too fast, was found to be dangerous. In fact, there were several deaths attributed to kidney failure caused by toxicity to EDTA.

Fortunately, these early problems have been worked out. EDTA chelation therapy that is used now is totally safe. There have not been any deaths or significant adverse reactions in well over 500,000 patients who have undergone EDTA chelation therapy in recent years. Because EDTA chelation improves blood flow throughout the body, the "side effects" are usually beneficial and only a few adverse effects are noticed.

There now exists a substantial body of scientific evidence on the use of EDTA chelation therapy in the treatment of angina, peripheral vascular disease, and cerebral vascular disease.[8] Since 1987, numerous FDA-approved studies have demonstrated some rather impressive results.

Still, if you mention EDTA chelation therapy to a cardiologist or heart surgeon, the surgeon will likely flush with anger, even though the science indicating that EDTA therapy is of benefit is far more convincing than the evidence for bypass surgery or angioplasty. It is a less expensive treatment, it can be done in the doctor's office, and it does not require the high-tech approach and hospitalization that comes with modern heart surgery.

Comparative costs speak eloquently: a coronary artery bypass surgery or angioplasty usually costs between $40,000 to $100,000. EDTA chelation therapy usually costs less than $2,500 for a full set of treatments. Yet physicians using EDTA chelation therapy are frequently challenged for its high costs!

The Argument Against Chelation

As the public has become aware of the failure of the surgical approach to angina and other conditions related to atherosclerosis, they have looked for alternatives. Unfortunately, alternatives are not easily or readily accepted by established practitioners of other methods. The current battle cry against EDTA is a "negative" study from Denmark, and a recent Harvard Medical School Health Letter.

The study in question was done by vascular surgeons, who were naturally biased against a nonsurgical therapy. Why would vascular surgeons, who depend upon fees from surgery to sustain their livelihood, be in favor of a study on chelation?

The study was not conducted on patients with angina. Instead, it featured patients with a condition known as "intermittent claudication." This is characterized by the presence of a painful leg cramp produced when walking.[9] Intermittent claudication is like "angina of the calf." It is an example of a peripheral vascular disease. Like coronary artery disease, intermittent claudication is caused by atherosclerosis. EDTA chelation therapy is as effective in intermittent claudication as it is in angina.

There are six major reasons why the public should question the results of this study:

1. The study is not consistent with other studies, which show EDTA chelation to be of considerable benefit to patients with symptoms from atherosclerosis. After forty years of clinical use and dozens of published clinical studies, this is the only study that has been negative.

2. The researchers were to randomly select 30 test subjects from a group of 153 patients. In this group of 153 subjects, there were 106 smokers. In the 30 subjects selected by the researchers, 29 were smokers. That certainly doesn't seem like a random selection. The odds of this happening randomly are about 1 in 15,000. It appears that smokers were specifically chosen because the researchers believed that cigarette smoking (which was allowed during the study) would interfere with some of the benefits of EDTA chelation therapy.

3. The study was supposed to be double-blind, meaning no one was to know who was getting what, until the end. Inexplicably, the surgeons broke the code six months early, and several patients stated that they knew what they were receiving. Also, surgeons failed to add magnesium to the EDTA solution; without it, the solution is acid and burns at the needle site. The placebo does not burn, so without magnesium added to EDTA, a double-blind study would be impossible. Inexplicably, neither group ever complained of a burning feeling upon injection, raising the possibility that EDTA was never given. In addition, according to patient interviews, patients appeared to have been switched randomly from the EDTA group to the placebo group, to make sure that there was no therapeutic difference between the two groups?

4. The statistical method used to report the results is unclear, especially in light of the fact that exactly who received EDTA and who did not is in question.

5. While the researchers stated that there was no therapeutic effect noted, in reality an effect was noted. Both groups noted a 51 percent increase in the walking distance that they could cover. If EDTA was given and patients were crossed over to placebo therapy during the study (as patient interviews indicate), this is the result that would be expected.

6. The surgeons may have falsified data. Patient Sonja Rosen reported to researchers that her legs felt better, but, according to the patient, researchers reported that she experienced no improvement.

In October of 1992, the Harvard Medical School Health Letter questioned chelation therapy with an article entitled, "Chelation Therapy, Risk Without Benefits?" They cited the Danish study (just discussed) as confirmation for taking action against doctors who recommended the therapy.

The authors of this newsletter did not cite any of the hundreds of studies showing EDTA to be beneficial. For example, they refused to note one double-blind study where the therapy relieved leg pain and markedly increased walking distance, a study that was co-authored by James Carter, M.D., Ph.D., a respected professor of nutrition at Tulane Medical School.

The Harvard Health Letter cited "potential risks" of EDTA, such as kidney damage and cardiac arrhythmia. The University of California at Berkeley Wellness Letter also cited risks, in October of 1990. But when those "experts" at Harvard and Berkeley wrote about the toxicity of EDTA, they neglected to mention that in 1987, the FDA assessed the toxicity of 10 to 15 million EDTA infusions used in half a million patients, over a 30-year period, and found none of the toxicity mentioned in either the Harvard or Berkeley letter. The writers of those letters must have known that.

The attitude of these newsletters and mainstream medicine against EDTA chelation therapy is unfounded. Why are they so vehement that it doesn't work? Could it be that they are trying to protect a $60 billion-a-year existing industry?

Chelation and the Tomato Effect

Modern medicine is often reluctant to employ beneficial therapies even when these therapies are proven to work. This is called the "tomato effect," alluding to the widely-held eighteenth century belief in North America that tomatoes were poisonous, though they were a dietary staple in Europe. It wasn't until 1820, when Robert Gibbon Johnson ate a tomato on the courthouse steps in Salem, Indiana, that the "poisonous tomato" barrier was broken.

In medicine, the tomato effect is the opposite of the placebo effect. The tomato effect describes a therapy that does work, but is widely scorned. EDTA chelation therapy is a classic example.

EDTA chelation therapy has flourished anyway, in the face of unbelievable odds: scorn from mainstream doctors, who say that "it doesn't work and it's dangerous;" refusal to pay for it by insurance companies; censure from peers and the threat of losing their medical license. In spite of this, over half a million Americans, attracted by word of mouth, have received the therapy from the thousand doctors who believe in it. EDTA works. The numbers are convincing.

I have seen many patients, hospitalized with severe chest pain and told that if they left the hospital without bypass surgery, they would die. But instead of accepting this "death sentence," these patients chose to investigate the Whitaker Wellness Institute, and began following our program of diet, exercise, nutritional supplements, and EDTA chelation therapy.

Did I guarantee them they would not have a heart attack following my program? Of course not. But I did educate these patients about the risk of invasive therapies versus our program. As pointed out earlier, in most cases, surgery is not the ideal option, when the high rate of mortality associated with coronary artery bypass is taken into consideration. In over 30,000 bypass operations in the state of California in 1989, the death rate was 5.73 percent (about one out of seventeen patients).[10] The risk of having a fatal heart attack in a patient with angina is reasonably estimated at between 1 percent and 2 percent, if they did not do anything. If they follow our program, they are choosing a course of action with the lowest risk and the greatest possibility of benefit.

Here are two examples of patients who went with the Whitaker Wellness Program:

Patient 1. At 61, "Richard" was hospitalized with severe chest pain and told that if he left the hospital without bypass surgery, he would die. Richard signed himself out of the hospital and came to me for EDTA chelation therapy. A year and a half later, he is pain-free and is taking no heart medications.

Patient 2. "Robert," 58, had severe blockage in two of the arteries to his heart. He was also given the "death sentence" unless he had surgery. He chose a better diet and EDTA therapy instead. Two years later, he is drug-free, pain-free, and jogging four miles a day.

These are just two examples of the over 500,000 people who have been successfully treated by EDTA chelation. If these patients had elected surgery, the total hospital bill would have likely been over $400,000. Both of my patients were treated for less than $7,500—roughly 2 percent of the cost if they had elected surgery. It is sad to think that many insurance companies will not pay for chelation therapy because "it is too expensive," but have no problem writing a check out to the surgeon, even if the patient dies on the operating table.

For more information on EDTA chelation therapy, there are three excellent books written for the layperson, available in your book store or from the American Preventive Medical Association (1-800-230-APMA). These books are *Bypassing Bypass* by Elmer Cranton, M.D.; *Forty Something Forever* by Harold and Arlene Brecher, and *Racketeering in Medicine: The Suppression of Alternatives* by James Carter, M.D.

Additional Measures for Angina

In addition to EDTA chelation therapy, it is very important to utilize nutritional measures designed to improve energy metabolism within the heart and improve blood supply to the heart. These goals are interrelated. An increased blood flow means improved energy metabolism—and vice versa.

Foremost in achieving this goal is dietary intervention. Atherosclerosis can be reversed. The best illustration of the tremendous therapeutic power of diet therapy in angina and atherosclerosis is the now-famous Lifestyle Heart Trial conducted by Dr. Dean Ornish.[11] In this study, subjects with heart disease were divided into a control group and an experimental group. The control group received regular medical care while the experimental group was asked to eat a low-fat vegetarian diet for at least one year. The diet included fruits, vegetables, grains, legumes, and soybean products. Subjects were allowed to consume as many calories as they wished. No animal products were allowed except egg white and one cup per day of nonfat milk or yogurt. The diet contained approximately 10 percent fat, 15 to 20 percent protein, and 70 to 75 percent carbohydrates, which were predominantly complex carbohydrates from whole grains, legumes, and vegetables.

The experimental group was also asked to perform stress-reduction techniques such as breathing exercises, stretching exercises, meditation, imagery, and other relaxation techniques for an hour each day and to exercise at least three hours a week.

At the end of the year, the subjects in the experimental group showed significant overall regression of atherosclerosis of the coronary blood vessels. In contrast, subjects in the control group showed progression of their disease. These controls were being treated with regular medical care and following the standard American Heart Association diet. They actually got worse. Ornish states: "This finding suggests that conventional recommendations for patients with coronary heart disease (such as a 30 percent fat diet) are not sufficient to bring about regression in many patients."

My program for the treatment of angina goes beyond diet. Several nutritional supplements and herbal extracts have been shown to improve angina. For example, carnitine and coenzyme Q10, essential compounds in normal fat and energy metabolism, are of extreme therapeutic benefit to sufferers of angina. These nutrients are manufactured in the body under normal circumstances. But due to lack of oxygen supply to the heart, nutrient deficiency, or some other reason, people with angina and other heart problems are typically deficient in one or both of these nutrients.

Carnitine and coenzyme Q10 function in preventing the accumulation of fatty acids within the heart muscle by improving the conversion of fatty acids and other compounds into energy. A deficiency of carnitine or coenzyme Q10 in the heart would be similar to trying to run an automobile without a fuel pump. There may be plenty of fuel, but there is no way to get it to the engine.

Several clinical trials have demonstrated that carnitine improves angina. Other clinical studies have demonstrated that coenzyme Q10 improves angina.[12] In fact, both carnitine and coenzyme Q10 have been shown to produce as good a result as standard drug therapy for angina.

Unfortunately, no studies have looked at what happens when both carnitine and coenzyme Q10 are used. Because of their overlapping mechanisms of action, I believe that combining them would produce much better results than using either separately.

The dosage of carnitine should be 500 milligrams, twice daily, and the dosage of coenzyme Q10 should be 30 to 100 milligrams, three times daily. It is important to use L-carnitine or acetyl-carnitine versus D,L-carnitine, which is a mixture of the D and L forms of carnitine. The body uses L-carnitine but the D form actually interferes with L-carnitine.

I recommend Rogenic (Enzymatic Therapy) to my patients with angina, high blood pressure, and other heart problems. Rogenic provides essential vitamins and minerals for the heart and vascular system, along with some special herbal extracts.

One additional, important supplement in Rogenic is magnesium. Magnesium supplementation alone has shown impressive results in the treatment of angina and acute myocardial infarction (heart attacks).[13] In the Whitaker Wellness Program, I recommend 1,000 milligrams of magnesium daily. A person with angina requires even more. Two tablets of Rogenic three times daily will provide an additional 450 milligrams of magnesium as magnesium aspartate.

Two of the herbal extracts in Rogenic deserve special mention, hawthorn (*Crataegus monogyna*) and khella (*Ammi visnaga*). Hawthorn extracts are widely used by physicians in Europe in their cardiovascular therapies. Studies have demonstrated hawthorn extract to be effective in reducing angina attacks. It improves the blood and oxygen supply to the heart by dilating the coronary vessels. It also improves the metabolic processes in the heart. It is a very useful herb in treating any heart condition, but especially angina and congestive heart failure.[14]

Khella is an ancient medicinal plant native to the Mediterranean region. It has been used in the treatment of angina and other heart ailments for thousands of years. Several of its components have demonstrated positive effects in dilating the coronary arteries. Its mechanism of action appears to be very similar to the calcium channel-blocking drugs often used in the treatment of angina.

Since the late 1940s, there have been numerous scientific studies on the clinical effectiveness of khella extracts in the treatment of angina. More specifically, khellin, a derivative of the plant, was shown to improve exercise tolerance and normalize EKG (electrocardiograph) tests. A study published in the *New England Journal of Medicine* in 1951 concluded: "The high proportion of favorable results, together with the striking degree of improvement frequently observed, has led us to the conclusion that khellin, properly used, is a safe and effective drug for the treatment of angina pectoris."[15]

Although most clinical studies used high dosages, several studies show that as little as 30 milligrams of khellin per day appears to offer just as good results with fewer side effects.[16] At higher doses, 120 to 150 milligrams per day, pure khellin was associated with mild side effects, such as loss of appetite, nausea, and dizziness. Taking six tablets of Rogenic per day will provide 36 milligrams of khellin, a safe and effective amount.

If you have angina and your cholesterol levels are high, follow the recommendations for cholesterol, page 191.

Anxiety

Dr. Whitaker's Prescription for Anxiety:

1. Follow recommendations for enhancing adrenal function in Chapter 6.
2. Follow the Whitaker Wellness Program.
3. Avoid alcohol, caffeine, and sugar.
4. Take one capsule Stress-End formula, three times daily.
5. Take L.72 Anti-Anxiety formula, 20 drops in 2 to 3 ounces of water, three to four times daily.
6. Take 750 to 1,000 milligrams of GABA daily.
7. If all the above produces little help, ask your physician for a prescription for Dilantin (100 milligrams three times daily).

Description

Anxiety is defined as "an unpleasant emotional state ranging from mild unease to intense fear." Anxiety differs from fear: fear is a rational response to a real danger; anxiety usually lacks a clear or realistic cause. Though some anxiety is normal and, in fact, healthy, higher levels of anxiety are not only uncomfortable, they can lead to significant problems.

Anxiety is often accompanied by a variety of symptoms. The most common symptoms relate to the chest. These include heart palpitations (awareness of a more forceful or faster heartbeat), throbbing or stabbing pains, a feeling of tightness and inability to take in enough air, and a tendency to sigh or hyperventilate. Anxiety can cause tension in the muscles of the back and neck and can lead to headaches, back pains, and muscle spasms. Other symptoms include excessive sweating, a dry mouth, dizziness, symptoms of irritable bowel syndrome (see page 293), and the constant need to urinate or defecate.

The anxious individual usually has a constant feeling that something bad is going to happen. They may fear that they have a chronic or dangerous illness. The symptoms of anxiety may reinforce this belief. For many, the symptoms lead to difficulty in getting to sleep and constant waking through the night.

When most people go to a medical doctor for relief of symptoms of anxiety, they are usually given a tranquilizer. Drugs like Valium, Xanax, Librium, and Tranxene are familiar prescriptions. These and a host of similar drugs work to repress symptoms. The goal is to make the patient "numb to the world." Drugs in this category are among the most widely prescribed. It is estimated that somewhere between 60 and 80 million prescriptions are written for these drugs each year.

Why are these drugs so often prescribed? The physician wants to do something about the presenting problem but is at a loss, he can't get to the bottom of the psychological or physiological factors that might be causing the anxiety. So the physician prescribes a "you'll feel better" drug, and the patient gets some relief, or at least a sense that something has changed. The physician gets to feel better, thinking that something helpful has been done.

A short-term benefit is gained from such prescriptions. Tranquilizers are often effective in reducing the anxiety. However, they do not address the underlying cause. The human spirit has a sort of "rebound" factor. When the effect of the suppressing pills wears off, the "cause" comes back. Sometimes it comes back worse for having been pushed away by the numbing drug. Not surprisingly, tranquilizers are highly addictive. The patient wants to keep the "cause" at a distance and so takes more pills.

This can be a vicious cycle which can go on for months or even years. I strongly recommend that before starting on this road that an alternative program be engaged. The anxious person should try non-drug treatment, including psychological counseling and the Whitaker Prescription for Anxiety.

Comments on Dr. Whitaker's Prescription for Anxiety

The basic decisions we make about what we eat and drink are strongly linked to the development of anxiety. To demonstrate this link, I am going to describe an important biochemical process.

Research has revealed some important physiological changes during times of clinical anxiety, including panic attacks. Individuals with anxiety have elevated blood levels of lactate. They also have higher ratios of lactate to pyruvate compared to control groups. Furthermore, an unpleasant but revealing study has shown that when patients with panic attacks are injected with lactate, severe panic attacks are produced. In normal individuals, nothing happens.

It appears from this research that individuals with anxiety may be sensitive to lactate. This sensitivity may guide us to a way to manage anxiety without resorting to drugs.

Nutritional choices can play a key role in reducing lactic acid levels. According to Melvyn Werbach, M.D., author of *Nutritional Influences on Mental Illness* (Third Line Press, 1991), there are at least seven nutritional factors which may be responsible for elevated lactate levels:

1. Alcohol
2. Caffeine
3. Sugar
4. Deficiency of niacin
5. Deficiency of thiamin
6. Deficiency of magnesium
7. Food allergies

Avoiding alcohol, caffeine, sugar, and foods to which you are allergic can go a long way in relieving symptoms of anxiety.[1] There is common sense here. Think about the effects you have felt from caffeine, sugar, and alcohol. Food allergies can cause similar symptoms.

In addition to these basic changes in food and drink choices, follow the Whitaker Wellness Program. The "fight or flight" response involved with panic attacks and the chronic stress from anxiety both argue that a person with these conditions give particular attention to adrenal support. (Follow the recommendations for supporting the adrenal glands given in Chapter 6.)

A specific nutritional formula can be helpful with anxiety. I recommend Stress-End from Enzymatic Therapy. This formula supplies a combination of key nutrients involved in dealing with stress and anxiety. It also includes concentrated herbal extracts of Siberian ginseng, valerian, passionflower, hops, and skullcap. Take one capsule, three times daily.

L.72 Anti-Anxiety Formula

As an alternative to tranquilizers, I recommend a special homeopathic combination. If you are not familiar with homeopathy, it is a system of medicine which originated in Germany 200 years ago. The founder of homeopathy, Samuel Hahnemann, was seeking an alternative to the "heroic" medical practices of bloodletting and mercury medicines which dominated medical practice at the time. Homeopathy became extremely popular in the United States until the early part of this century. But as the drug companies rose in prominence, they effectively suppressed this form of medicine. Homeopathy continued to grow in popularity in many parts of the world, especially Europe and India. It is now experiencing a tremendous rise in popularity in the United States. In fact, homeopathic preparations are recognized by the FDA.

The word "homeopathy" comes from the Greek word *homios*, which means like, and *pathos*, which means suffering. Homeopathy is based on the principle that "like cures like." Hahnemann's study showed that a substance that can cause a certain symptom in a healthy person may treat the same symptom in a sick person. Only the treatment uses minute quantities of these substances. (Anyone wishing more information on this form of medicine can contact Homeopathic Educational Services, 2124 Kittredge St., Berkeley, CA 94704, 510-649-0294. They have an impressive catalog. If you are looking for a good book on homeopathy, read any of the many books on the subject written by Dana Ullman.

The homeopathic preparation I recommend for anxiety is called L.72 Anti-Anxiety. This combination remedy has been shown to be as effective as diazepam (Valium).[2] In the study, thirty women received L.72 and thirty women received 2 milligrams of diazepam. The patients were evaluated before and after a 30-day treatment. The study used a special scoring scale, known as the Hamilton scale, which is often used to evaluate anxiety. The results indicated that L.72 was as effective as diazepam in reducing anxiety, phobia, and emotional instability. The same held true for symptoms that often accompany anxiety, including hot flashes, rapid heartbeat (tachycardia), shortness of breath, intestinal problems, frequent urination, and dizziness.

Subjects in both groups showed spectacular gains in the number of hours of sleep and a considerable decrease in pulse rates. On day one, patients using L.72 had an average pulse rate of 93. At the end of the 30-day study, this had been reduced to 83. The overall assessment of the patients and physicians who participated in the study was that L.72 was as effective as diazepam in reducing symptoms of anxiety and depression.

The big difference occurs when nonconventional therapies are compared with drug therapies—side effects. Diazepam is associated with significant toxicity and addiction. L.72, on the other hand, is without side effects and is nonaddictive. It is also much less expensive.

L.72 Anti-Anxiety formula is manufactured by Lehning Laboratories, one of the leading manufacturers of homeopathic medicines in France. It is distributed in the United States by Enzymatic Therapy. L.72 is composed of the following homeopathic medicines: *Cicuta virosa* 4X, *Ignatia* 4X, *Staphysagria* 4X, *Asfoetida* 3X, *Corydalis formosa* 3X,

Sumbulus moschatus 3X, *Loei gaultheria procubens* 4X, *Valeriana offi-cianalis* 3X, *Hyoscyamus* 3X, and *Avena sativa* 1X.

Take L.72 Anti-Anxiety formula by placing twenty drops in two to three ounces of water, three to four times per day.

A note of caution: This anxiety program can be helpful to a person who is already using a tranquilizer or antidepressant. But you will need to work with a physician to get off the drug first and then to begin the wellness program. Stopping the drug on your own can be dangerous. You absolutely must have proper medical super-vision.

GABA

Benzodiazapine drugs like Valium work by stimulating receptors in the brain for gamma-aminobutyric acid (GABA)—the brain's natural calming agent. GABA is a nonessential amino acid. This means our bodies have the capacity to manufacture what we need. However, sometimes the brain does not have enough.

I have used GABA as a "natural tranquilizer" with much suc-cess. Here is an illustrative case:

Linda B. worked in a pressure cooker. She felt a certain degree of anxiety, but assumed it was just part of the job. However, these episodes of anxiety were getting more intense and happening more frequently. She heard about GABA and got a bottle. The following week, she had a full-fledged panic attack with extreme anxiety, sweat-ing, muscular tightness, and shakiness. She emptied a 750-milligram GABA capsule into a half-cup of water and drank it. She immediately felt calmer.

Linda doesn't take GABA regularly, but she keeps it with her and at the first signs of anxiety, or when things get particularly hectic at work, she takes half a capsule in water. She also notes that she has al-ways been prone to muscle tightness in her neck and shoulders as a re-sult of stress, and that since she has been using GABA, this has improved.

My usual prescription for GABA in anxiety is 750 to 1,000 mil-ligrams per day.

Dilantin

If all else fails, I turn to the prescription drug Dilantin (phenytoin). If you read the *Physician's Desk Reference* about this drug, you will find it listed as an anticonvulsant in the treatment of epilepsy. This limitation is imposed by the FDA for a drug that has been reported by thousands of physicians throughout the world to be useful for over fifty symp-toms and disorders, including anxiety.

Have you heard of Dreyfus mutual funds? This highly succesful family of mutual funds was founded by Jack Dreyfus. In 1963, Mr. Dreyfus was suffering from depression which resolved immediately upon taking Dilantin. He was so grateful to be taken out of his miserable condition that he felt a tremendous obligation to investigate its potential for others. He then formed the Dreyfus Medical Foundation, a charitable foundation designed to study the effects of Dilantin. Mr. Dreyfus believes the misunderstandings of the broad clinical applications for Dilantin amounts to a great catastrophe. To back up this belief, one need only examine the impressive bibliography and reviews that the Dreyfus Medical Foundation has put together. To learn more about the work of this foundation, and the over 10,000 studies that have been performed on this medicine, contact the organization:

Dreyfus Medical Foundation
767 Fifth Avenue
New York, NY 10153
212-752-6383

If Dilantin is going to work for you, the results will be noticeable almost immediately, or well within the first two weeks of use. The dosage I recommend is 100 milligrams, three times daily. Dilantin is available only by prescription.

Arthritis (see Gout, Osteoarthritis or Rheumatoid Arthritis)

Arthritis is a nonspecific term used to describe general inflammation and pain in a joint. The most common forms of arthritis share some common features. They also have some important differences. Each type is discussed individually: osteoarthritis, gout, and rheumatoid arthritis. If you are not sure which form you have, read the description of the major signs and symptoms of each, and you should be able to self-diagnose. Osteoarthritis is the most common form of arthritis.

Asthma

Dr. Whitaker's Prescription for Asthma:

1. Eliminate food allergies.
2. Avoid airborne allergens.
3. Follow a vegetarian diet.

4. Take 750 to 1,000 milligrams of magnesium citrate daily.
5. Support the body's anti-allergy mechanisms with vitamin C, other antioxidants, quercetin, vitamin B12, and vitamin B6.
6. If needed, use ephedra-based herbal products.
7. If mucus is a problem, use Air-Power (Enzymatic Therapy).
8. If needed, use extracts of adrenal cortex to boost natural cortisone.
9. If needed, use the following prescription items, in order of least toxicity and greatest long-term benefit:
    a. Inhalants containing cromolyn
    b. Inhalants containing beta-blockers
    c. Inhalants containing corticosteroids
    d. Theophylline-containing products
    e. Oral corticosteroids like prednisone

Description

Asthma is an allergic disorder characterized by spasm of the bronchial tubes and excessive excretion of a viscous mucus in the lungs. This can lead to difficult breathing. Asthma occurs as recurrent attacks, from mild wheezing to a life-threatening inability to breathe.

The number of Americans suffering from asthma and other allergies has risen dramatically over the last fifteen years.[1] Some possible reasons include: increased stress on the immune system due to greater chemical pollution in our air, water, and food; earlier weaning of infants and earlier introduction of solid foods; food additives; and genetic manipulation of plants, resulting in food components with greater allergenic tendencies.

Conventional treatment of asthma addresses its symptoms. Prescriptions may bring short-term benefits. More often, one prescription leads to another. Soon an individual has multiple prescriptions, each stronger than the last. The underlying problems are not addressed. Yet the asthma is not caused, to paraphrase a statement familiar to many nutrition-oriented physicians, "by lack of medication."

What are the long-term effects of this symptom-masking, disease-management strategy? Asthma is a serious health problem that is getting worse. Mortality more than doubled during the 1980s alone.[2]

This escalating problem amidst ever-more aggressive treatment reminds me of a historic note from a century and a half ago. At that time "heroic" medicines like mercury and bloodletting, with their awful, killing side effects were common treatments. It is said that physicians often mistook the side effects of their medicines for the disease itself.

Are conventional asthma strategies responsible for the horrendous increase in this health problem, including the incidence of death?

My clinical understanding and my reading of the scientific literature suggest that the answer may be yes. Asthma drugs can be extremely harmful. Appropriate treatment of asthma must focus on correcting underlying problems.

Comments on Dr. Whitaker's Prescription for Asthma

Have you ever heard the expression "the straw that broke the camel's back?" The natural approach to asthma and other allergies can be viewed as an attempt to: (1) remove as many straws as possible and (2) strengthen the camel's back. "Removing straws" means avoiding allergens in the food and air. "Strengthening the camel's back" means using natural substances which can help reduce the allergic response.

This twofold approach typifies many natural approaches. First, remove the obstacles to cure. Second, assist the body's healing abilities.

Food allergies are a major cause of asthma, especially in children.[3] Milk, corn, wheat, citrus, peanuts, eggs, chocolate, food colorings, and food additives are the major culprits. In childhood asthma, eliminating food allergies and food additives is often all that is needed. (To learn how to identify and eliminate food allergies, see page 242.)

Airborne allergens such as pollen, dander, and dust mites are often difficult to avoid entirely. Measures can be taken to reduce exposure. A great first step is to treat dogs and cats like a high-fat diet and get them out of your life! Cleaning or removing carpets, rugs, upholstered furniture, and other surfaces where allergens can collect is also a good step.

Cleansing cannot be done perfectly, but do pay special attention to the bedroom. Make it as allergy-proof as possible. Encase the mattress in an allergen-proof plastic; wash sheets, blankets, pillowcases, and mattress pads every week; and consider using bedding material made from Ventflex, a special hypoallergenic synthetic material.

Install an air purifier. The best mechanical air purifiers are HEPA (high-efficiency particulate-arresting) filters that can be attached to central heating and air-conditioning systems. These units are available from suppliers of heating and air-conditioning units. Portable HEPA air purifiers are less effective, but may still provide good results. These units typically cost $300 to $500.

If you have rugs and upholstery in the house, it is important to use a vacuum cleaner that has an efficient filtering system, such as those which trap dust in water or HEPA filters. Most vacuum cleaners have health-damaging side effects for asthma sufferers. They do not trap all the material they collect; they actually spread allergens throughout the air. Vacuum cleaners with efficient filtering units are the only types an allergic person should use.

All of the special products described above are available from supply houses that deal specifically with products designed for allergy sufferers:

Allergy Control Products
89 Danbury Road
Ridgefield, CT 06877
1-800-422-DUST

National Allergy Supply
4579 Georgia Highway 120
Duluth, GA 30136
1-800-522-1448

If you have asthma, buy indoor plants: houseplants, and plants for your office. This step toward health may be particularly important if you work in a large office building. Plants are phenomenal air filters. Much of the pollution that is generated in a large office building is the out-gassing of the material used in building or in maintaining the structure. Machines or cleaners used inside can also create this out-gassing. There are many sources, including foam insulation, plywood, particulate fibers, plastics, inks, and oils, as well as out-gassing from business machines, such as fax machines and copiers.

These indoor pollutants are becoming much more serious as energy-efficient buildings generally cut out circulation from the outdoor air. The pollutants are trapped. Have you ever heard of the "sick building syndrome?" It is a condition where people literally feel sick when they are at work because of the increased exposure to indoor air pollution.

Plants may be the answer to this problem. We have the Central Intelligence Agency (CIA) and the National Aeronautics and Space Administration (NASA) to thank for this solution.

In 1973, NASA found that the tightly contained air inside Skylab was contaminated with more than 100 toxic chemicals. Without effective purification, space travel would be impossible. Fortunately, NASA was tipped off by the CIA that the Russians were experimenting with plants as air purifiers. The space agency then started a crash course on researching this potential. NASA hired Dr. Bill Wolverton, former research scientist with NASA's John C. Stennis Space Center, to head up the research team.

The results were phenomenal. NASA scientists learned that virtually all indoor plants clean the air of almost all known contaminants. The contaminants are sucked into the leaves and migrate into the soil, where microorganisms associated with the roots break them down and turn them into plant food.

Using sealed growth chambers, Dr. Wolverton demonstrated that common houseplants were the most effective purifiers of our most common pollutants, nasty chemicals, such as trichloroethylene, formaldehyde, and benzene. Common plants like Peace Lily, Lady Palm, Areca Palm, Corn Plant, and Tricina Marginada, all plants used to decorate interior environments, were found to be effective air purifiers. Essentially, any one of these plants could purify the air in 100 square feet. The more plants you have in the office building or house, the more pure the air becomes.

This is a bit of natural wonderment that is worth pausing to behold: the Peace Lily vs. trichloroethylene. Which one would you bet on? The Peace Lily is a strong, hungry plant and could comfortably give this pre-fight boast to pollutants: "I'll eat you for breakfast!"

Plants work well by themselves, and if you are interested in potentiating their effects, call the Hall Environment Group (1-800-285-5723). Request information on Nature's Air Filter, a system patented by Dr. Wolverton that consists of a 15 1/2-inch high, 12 inch diameter pot with a built-in two-speed fan. It comes with potting soil containing activated carbon and zeolite, the same materials used in HEPA mechanical filters.

Strengthening the Camel's Back

Here are some ways to strengthen the body and reduce the allergic response. Perhaps the most important way is also basic to my overall Prescription for Wellness: Decrease the intake of animal fats while simultaneously increasing consumption of omega-3 oils. Use flax oil, fish, and fish oil supplements of a combination. The net effect of this simple dietary change is a significantly reduced inflammatory-allergic response.

I think an entirely vegetarian diet is the best diet for asthma. In one long-term trial of a vegan diet in which all animal products were eliminated, a significant improvement was noted in 92 percent of the twenty-five treated patients who completed the study. Note that some patients seemed to have trouble with the strictness of the diet. Nine dropped out within the first two months.[4] The diet excluded all meat, fish, eggs, and dairy products. Drinking water was limited to spring water. Chlorinated tap water was specifically prohibited. Coffee, caffeinated tea, chocolate, sugar, and salt were excluded.

One key point that needs to be made is that it is important to stay on the diet for at least a year. In the study we are discussing, while 71 percent of the patients responded within four months, one year of therapy was required before the 92 percent level was reached. It takes time to change the essential fatty acid components of the body. This is a commitment. But when you consider the seriousness of the problems associated with asthma medications, such a commitment is easier to make.

Magnesium

Magnesium promotes relaxation of the bronchial smooth muscles; as a result, airways open and breathing is made easier. Intravenous magnesium (2 grams of magnesium sulfate infused every hour, up to a total of 24.6 grams) is a well-proven and clinically accepted measure to halt an acute asthma attack. For preventive measures and long-term care, I recommend supplementing the diet with 750 to 1,000 milligrams of magnesium as magnesium citrate or Krebs cycle magnesium.

Antioxidants

Antioxidant nutrients are extremely important in all allergic and inflammatory conditions. The levels given in the Whitaker Wellness Program (see Chapter 2) are sufficient in most cases. Vitamin C, vitamin E, and selenium have all demonstrated significant anti-allergy effects in experimental and clinical studies. Antioxidants are thought to provide important defense against allergies and asthma. The reason is that oxidizing agents can both stimulate constriction of airways and increase allergic reactions to other agents.

Simply increasing vitamin C intake to the levels recommended in Chapter 3 may offer significant benefit to many asthma sufferers. Asthmatic patients have been shown to have significantly lower levels of vitamin C in the blood and white blood cells.[5] Studies have shown that increased vitamin C intake can be beneficial: Vitamin C has been shown to inhibit bronchial constriction in both normal and asthmatic subjects.[6] Vitamin C also reduces histamine production and hastens its detoxification.[7]

Quercetin

The bioflavonoid known as *quercetin* appears to offer some benefit in the treatment of asthma. Quercetin has consistently displayed the highest degree of activity in models of allergy and inflammation. Unlike antihistamine drugs that block the binding of histamine to cellular receptors, quercetin actually inhibits the release of histamine and other inflammatory compounds.[8] By inhibiting the release of histamine and other inflammatory compounds, quercetin greatly reduces the allergic-inflammatory response.

Quercetin has further anti-allergy action due to its potent antioxidant activity and its ability to inhibit the formation of inflammatory compounds like leukotrienes.[9] These compounds are 1,000 times more potent in stimulating inflammatory processes than histamine.

A problem with quercetin is that it is not absorbed well. Michael T. Murray, N.D., coauthor of the *Encyclopedia of Natural Medicine*, originated an approach to quercetin supplementation that helps get around this problem. He recommended that quercetin be combined with an equal amount of bromelain, the anti-inflammatory enzyme from pineapple. Bromelain has been shown to increase the absorption and tissue concentrations of a variety of compounds and may produce a similar effect with quercetin.[10] A good dosage for quercetin is 250 to 500 milligrams, five to ten minutes before meals.

Herbal Formulas

If additional support is needed to throw off asthma, I recommend ephedra-containing herbal formulas. Ephedra has been used in Chinese medicine for over 5,000 years.[11] Its use in modern medicine began in 1923 with the "discovery" of the alkaloid compound *ephedrine.*

The old-time herbal treatment of asthma and hayfever involved the use of ephedra in combination with herbal expectorants. Expectorants are herbs that modify the quality and quantity of secretions of the respiratory tract. This results in the expulsion of the secretions and improvement in respiratory tract function. Examples of commonly used expectorants include: lobelia (*Lobelia inflata*), licorice (*Glycyrrhiza glabra*), and grindelia (*Grindelia camporum*). Many suppliers offer ephedra-based asthma formulas featuring these or similar herbs.

The optimum dosage of ephedra depends on the alkaloid content in the form used. Standardized preparations are often preferred, as they have more dependable therapeutic activity. The dose should have an ephedrine content of 12.5 to 25 milligrams, and may be taken two to three times daily.

Ephedra can produce the same side effects that ephedrine can, such as increased blood pressure and heart rate, insomnia, and anxiety. However, the American Pharmaceutical Association states: "There is far more discussion of ephedrine tachyphylaxis (rapid decrease in effectiveness) or tolerance than is evidenced as a significant problem in the scientific literature."[12] In addition, a 1977 study of ephedrine therapy in asthmatic children (published in JAMA) concluded: "Ephedrine is a potent bronchodilator that, in appropriate doses, can be administered safely along with therapeutic doses of theophylline without the fear of progressive tolerance or toxicity."[13]

The FDA advisory review panel on over-the-counter drugs recommended that ephedrine not be taken by patients with heart disease, high blood pressure, thyroid disease, diabetes, or difficulty in urination due to enlargement of the prostate gland. Nor should ephedrine be used in patients on antihypertensive or antidepressant drugs.

Adrenal Cortex Extracts

If even more support is needed or if a patient has been on corticosteroids like prednisone, the next step is using products containing adrenal (bovine) cortex tissue concentrates. They function to boost natural cortisone levels. If fatigue is a problem, I recommend Enzymatic Therapy's Raw Adrenal at a dosage of one to two capsules with meals. If fatigue is not an issue, I recommend Enzymatic Therapy's Adrenal Cortex Complex at an initial dosage of one capsule, three times daily. Take adrenal products with meals, as they can cause slight stomach irritation when taken on an empty stomach.

Mucolytic Therapy

Asthma patients will often need "mucolytic" therapy, especially if they live in areas where air pollution is a problem. In Southern California, where I live, the air is often filled with what we natives kindly call a "coastal haze." This term is much easier for us to live with than "smog." Poor air quality tends to aggravate asthma. One of the ways it does this is by increasing the secretion of mucus (phlegm) or causing the mucus to become thick. If mucus is a problem, use Enzymatic Therapy's Air-Power. This product contains a natural plant expectorant that helps thin mucus and loosen phlegm and bronchial secretions. Air-Power is very effective at removing bothersome mucus and phlegm from the airways. Take one or two tablets, three times daily, for an effective dosage.

Prescription Medications

In some cases of asthma, prescription medications may be necessary. Here is the order in which I recommend asthma drugs, in the order of safety of long-term use.

1. Inhalants containing cromolyn
2. Inhalants containing beta-blockers
3. Inhalants containing corticosteroids
4. Theophylline-containing products
5. Oral corticosteroids like prednisone

Bladder Infection

Dr. Whitaker's Prescription for Bladder Infection:

1. Drink plenty of water, 3 quarts or more per day, to help flush out infection.
2. Try to urinate as soon after sex as possible.
3. Drink 8 ounces of pure cranberry juice, or take two tablets of Cran-Uti (Ecological Formulas), or two capsules of CranActin (Solaray) daily.
4. Drink an additional 8 ounces of pure cranberry juice, or take two tablets of Cran-Uti, or two capsules of CranActin, before and a few hours after sex, bike riding, horseback riding, or any activity that manipulates or puts pressure in the pelvic area.
5. At the first hint of burning urination, drink 8 ounces of cranberry juice, or take two tablets of Cran-Uti, or two capsules of CranActin; repeat in 3 to 4 hours.

Description

Cystitis, or urinary tract infections, are felt as pain in the bladder. Over 20 percent of women have some form of cystitis at least once a year, and these infections hit many women as frequently as the common cold. If not treated early and well, the infection may become chronic and spread to the kidneys.

Cystitis is almost always caused by fecal bacteria, usually E. coli, that migrate up the urethra and into the bladder where they can multiply and cause infection. The most common symptoms of a bladder infection are severe pain with urination and "urgency," a constant sensation that one needs to urinate.

Urinary tract infections in men and women are frequently associated with sexual activity. In fact, the condition "honeymoon cystitis" is self-explanatory. However, cystitis is not a sexually transmitted disease. Sexual activity simply facilitates migration of bacteria into the bladder.

Considering that E. coli and other bacteria almost routinely migrate into the bladder, it is a wonder that we are not constantly suffering with cystitis. However, for cystitis to occur, the bacteria must anchor themselves to the walls of the bladder. The overwhelming majority are washed out with urination.

Comments on Dr. Whitaker's Prescription for Bladder Infections

For years I have recommended that men and women with urinary tract symptoms drink copious amounts of water to increase urine flow, and to drink cranberry juice. I had thought, as I suspect many other physicians did at the time, that cranberry juice helped by making urine more acidic and less hospitable for the bacteria.

This was an example of having the right therapy—for the wrong reason. As noted, for bacteria to stay in the bladder, they must anchor themselves to the cells of the bladder. The surface of the bacteria is dotted with special substances called *lectins* that form strong bonds with the sugar components of the mucopolysaccharides on the surface of cells lining the bladder.

Cranberry juice contains substantial quantities of alpha D mannopyranoside, a derivative of the sugar D-mannose. This sugar attaches to the lectins of the bacteria and thus prevents bacteria from attaching to the bladder wall. The bacteria have fewer places to grip on.

In one study, urine from either mice or humans given cranberry juice inhibited attachment of bacteria to bladder cells in the test tube.[1] Another study showed that 16 ounces of cranberry juice per day eliminated cystitis in 73 percent of 44 women and 16 men.[2] And finally, the *Journal of the American Medical Association*, in a double-blind, placebo-controlled study, recently "discovered" the ability of daily ingestion of 16 ounces of cranberry juice to significantly inhibit the growth of bacteria in the urine.[3]

In the JAMA study, saccharin-sweetened cranberry juice was used because the presence of sugar was thought to nullify some of the effects of cranberry juice. Unfortunately, most cranberry juice products on the market are loaded with sugar. For this reason, I recommend that you get your daily quota of cranberry juice in pill form if you suffer from recurrent bladder infections.

Try either Cran-Uti from Ecological Formulas, or CranActin from Solaray. Cran-Uti is a chewable tablet; CranActin is a capsule. For either product, take two tablets or capsules twice daily if you have symptoms. For prevention, take two daily. This will provide the equivalent of 16 ounces of cranberry juice—without the sugar.

Boils

Dr. Whitaker's Prescription for Boils:

1. Apply a hot compress over the area every two hours.
2. Apply tea tree oil topically, two to three times daily.
3. Take 100 to 150 milligrams of zinc daily for one month.

Description

A boil is an inflamed, pus-filled area of skin, usually due to a hair follicle (the tiny pit from which a hair grows) becoming infected with the bacteria *Staphylococcus auereus.* A boil will usually start as a painful, red lump. As it swells it fills with pus and becomes rounded, with a yellowish tip (head). Common sites include the back of the neck and moist areas such as the armpits and groin. A more severe and extensive form of a boil is a *carbuncle.*

Common measures should be taken to prevent the spread of infection, such as cleaning the affected area, taking showers instead of baths, and washing the face and hands several times a day. Towels, linens, and clothing should be kept away from other family members, to avoid spreading to others. Do not burst a boil. This may spread infection to deeper tissues. A hot compress applied every two hours will relieve discomfort and hasten drainage and healing. If the boil is especially large or painful, consult your physician for proper drainage.

Comments on Dr. Whitaker's Prescription for Boils

In addition to the general measures discussed above, I recommend applying tea tree oil to the boil at least two times daily. Australian tea tree oil has significant antiseptic properties and is regarded by many as the ideal skin disinfectant. It is active against a wide range of organisms. It also possesses good penetration and is nonirritating to the skin.[1]

Because a boil is an infectious disease, the recommendations given in Chapter 7 about enhancing the immune system are appropriate. The prescription for acne (see page 141) can also be followed. Specifically, I recommend a daily zinc intake of 100 to 150 milligrams for one month. Zinc has been shown in several studies to be quite useful in skin infections.

In one zinc study, Dr. Isser Brody of the General Hospital of Eskiltuna, Sweden, found that all fifteen patients seen in the dermatology clinic who suffered from recurrent boils had low serum zinc levels.[2] He divided these fifteen patients into two groups. In the first group, eight patients (four males and four females) had their boils lanced and were prescribed antibiotics. During the next three months all of these patients had recurrences. In the other group, Dr. Brody prescribed 45 milligrams of zinc three times per day. Their boils quickly regressed and none of these patients experienced a new lesion within the three-month study. In all eight patients, blood levels of zinc reached normal limits within one month of therapy.

Because the zinc levels were normalized within one month in these patients, I recommend the high dosage of zinc be taken only for thirty days. After a month, the dosage should be reduced to 30 to 45 milligrams per day.

Bronchitis and Pneumonia

Dr. Whitaker's Prescription for Bronchitis and Pneumonia:

1. Follow recommendations for thymus extracts and echinacea given in Chapter 7.
2. Take 1,000 milligrams of vitamin C, or as much as your bowel will tolerate (see page 41), every waking hour.
3. Take 750 to 1,000 milligrams of magnesium per day.
4. Use goldenseal and bromelain in combination at levels recommended in this section.
5. Use postural drainage techniques and herbal expectorants to promote the elimination and breakdown of mucus.

Description

Bronchitis and pneumonia often follow the common cold. Bronchitis refers to an infection or irritation of the bronchial tree; pneumonia refers to infection or irritation of the lungs. Both are characterized by chills, fever, and chest pain. Pneumonia will show more signs of lung involvement (shallow breathing, cough, abnormal breath sounds). X-rays of patients with pneumonia will show infiltration of fluid and lymph in lungs. Of the two conditions, pneumonia is by far the more serious.

Although pneumonia may appear in healthy individuals, it is usually seen in individuals with low immune function, particularly the elderly, patients on immunosuppressive drugs, AIDS patients, and drug and alcohol abusers. Pneumonia is still the fifth leading cause of death in the United States. It is particularly dangerous in the elderly.

Comments on Dr. Whitaker's Prescription for Bronchitis and Pneumonia

Pneumonia can be quite serious. If you have symptoms suggestive of pneumonia, see a physician. The recommendations given below are for all types of pneumonia and bronchitis. They are of a general nature, and are to be used along with those recommendations for enhancing the immune system in Chapter 7.

Here are some specific supplement recommendations: Take two tablets of ThymuPlex (see page 118), three times daily; 1,000 milligrams of vitamin C every hour until symptoms pass; and 750 to 1,000 milligrams of magnesium as magnesium citrate per day.

Another good recommendation for bronchitis and pneumonia is the use of combinations of goldenseal (*Hydrastis canadensis*) and bromelain. The medicinal value of goldenseal is due to its high content of alkaloids, of which berberine has been the most widely studied. Berberine has broad antibiotic effects. It also has anti-infective and immune-stimulating actions. Together, these support the historical use of goldenseal in infections of the mucous membranes: the linings of the oral cavity, throat, sinuses, bronchi, lungs, genitourinary tract, and gastrointestinal tract.[1]

For best results, goldenseal extracts standardized for berberine or hydrastine content are preferred. For an extract standardized at 5 percent hydrastine, the dosage in the case of bronchitis or pneumonia would be 400 to 800 milligrams, three times daily.

The beneficial effects may be increased by bromelain, a protein-digesting enzyme complex from pineapple. Bromelain has been shown to be quite useful in the treatment of bronchitis and pneumonia.[2] Bromelain exerts some direct antibiotic effects, as well as helping to break down thick mucus to allow for easier expectoration. As a bonus, bromelain has been shown to enhance the absorption of antibiotics into the lungs and respiratory tracts, and may also do the same for the berberine component of goldenseal.[3] A good therapeutic dosage for bromelain (in bronchitis or pneumonia) is 200 to 400 milligrams of 1,800 m.c.u. bromelain, three times daily on an empty stomach.

Enzymatic Therapy is the only company that I know of that has put goldenseal and bromelain together in one capsule. Their product, Hydrastine, provides 200 milligrams of an 8 percent alkaloid extract of goldenseal, along with 100 milligrams of bromelain and 100 milligrams of vitamin C. This product is super for upper respiratory infections. Take two to four capsules three times daily between meals.

One of our main treatment goals in bronchitis and pneumonia is to help the lungs and air passages get rid of excessive mucus. Here is what I recommend you do at least twice daily:

1. Apply a heating pad, hot water bottle, or a mustard poultice to the chest for up to twenty minutes. A mustard poultice is made by mixing one part dry mustard with three parts flour and adding enough water to make a paste. The paste is then spread on thin cotton (old pillowcases work well) or cheesecloth, folded, and then placed on the chest. If you are using a mustard poultice, be sure and check it periodically. The mustard can cause blisters if left on too long.

2. After the hot pack, perform postural drainage by lying with the top half of the body off the bed using the forearms as support (see figure). The position should be assumed for a 5 to 15 minute period while you try to cough and expectorate into a basin or newspaper on the floor. Postural drainage can be hard work, so it is a good idea to have a helper.

Position for Postural Drainage

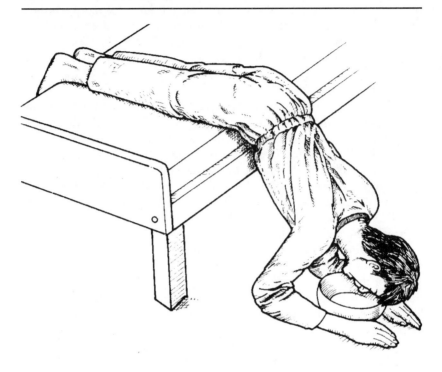

3. In addition to these physical measures, try to stay away from using cough suppressants. I recommend instead that you use an expectorant. Expectorants thin the mucus and promote its elimination. Read the description of Air-Power in the prescription for asthma (see page 163). It is a good herbal expectorant formula. If you are an adult, take two tablets, three times daily. For children 6 to 12, take one tablet three times daily. Air-Power, or a similar expectorant, will help relieve a cough by eliminating the irritation that is causing it—rather than simply suppressing it.

Candidiasis

Dr. Whitaker's Prescription for Candidiasis:

1. Eliminate the use of antibiotics, steroids, immune-suppressing drugs, and birth control pills (unless there is absolute medical necessity).
2. Follow the following special dietary guidelines:
   a. Do not eat foods high in sugar.

    b. Do not eat foods with a high content of yeast or mold, including alcoholic beverages, cheeses, dried fruits, melons, and peanuts.

    c. Do not eat milk and milk products due to their high content of lactose (milk sugar) and trace levels of antibiotics.

    d. Avoid all known or suspected food allergies.

3. Follow the Whitaker Wellness Program.
4. Enhance digestive function with the use of hydrochloric acid and pancreatic enzymes (as detailed in Chapter 3).
5. Enhance detoxification (as detailed in Chapter 4).
6. Enhance immune function (as detailed in Chapter 7).
7. Use nutritional and herbal supplements to help control against yeast overgrowth and promote a healthy bacterial flora.
8. Use *Lactobacillus acidophilus* products.
9. Promote the elimination of candida toxins by using a water-soluble fiber source such as guar gum, psyllium seed, or pectin, which can bind to toxins in the gut and promote their excretion.

Description

When most people think "bacteria" they think "Bad! Bad! Bad!" It's unfortunate. Bacteria are not only pathogens, they are also essential for healthy functioning. We need bacteria for healthy soils. For instance, it is these microscopic biota that help plants convert chemicals associated with "sick building syndrome" into plant food. (See Asthma, page 163.) Chemical agents used in farming, and by many of us in our yards, will not only kill the insect or fungus that is targeted. The healthy biota is also harmed.

    A similar process takes place in our "internal soils," or the *terrain interieur,* as the nineteenth century French scientist Claude Bernard called it (see Chapter 7). The gastrointestinal tract is home to helpful bacteria that are necessary for proper digestion. Unfortunately, systemic antibiotics are as nondiscriminating as chemical fungicides. The good bacteria is also killed. A void is created. This void, created indirectly by extensive antibiotic treatment, can become the playfield for candida.

    Candida overgrowth is now becoming recognized as a complex medical syndrome known as the *yeast syndrome* or *chronic candidiasis* (see profile). This overgrowth is believed to cause a wide variety of symptoms in virtually every system of the body: the gastrointestinal, genitourinary, endocrine, nervous, and immune systems are the most susceptible.

    Although chronic candidiasis has been clinically defined for a long time, it was not until Orion Truss published *The Missing Diagnosis* and William Crook published *The Yeast Connection* that the public and many physicians became aware of the magnitude of the problem.[1]

Typical Chronic Candidiasis Patient Profile

Sex: Female
Age: 15 to 50
General symptoms:
  Chronic fatigue
  Lack of energy
  General malaise
  Decreased libido
Gastrointestinal symptoms:
  Thrush
  Bloating, gas
  Intestinal cramps
  Rectal itching
  Altered bowel function
Genitourinary system complaints:
  Vaginal yeast infection
  Frequent bladder infections
Endocrine system complaints:
  Primarily menstrual complaints
Nervous system complaints:
Depression
  Irritability
  Inability to concentrate
Immune system complaints:
  Allergies
  Chemical sensitivities
  Low immune function
Past history:
  Chronic vaginal yeast infections
  Chronic antibiotic use for infections or acne
  Oral birth control usage
  Oral steroid hormone usage
Associated conditions:
  Premenstrual syndrome
  Sensitivity to foods, chemicals, and other allergens
  Endocrine disturbances
  Psoriasis
  Irritable bowel syndrome
Other:
  Craving for foods rich in carbohydrates or yeast

The diagnosis of chronic candidiasis is often quite difficult. There is no single specific diagnostic test. Stool cultures and elevated antibody levels of candida are useful diagnostic aids, but they should not be relied upon for diagnosis. The best method for diagnosing chronic candidiasis is a detailed medical history and patient questionnaire (see figure), which is the questionnaire that I use (adapted from Crook WG: *The Yeast Connection,* 2nd edition. Professional Books, Jackson, TN, 1984).

Candida Questionnaire

History   Point Score

1. Have you taken broad-spectrum or other antibiotics for acne for one month or longer?   25
2. Have you, at any time in your life, taken other "broad-spectrum" antibiotics for respiratory, urinary, or other infections for two months or longer, or in short courses four or more times, in a one-year period?   20
3. Have you ever taken a broad-spectrum antibiotic—even a single course?   6
4. Have you, at any time in your life, been bothered by persistent prostatitis, vaginitis, or other problems affecting your reproductive organs?   25
5. Have you been pregnant . . .

    One time?   3
    Two or more times?   5

6. Have you taken birth control pills . . .

    For six months to two years?   8
    For more than two years?   15

7. Have you taken prednisone or other cortisone-type drugs . . .

    For two weeks or less?   6
    For more than two weeks?   15

8. Does exposure to perfumes, insecticides, fabric shop odors, and other chemicals provoke . . .

    Mild symptoms?   5
    Moderate to severe symptoms?   20

9. Are your symptoms worse on damp, muggy days, or in moldy places?   20
10. Have you had athlete's foot, ringworm, "jock itch," or other chronic infections of the skin or nails?

    Mild to moderate?   10
    Severe or persistent?   20

11. Do you crave sugar?   10
12. Do you crave breads?   10
13. Do you crave alcoholic beverages?   10
14. Does tobacco smoke really bother you?   10

Total Score   _____

Major Symptoms

For each of your symptoms, enter the appropriate figure in the Point Score column.
Score column:

    If a symptom is occasional or mild, score 3 points.
    If a symptom is frequent and/or moderately severe, score 6 points.
    If a symptom is severe and/or disabling, score 9 points.

	Point Score
1. Fatigue or lethargy	_____
2. Feeling of being "drained"	_____
3. Poor memory	_____
4. Feeling "spacey" or "unreal"	_____
5. Depression	_____
6. Numbness, burning or tingling	_____
7. Muscle aches	_____

8. Muscle weakness or paralysis ——————
9. Pain and/or swelling in joints ——————
10. Abdominal pain ——————
11. Constipation ——————
12. Diarrhea ——————
13. Bloating ——————
14. Persistent vaginal itch ——————
15. Persistent vaginal burning ——————
16. Prostatitis ——————
17. Impotence ——————
18. Loss of sexual desire ——————
19. Endometriosis ——————
20. Cramps and/or other menstrual irregularities ——————
21. Premenstrual tension ——————
22. Spots in front of eyes ——————
23. Erratic vision ——————

      Total Score ——————

Other Symptoms

For each of your symptoms, enter the appropriate figure in the Point Score column.
Score column:

    If a symptom is occasional or mild, score 1 point.

    If a symptom is frequent and/or moderately severe, score 2 points.

    If a symptom is severe and/or disabling, score 3 points.

	Point Score
1. Drowsiness	——————
2. Irritability	——————
3. Incoordination	——————
4. Inability to concentrate	——————
5. Frequent mood swings	——————
6. Headache	——————
7. Dizziness/loss of balance	——————
8. Pressure above ears, feeling of head swelling and tingling	——————
9. Itching	——————
10. Other rashes	——————
11. Heartburn	——————
12. Indigestion	——————
13. Belching and intestinal gas	——————
14. Mucus in stools	——————
15. Hemorrhoids	——————
16. Dry mouth	——————
17. Rash or blisters in mouth	——————
18. Bad breath	——————
19. Joint swelling or arthritis	——————
20. Nasal congestion or discharge	——————
21. Postnasal drip	——————
22. Nasal itching	——————
23. Sore or dry throat	——————
24. Cough	——————
25. Pain or tightness in chest	——————
26. Wheezing or shortness of breath	——————
27. Urinary urgency or frequency	——————
28. Burning on urination	——————

29. Failing vision   _____
30. Burning or tearing of eyes   _____
31. Recurrent infections or fluid in ears   _____
32. Ear pain or deafness   _____

   Total Score   _____

   Total Score (all three sections)   _____

Interpretation	_Women_	_Men_
Yeast-connected health problems are almost certainly present	>180	>140
Yeast-connected health problems are probably present	120–180	90–140
Yeast-connected health problems are possibly present	60–119	40–89
Yeast-connected health problems are not likely present	<60	<40

Comments on Dr. Whitaker's Prescription for Chronic Candidiasis

In most cases, chronic candidiasis is the outcome of a vicious cycle. Something gets the snowball rolling. Once it starts, it builds up momentum of its own. (See figure for an illustration of the positive feedback cycle of chronic candiasis.)

In order to get a handle on candida overgrowth, it is critical to eliminate the factors that are triggering the overgrowth. In the case of chronic candidiasis, trying to kill off the candida with the use of nystatin, ketoconazol, or other antifungal drugs, rarely produces significant long-term results. This approach fails to address the underlying factors that promote candida overgrowth. It is like trying to weed your garden by cutting the top off the weed: The roots remain, and the weed sprouts up again.

To "get to the root" of the candida problem, a comprehensive approach is necessary. If my recommendations for this condition seem overwhelming, it is because systemic candidiasis affects so many areas of healthy functioning. It is a tough condition to resolve. Lesser strategies often fail. The infection seems to have the ability to retreat and wait out attacks if only portions of this comprehensive approach are engaged. Candida can bounce back from natural therapeutics, just as it does from antibiotics. I strongly urge you to employ the comprehensive approach, if you really want to get rid of this problem.

An extra benefit of embracing this comprehensive plan is that other health concerns will also clear up. You will not only be combating candida. You will gain health.

Positive Feedback Cycle of Chronic Candidiasis

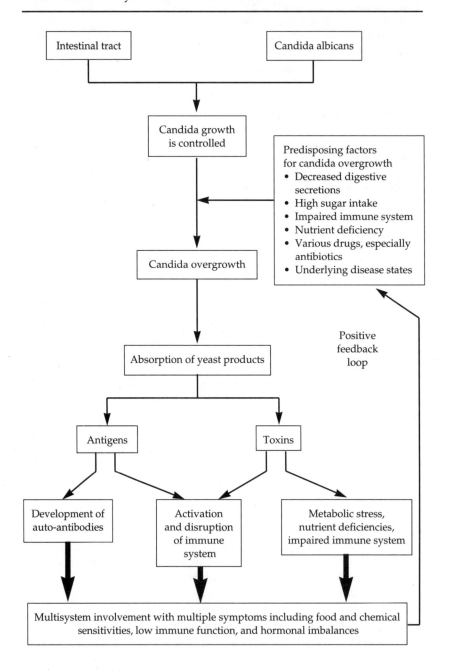

Diet

Diet is the first step. Avoid those foods which promote candida growth, including high-sugar foods, alcohol, foods with a high content of yeast or mold (cheeses, dried fruits, and peanuts), milk, and milk products. In addition, it is important to avoid food allergies (see page 242).[2]

Digestion

The next step is usually improving digestion. Digestive secretions, such as gastric acid, pancreatic enzymes, and bile, are all potent natural factors that inhibit the overgrowth of candida.[3] Promoting improved digestion with the aid of hydrochloric acid and pancreatic enzyme preparations is extremely important in relieving chronic candidiasis.[4] (These are detailed in Chapter 3.)

Detoxification

Candida patients usually exhibit multiple chemical sensitivities and allergies. This is an indicator that detoxification reactions are stressed. Therefore, those measures discussed in Chapter 4 are quite important. At the very least, the candida patient should be on a good lipotropic formula like Liv-A-Tox or Lipotropic Complex (see page 82). This recommendation is reinforced by animal research. Studies have shown that, in mice, damaging the liver leads to candida overgrowth.[5] Improving the health of the liver may be one of the most critical factors in the successful treatment of candidiasis.

Immune System

Another crucial step in the campaign against candida overgrowth is to enhance the immune system. I recommend ThymuPlex as a general immune-enhancing formula. My initial recommendation is two tablets three times a day for one month, then drop the dosage to two tablets daily for long-term maintenance.

Supplements

The next step is using any of a number of nutritional and herbal substances that are designed to kill off the organism. Caprylic acid and garlic preparations have now been used for many years by alternative healthcare professionals in the treatment of candida overgrowth. Garlic has been shown to be more potent than nystatin, gentian violet, and many other anti-candida agents in experimental studies.[6] Garlic preparations producing a high allicin-potential may offer the greatest benefit.

Consider using commercial preparations concentrated for allicin because allicin is relatively "odorless" until it is converted to allicin in the body. For best results, products standardized for allicin content are preferred. The dosage should provide a daily dose of 8 milligrams allicin.

Caprylic acid has also demonstrated good anti-candida effects. Since caprylic acid is readily absorbed in the intestines, it is necessary to take timed-release or enteric-coated caprylic acid formulas. This will allow for gradual release throughout the entire intestinal tract.[7] Many manufacturers offer such products, including Solgar, Arteria, and TwinLab.

Recently, many alternative healthcare physicians began using stronger natural anti-candida agents. One is grapefruit seed extract. (I like Grapefruit Seed Extract from NuBiotic, ParaMicrocidin from Allergy Research Group, and Citronex from Murdock Pharmaceuticals.) Others use specially-prepared volatile oil preparations, like emulsified oregano oil (ADP from Biotics Research Laboratories) and enteric-coated peppermint oil (Peppermint Plus from Enzymatic Therapy). Many physicians who are using these "new wave" natural anti-candida formulas find them more effective than caprylic acid and garlic products. The volatile oil products are especially promising. Follow the recommendations given on the bottle or those recommended by your physician.

It is a good idea to use *Lactobacillus acidophilus* products to replenish the gut flora with health-promoting bacteria. *L. acidophilus* has been shown to retard the growth of candida in culture media. It is thought to be one of the natural protective measures against candida overgrowth.[8] There are many companies marketing *L. acidophilus* products, and many different opinions among physicians as to which company offers the best product. Here are some of the more popular products available in health food stores: Superdophilus from Natren, Prime-Dophilus from Klaire Laboratories, Primadophilus from Nature's Way, and EnzyDophilus from Enzymatic Therapy. Follow the directions on the label.

To promote the elimination of candida toxins, take three to five grams of a water-soluble fiber source such as guar gum, psyllium seed, or pectin at night before going to bed. These fibers can bind to candida toxins in the gut and promote their excretion.

Canker Sores

Dr. Whitaker's Prescription for Canker Sores:

1. Follow the Whitaker Wellness Program.
2. Identify and eliminate food allergies.
3. Take two chewable tablets of either DGL (Enzymatic Therapy) or

DGL-Power (Nature's Herbs), twenty minutes before meals, three times daily.

Description

Canker sores are shallow, painful ulcers found anywhere in the mouth cavity. They can be single or clustered and anywhere from 1 to 15 millimeters in diameter. The ulcers are surrounded by a reddened border, and are often covered by a white membrane.

An occasional canker sore may be the result of trauma from your toothbrush. Such ulcers will usually resolve in seven to twenty-one days. But in many people, canker sores are recurrent. In fact, recurrent canker sores are an extremely common condition, estimated to affect 20 percent of the population. Based on studies of initiating factors, the cause of recurrent canker sores appears to be related to food sensitivities, stress, and/or nutrient deficiency.

Canker sores are often confused with cold sores (see page 206). However, cold sores most often occur on the border of the lips and are linked to the herpes virus.

Comments on Dr. Whitaker's Prescription for Canker Sores

Any of a number of nutrient deficiencies can lead to canker sores. The cells of the mouth reproduce themselves every one to four days. They need a constant supply of nutrients. The nutrients most often linked to canker sores are iron, zinc, vitamin B12, and folic acid. Supplementation with these nutrients at the levels given in Chapter 3 has been shown to eliminate the recurring problem of canker sores in some patients.[1]

Another possible cause of recurrent canker sores is food allergy.[2] Identifying and eliminating food allergies is imperative if you really want to stop canker sores from recurring.[3] The big culprits are wheat and milk. You may want to simply eliminate wheat and milk for one month to find out.

DGL (deglycyrrhizinated licorice) in chewable tablets is very effective in oral ulcers just as it is in peptic ulcers (see page 349). In one study, DGL was shown to lead to complete healing within three days in fifteen out of twenty patients.[4] One of these patients had recurrent canker sores for over ten years without an ulcer-free period for the past year. He had multiple ulcers on the tongue, lips, inside of the cheek, palate, and back of the throat. By the seventh day of treatment with DGL, the patient was completely free of any mouth ulcers. Can you imagine having a mouth full of canker sores for over a year and then having them all gone? This patient remained on DGL for one year, and after battling recurrent canker sores for over 10 years, did not have one single recurrence. I have had similar experiences with my patients. DGL is completely safe and there are no known side effects.

DGL is available from Enzymatic Therapy (DGL) and Nature's Herbs (DGL-Power). Take two tablets of either product twenty minutes before meals, three times daily.

Carpal Tunnel Syndrome

Dr. Whitaker's Prescription for Carpal Tunnel Syndrome:

1. Follow the Whitaker Wellness Program.
2. Take a total of 150 milligrams per day of vitamin B6.
3. Use bromelain or Curazyme (Enzymatic Therapy) to reduce inflammation.

Description

Carpal tunnel syndrome is a common, painful disorder caused by compression of the median nerve as it passes between the bones and ligaments of the wrist. Compression of the nerve causes weakness, pain when gripping, and burning, tingling, or aching. The sensation may radiate to the forearm and shoulder. Symptoms may be occasional or constant. They usually occur the most at night. Carpal tunnel syndrome is found most often in people who perform repetitive, strenuous work with their hands, such as grocery store checkers and carpenters.

Comments on Dr. Whitaker's Prescription for Carpal Tunnel Syndrome

Vitamin B6 (pyridoxine) deficiency is a common finding in carpal tunnel syndrome. In double-blind, placebo-controlled clinical studies, John Ellis, M.D., Karl Folkers, Ph.D., and their coworkers at the University of Texas successfully treated hundreds of patients suffering from carpal tunnel syndrome with vitamin B6.[1] The effectiveness of vitamin B6 in carpal tunnel syndrome has been confirmed by other researchers as well.[2] Even the famed surgeon George Phalen, M.D., the man who pioneered the surgical treatment for carpal tunnel syndrome, believes that pyridoxine may be the "treatment of choice."[3]

Alan Gaby, M.D., author of *The Doctor's Guide to Vitamin B6*, has posed a fascinating link. Dr. Gaby suggests that the increased rate of carpal tunnel syndrome since its initial description by Dr. Phalen in 1952 parallels the increased levels of vitamin B6 antagonists in both the food supply and drugs. These antagonists include the hydrazine dyes (FD&C yellow #5), drugs (isoniazid, hydralazine, dopamine, and penicillamine), oral contraceptives, and excessive protein intake.[4] Therefore, avoid foods containing yellow dyes. Limit protein consumption to 50 grams per day. And take a total of 150 milligrams of vitamin B6 daily.

It may take as long as three months to produce a benefit. Remember, natural therapies often take time to resolve chronic conditions that have developed over time. The treatment will work in most cases, and is a lot better than having surgery. In fact, most often the surgery does not work because scar tissue forms around the carpal tunnel. The nerve passageway can be narrowed even further, thus increasing likelihood of the recurrence of the syndrome.

During the time it may take for vitamin B6 to work, you may want to use Enzymatic Therapy's Curazyme. This formula is composed of curcumin and bromelain. These are two herbal substances with confirmed anti-inflammatory activity in clinical trials (see Rheumatoid Arthritis, page 335). Take two to four capsules twice daily on an empty stomach.

Cataract

Dr. Whitaker's Prescription for Cataracts:

1. Follow the Whitaker Wellness Program.
2. Take the necessary amounts of antioxidant nutrients, as directed in the Whitaker Wellness Program.
3. Consider using bilberry extracts or pycnogenols, especially if you are a diabetic or there is evidence of macular degeneration.

Description

A cataract describes a loss of transparency of the lens of the eye. The origin of cataract formation is free radical damage to some of the sulfur-containing proteins in the lens. These delicate protein fibers form white spots when they are damaged, in a similar manner to the way sulfur-rich proteins of eggs are damaged when they are fried or boiled. The damaged lens will not be able to transmit light effectively to the retina.

Cataracts affect approximately 4 million people in the United States. At least 40,000 Americans are blind due to cataracts. For individuals on Medicare, cataract surgery is the most common major surgical procedure done in the United States each year (600,000 per annum).

Comments on Dr. Whitaker's Prescription for Cataracts

As with most chronic degenerative diseases, prevention or treatment at an early stage is most effective. Progression of cataracts can be stopped, and early cataracts can be reversed by following my recommendations. However, do not expect a miracle if you have a well-developed cataract.

The first thing you should do to prevent cataracts is avoid direct sunlight hitting the lens of the eye. Wear sunglasses when outdoors and make sure they block ultraviolet rays. The second step is to make sure that your intake of antioxidant nutrients is high. Eat an abundance of fresh fruits and vegetables (rich in carotenes, flavonoids, and numerous other antioxidants). Individuals desiring to prevent cataracts or halt their progression should take additional vitamin C, beta-carotene, selenium, zinc, and vitamin E. Follow the general guidelines given in Chapter 2. Individuals with higher dietary intakes of vitamins E and C, and carotenes have a much lower risk for developing cataracts.[1]

These antioxidant nutrients may offer some additional therapeutic effects. Several clinical studies have demonstrated that vitamin C supplementation can halt cataract progression and, in some cases, significantly improve vision. For example, in one study, 450 patients with cataracts were placed on a nutritional program that included 1 gram of vitamin C per day. This resulted in a significant reduction in cataract development.[2] Similar patients had required surgery within four years. But in the vitamin C-treated patients, only a handful required surgery. In most patients there was no evidence that the cataract progressed over the 11-year period of the study.

It appears that the dosage of vitamin C necessary to increase the vitamin C content of the eye and improve cataracts is 1,000 milligrams.[3] Take at least 1,000 milligrams of vitamin C three times daily if you have a cataract forming.

If you are a diabetic or there is evidence of macular degeneration, see page 299 and follow the recommendations given there for the use of bilberry extracts and pycnogenol products.

Cerebral Vascular Insufficiency

Dr. Whitaker's Prescription for Cerebral Vascular Insufficiency:

1. If symptoms or blockage is severe, consider EDTA chelation therapy (see page 150).
2. Follow the Whitaker Wellness Program.
3. Take *Ginkgo biloba* extract (24 percent ginkgo flavonglycosides) at a dosage of 40 milligrams, three times daily.
4. If cholesterol levels are high, follow recommendations on page 191.

Description

Cerebral vascular insufficiency means that there is a lack of blood flow to the brain. This extremely common condition in the United States is due to the high rate of atherosclerosis. The atherosclerotic plaque pinches off the flow of blood to the brain. The major symptoms of cerebral vascular insufficiency are impaired mental performance, short-term memory loss, dizziness, headache, ringing in the ears, and depression. These symptoms are extremely common in the elderly and are often referred to as "symptoms of aging."

Comments on Dr. Whitaker's Prescription for Cerebral Vascular Insufficiency

Some general aspects of cerebral vascular insufficiency were discussed in Chapter 5. The most important step is to prevent atherosclerosis altogether by adopting a healthful diet.

A therapeutic agent of particular value (discussed in Chapter 5) is *Ginkgo biloba* extract (GBE). Because of its multitude of vascular effects, GBE offers effective treatment for the signs, symptoms, and underlying disease-state that causes cerebral vascular insufficiency. More than forty double-blind studies have shown it effective in cerebral vascular insufficiency, as well as preventing strokes.[1] Take 40 milligrams of the 24 percent ginkgo flavonglycoside extract three times daily. Most often, results will be apparent within two to four weeks. But if improvements are not noted in this time period, do not stop the GBE. In some cases, improvements may not be apparent for up to six months.

If the blockage or the symptoms are severe, EDTA chelation therapy is definitely indicated. This therapy was fully discussed under Angina (see page 145). Cerebral vascular insufficiency and angina share many common features. Both thrive on the standard American high-fat diet. They are usually caused by the accumulation of atherosclerotic plaque. Both can lead to serious consequences. In the case of angina, this is a heart attack; in the case of cerebral vascular insufficiency, a stroke.

The medical treatment of either usually involves dangerous and largely unsuccessful surgeries. For angina, the surgery is the coronary bypass operation. For cerebral vascular insufficiency the surgery is called "carotid endarterectomy." Studies have shown that these expensive surgeries are not only of limited value, they are most often performed unnecessarily and can be extremely dangerous. By dangerous, I mean they can kill you.

Carotid endarterectomy involves the removal of the atherosclerotic plaque from the carotid artery, the main artery that delivers oxygen-rich blood to the brain. An angiograph of the carotid artery is taken. This procedure produces a stroke in about 1 out of 100 patients.[2] The surgery is even more dangerous. Approximately 6 to 10 percent of the patients will either die or suffer severe neurological damage as a result of a stroke.[3,4] All in all, approximately 7 to 11 percent of the patients will die in the surgical treatment of cerebral vascular insufficiency.

Most of these patients are dying in vain. Like coronary bypass, the majority of patients having carotid endarterectomy do not need it. A 1988 article published in the *New England Journal of Medicine* showed the results from a panel of nationally known experts who rated the appropriateness of carotid endarterectomy. In a random sample of 1,302 Medicare patients, they found that only 35 percent of the patients had carotid endarterectomy for appropriate reasons.[4] This same study found that approximately 9.8 percent of the patients undergoing carotid endarterectomy will die of a stroke within 30 days of the operation, or suffer permanent neurological damage.

Keep in mind that these dismaying results were from a panel of peers, and are not made up to scare you by alternative practitioners or nutrition-oriented physicians.

Carotid endarterectomies are of no value in patients with less than 70 percent blockage, as determined by angiograph.[5] Again, like coronary bypass, it appears that most patients not electing to have the surgery will outlive the patients who do have the surgery. Even in those patients with blockage greater than 70 percent, the long-term survival rate after carotid endarterectomy is not that much better, especially when risk is considered. In my opinion, carotid endarterectomy is extremely risky and provides very little benefit.

Approximately 100,000 endarterectomies are performed each year in the United States, as a cost of roughly $25,000 each time. That's a total of over $2.5 billion, money that could be better spent.

If you have symptoms of cerebral vascular insufficiency, you may want to consult a qualified EDTA chelation specialist. Contact the American College of Advancement in Medicine (ACAM), 23121 Verdugo Drive, Suite 204, Laguna Hills, CA, 92653, 1-800-532-3688 (outside California) or 1-800-435-6199 (inside California). For a discussion of EDTA, see Angina, page 150.

If cholesterol levels are high, follow guidelines under Cholesterol below.

Cholesterol

Dr. Whitaker's Prescription for Lowering Cholesterol:

1. Follow the Whitaker Wellness Program and specific dietary suggestions given below.
2. Take niacin in the form of inositol hexaniacinate at a dosage of 500 to 1,000 milligrams, three times daily, with meals.
3. After one to two months ask the following: Have blood cholesterol levels dropped at least 20 percent? Is the total cholesterol level still above 200? Is the total cholesterol to HDL cholesterol ratio greater than 4.5? Is your LDL to HDL cholesterol ratio greater than 3? If the answer is "yes" to any of these, add to the program an odor-free garlic preparation. It should be at a high enough dosage to provide 8 milligrams of allicin, or an allicin yield of 4,000 micrograms per day.
4. If after another month, you still haven't achieved your goals, add gugulipid at a dosage sufficient enough to provide 25 milligrams of guggulsterone three times daily.
5. If after a month you still need extra support, add 1,000 milligrams of carnitine per day to the program.
6. If another month goes by and your total cholesterol level is still elevated, stay on the above program for a minimum of three more months. If there is still no change, shift strategies. The level of antioxidant nutrients in your blood may be a more significant factor than cholesterol. Also, you may need to work with your liver to help it realize it is overproducing cholesterol. Follow the recommendations for detoxification given in Chapter 4.
7. Because the drugs Mevacor, Pravachol, or Zocor lower coenzyme Q10 levels, if you have taken any of these drugs, take 60 milligrams of coenzyme Q10 daily for one month.
8. For more information, get my book *Reversing Heart Disease* (Warner Books, 1985).

Description

Why is everyone so concerned about cholesterol? Because there is substantial evidence that elevated cholesterol levels greatly increase the risk of death due to heart disease, cancer, and stroke. These are the three leading killers of Americans.[1] Cholesterol contributes to the process of atheroscerolosis, a hardening of the artery walls due to a buildup of plaque-containing cholesterol, fatty material, and cellular debris.

Cholesterol is not the only thing to be concerned about if you want to prevent atherosclerosis, but it is certainly one of the most important factors. Other important factors include the level of antioxidants in the blood, like vitamin E, vitamin C, and beta-carotene; smoking; obesity; diabetes; high blood pressure; and lack of exercise.

Cholesterol is a white, waxy, fatty substance that is manufactured by the body and is also found in animal foods. Cholesterol is not found in plant foods. While we tend to think of all cholesterol as being bad, without cholesterol many body processes would not function properly. Cholesterol is used to build cells, sex hormones, and bile acids, among other things. Furthermore, there is substantial evidence that a certain form of cholesterol actually prevents atherosclerosis, and, as a result, heart disease and stroke. However, we do not need to eat cholesterol because the liver can make all the good cholesterol that our bodies require.

Cholesterol circulates in the blood attached to transport molecules known as lipoproteins. Because oil and water do not mix, cholesterol must be bound to lipoproteins to remain in solution in the blood. There are different types of lipoproteins. LDL, or low-density lipoprotein, is often referred to as the "bad" cholesterol. Cholesterol bound to HDL, or high-density lipoprotein, is referred to as the "good" cholesterol. LDL cholesterol increases the risk for heart disease, stroke, and high blood pressure. HDL cholesterol actually protects against heart disease.[2] There is also a cholesterol called VLDL, which is a very low-density lipoprotein. VLDL carries primarily triglycerides, another blood fat to be concerned about.

In simple terms, LDL transports cholesterol to the tissues while HDL transports cholesterol to the liver for metabolism and excretion from the body. Therefore the HDL-to-LDL ratio largely determines whether cholesterol is being deposited into tissues or broken down and excreted. The risk for heart disease can be reduced dramatically by lowering LDL cholesterol while simultaneously raising HDL cholesterol levels. Research has shown that for every 1 percent drop in the LDL cholesterol level, the risk for a heart attack drops by 2 percent. Conversely, for every 1 percent increase in HDL levels, the risk for a heart attack drops 3 to 4 percent.[2] From these numbers you can see that HDL levels are more important than total cholesterol levels.

When you have your cholesterol level checked, make sure they measure the HDL levels.

RECOMMENDED BLOOD CHOLESTEROL AND TRIGLYCERIDE LEVELS

Total cholesterol	less than 200 mg/dl
LDL cholesterol	less than 130 mg/dl
HDL cholesterol	greater than 35 mg/dl
Total cholesterol-to-HDL ratio	less than 4.5
LDL cholesterol-to-HDL ratio	less than 3.0
Triglycerides	50–150 mg/dl

Comments on Dr. Whitaker's Prescription for Lowering Cholesterol

It is said that clinical practice always lags behind scientific research. One way that the health of Americans is dramatically affected is that the medical education preparing physicians for clinical practice also lags well behind research.

I think of this when I reflect on the fact that most physicians immediately recommend drug treatment for elevated cholesterol levels. Yet research evidence irrefutably supports a non-drug approach to cholesterol problems. Unfortunately, even today, 75 percent of medical schools don't require a single course in nutrition.

Regardless of this deficiency in formal medical education, I hope that most of the research I am about to share will reach most of these drug-prescribing physicians. They must have felt the barrage of advertising from Quaker and other interested parties on the cholesterol-lowering effects of oats. They must have seen the journal articles and news reports on fats and atherosclerosis.

"Progressive" conventional physicians may therefore prescribe oats, or oat bran, to patients. But they do it as though oats were a drug. Or they may simply say: "You should eat more oats and less meat. Meantime, I'll give you a cholesterol-lowering drug."

The saturation of medical education in drug administration has shut the minds of physicians to the therapeutic directions that most current knowledge about cholesterol suggests. No room may exist in the physician's mindset or schedule for the multi-dimensional therapeutic strategies optimal for addressing elevated cholesterol. Most physicians don't embrace the need to be activists for change in the habits of their patients. Perhaps it is because it is difficult for physicians themselves to change the habits of their medical practice.

The health of Americans is the worse for it. So are the pocketbooks of individuals. And so is our national budget.

Let's take the research from the top. An Expert Panel of the National Cholesterol Education Program concluded simply: "Dietary therapy is the primary cholesterol-lowering treatment."[3] The quote is from the Panel's report on "Detection, Evaluation, and Treatment of High Cholesterol in Adults." In short, the first step in dietary therapy is to reduce the amount of cholesterol in the diet.

Start with a healthy breakfast. This mundane addition to this high-level recommendation grew out of a national survey of the nutrition and health practices of Americans. The study was called the "National Health and Nutrition Examination Survey II." It found that people who skip breakfast altogether have the highest cholesterol levels. Conversely, those who ate whole grain, fiber-rich cereals for breakfast had the lowest cholesterol levels.[4]

Resolving "serious chronic health problems" and "budget-breaking healthcare costs" can commence with such simple solutions as eating a good breakfast.

The Whitaker Wellness Program in Chapter 2 describes the basic dietary choices that will lower cholesterol levels. This is the foundation for a nondrug treatment. Research has shown that some foods deserve special attention: animal foods, butter and margarine, fish and fish oils, oats and fiber sources, and garlic and onions.

Animal Foods

There is no cholesterol in plants. This bears repeating because it gives some direction on how to easily lower cholesterol levels.

Animal foods are high in saturated fats, which seem to give the liver a message: "manufacture cholesterol." The liver gets the message and goes to work. If the message comes often enough, blood cholesterol levels are likely to end up dangerously elevated. Lowering dietary cholesterol may not, alone, reduce blood cholesterol levels. But studies have shown that people on low-cholesterol diets will live nearly three and a half years longer.[5] Over three full years in our lives and the lives of the children, grandchildren, and friends dear to us, simply by cutting back on eating most animal foods.

Butter or Margarine?

The high level of saturated fats in butter has landed this animal food in the same "don't" column with meats. Unfortunately, margarine, the accepted alternative to butter, does not have the clear multitude of benefits that we find in substituting a plant alternative for animal foods. In fact, margarine is one of the most damaging foods a person can eat.

Studies have shown that margarine has a double-whammy effect on cholesterol. It raises LDL levels; it lowers protective HDL levels.

Moreover, margarine interferes with the metabolism of essential fatty acids.[6] Recent studies have suggested that certain cancers may even be caused by margarine and other foods like shortenings, which share with margarine a processing characteristic.

The common denominator in these foods is that the vegetable oils from which they are made are first converted to a solid or semi-solid form. One can almost picture them collecting in and "hardening" our arteries. The conversion process is known as "hydrogenation." A hydrogen molecule is added to the natural unsaturated fatty acid molecule of the vegetable oil. The result is an "unnatural" form of the oil, which is more saturated and more solid.

My recommendation is to substitute polyunsaturated oils which lower cholesterol levels. Flax oil is the best choice. (See Chapter 2). Canola oil and olive oil, which hold up well to heat, are also much better than margarine or butter for cooking. Both butter and margarine intake should be restricted in any good diet.

Fish and Fish Oils

Which is better, the whole fish or the "fish extract," the supplemental omega-3 fish oils? In Chapter 1, I noted the refusal of the FDA to allow a health claim linking omega-3 fatty acid supplements with lowering heart disease. Hundreds of carefully controlled studies have shown that omega-3 fatty oils from fish are beneficial for the heart.[7] The FDA's action on omega-3 oils is one of the clearest cases in point of the agency's harmful bias.

The evidence is also clear that actually eating cold water fish like salmon, herring, and mackerel is better than taking omega-3 supplements. A recent study looked at twenty-five men with high cholesterol and followed them over a five-week period.[8] They consumed equivalent amounts of omega-3 oils, some in whole fish; others took the oils as a supplement. Though overall cholesterol levels were unchanged for both groups, benefits were found. Both dietary fish and omega-3 supplements raised HDL. Each also lowered triglyceride levels. But in addition, those who ate whole fish were found to have a benefit in reducing a clotting process in the blood which can lead to heart attacks and stroke. The whole fish reduced the stickiness of the platelets in the blood.

Omega-3 fatty acids are important parts of an anti-cholesterol diet. I recommend making cold water fish a dietary staple. For a supplement, flax oil is more economical than fish oils. Flax oil has the added benefit that it can be used directly, in dressing, as a food. If fish oils are your choice, take at least 10 grams each day. Usually, since most capsules are 1,000 milligrams, this means ten capsules a day.

Oats, Oat Bran, and Fiber Sources

A bowl of oat bran cereal or oatmeal sits before a person whose cholesterol is over 200 milligrams per deciliter. That bowl could mean a great deal. In fact, eating such a bowl daily could reduce your heart disease risk by nearly 50 percent.

We can reasonably estimate the value of the daily bowl of oatmeal because we know a lot about oats, oat bran, and cholesterol. In the last thirty years, over twenty major studies have examined these relationships.[9] Many variations on the theme have been investigated: bran muffins, entrées, breads, cereals. We know that a bowl of oatmeal has roughly three grams of fiber. Three grams of water-soluble oat fiber will lower cholesterol 8 to 23 percent. Because, every 1 percent drop in cholesterol levels brings the risk of heart disease down by 2 percent, the habit of a daily bowl of oatmeal lowers your risk by between 16 and 46 percent.

For individuals with normal or low cholesterol levels, however, frequent oat consumption will produce little or no change in cholesterol levels.

Studies that compare the value of oatmeal to oat bran have concluded that they have roughly the same cholesterol-lowering effectiveness. The polyunsaturated fatty acids in oatmeal have been found to contribute as much to its cholesterol-lowering abilities as its fiber content. So while oatmeal's 7 percent fiber content compares unfavorably to the 15 to 26 percent fiber in oat bran, the benefits are similar.

Oats and oat bran have become famous for their water-soluble fiber. But we can find dietary fiber in many foods. The high-fiber content of many fresh fruits is particularly surprising to some. Whole grains and beans are also excellent sources.

Another way to enrich the fiber content of your diet is to supplement it with fiber. Guar gum, psyllium, and pectin are sources which have been shown to reduce cholesterol levels. If you choose to use fiber supplements, please review the considerations in the section on fibers in Chapter 8. I recommend three grams per day of one or more of these products.

Garlic and Onions

Garlic and onions both have demonstrated beneficial effects on the cardiovascular system. They can lower overall cholesterol levels.[10] They both positively affect HDL-to-LDL ratios. HDL levels go up. LDL levels are lowered. In addition, garlic and onions prevent platelets from clumping together and forming blood clots, as well as acting as antioxidants.[11] The effect of garlic is stronger than that of onions. But people tend to eat more onions, so their benefits tend to be recognized as quite similar.

High dietary levels of these foods in populations where they are staples are associated with healthy epidemiological data on heart disease. To many population groups in the United States, however, the odor of garlic and onions is not socially acceptable. These foods aren't used as extensively as good cardiovascular health would recommend. To those with elevated cholesterol I say: "Explore cooking options which use more garlic and onions. Advertise your personal campaign for healthy blood. Eat more garlic and onions!"

If you are not ready to make this healthy but "stinky" fashion statement, the section on garlic supplements (see page 200) is for you.

Lifestyle Changes

The optimal cholesterol-lowering program is not limited to dietary changes. Here are a couple of lifestyle suggestions:

1. Cut back or eliminate coffee consumption. Drinking decaffeinated coffee won't work. Both caffeinated and decaffeinated beverages have been linked to elevated cholesterol levels.
2. Stop smoking. Continuation of this habit bedevils virtually all health efforts, cholesterol levels included.
3. Be physically active.

Exercise

Two recent studies published in the *New England Journal of Medicine* confirm what most of us already know: Exercise lowers cholesterol levels and prevents heart attacks. In a study from Norway, 1,960 healthy men 40 to 59 years of age were first evaluated in 1972 and followed for sixteen years.[12] They were divided into four groups according to physical activity. At the end of sixteen years, the heart death rate of the least active group was four times higher compared to the most active group. The death rate from cardiovascular disease went down in a smooth, graded fashion, with the least active highest and the most active lowest. In addition, physical activity reduced death from all causes, not just cardiovascular disease. The researchers pointed out that regular physical exercise lowers the blood cholesterol and triglyceride levels as well as blood pressure. Regular exercise also enhances the body's sensitivity to insulin. This improves the use of glucose, and increases the fluidity of the blood as a protection against abnormal blood clots.

In addition, exercise increases the body's ability to extract oxygen from the blood and actually enlarges the normal arteries carrying blood to the heart. Rather than simply saying the exercise was protective, the researchers implied that inactivity, like an elevated blood cholesterol level, greatly increases the risk for having a heart attack.

The second study of exercise and cholesterol is an interim report on a long-term study of 10,269 Harvard graduates who have been followed intermittently for over twenty years now.[13] Again, the benefits of physical activity are obvious. The men who began a moderately vigorous physical activity program after graduating from college experienced a 41 percent lower risk of death from heart disease, and a 23 percent reduction in all causes of death. The conclusions of the researchers in this study were the same as in the Norwegian study. Physical activity reduced death rates, and lack of physical activity increased them.

We are routinely advised to get a physical exam before starting an exercise program as if physical activity were dangerous. Actually, you should get a physical exam to see if you can withstand the dangers of the stresses of inactivity! Physical exams for all couch potatoes!

Additional Support

The best approach to lowering cholesterol levels is through diet and lifestyle modifications, but sometimes additional support is needed.

I strongly urge you to avoid the use of cholesterol-lowering drugs. As a rule, these drugs have not been shown to increase lifespan; and in fact, some of the drugs have actually been shown to harm people more than if they had not lowered their cholesterol levels. The side effects of these drugs can be quite serious and are relatively common. In addition, these drugs tend to be fairly expensive. Therefore, given their questionable long-term benefits, the risk of serious, potentially deadly side effects, and the expense, these drugs should not be used.

Fortunately, a number of natural substances can produce similar effects on blood cholesterol and triglyceride levels to those which these drugs target. The natural substances are more effective, safer, and less expensive than the standard drugs. These natural alternatives can be taken individually or in combination with one another.

Before we discuss these substances, I first want to share a study conducted by Mark Kelley, M.D., of the Department of Internal Medicine at the University of Alabama School of Medicine.[14] Dr. Kelley sought to answer two very important questions: (1) Would the money spent on treating high cholesterol levels save more lives if spent elsewhere? (2) How many dollars must be spent on a treatment to make one person live one year longer?

To answer these questions, Dr. Kelley constructed an elaborate formula. His aim was to compute the cost of medical treatment for elevated cholesterol levels which would result in increasing a person's lifespan by one year. In short: "What does it cost us to buy a person one year more of life?"

Dr. Kelley's final cost figure was based not only on the cost of the treatment; he also included the cost of side effects. Then he subtracted the cost of illnesses averted and added the extra income that would result from this continued good health. Here are the results:

Dietary advice	–$2,536
Niacin	–$1,234
Psyllium husk	–$642
Mevacor (lovastatin)	$50,510
Colestid (colestipol)	$73,406
Questran (*cholestyramine*)	$92,603
Lopid (*gemfibrozil*)	$108,826

The first three figures have minus signs. The negative dollars reflect net savings due to the illnesses prevented and the extra income earned as a result. In other words, reducing cholesterol by changing your diet, and/or taking niacin or a fiber supplement can not only save your life, it can save you a great deal of money as well.

Niacin

The best single "magic bullet" for high cholesterol levels is a special form of niacin known as *inositol hexaniacinate*. This form of niacin will also save you from the side effects associated with niacin in its standard form.

If niacin were a patentable drug, this message would have been blasted over the airwaves. Magazines would have full-color advertisements. Physicians would be barraged with ads in their journals.

But niacin is not patentable. So, unfortunately, most people working to control their cholesterol levels will probably never hear it. Here's the fine print for the never-to-be-printed ad:

"It's a simple prescription. It's simple to take. You can find this form of niacin in a health food store. Individuals with cholesterol levels above 280 should start with 500 milligrams, three times a day with meals, for two weeks. Then increase it to 1,000 milligrams three times per day thereafter. For individuals with elevated cholesterol levels below 280, the lower dose is all that is needed. After two months, check your cholesterol levels. They may already be in the target range. If so, reduce the inositol hexaniacinate dose by half, or just take it every other day. Check your levels in a month. If the levels have stabilized or are improving, you may no longer need this supplement. If they are rising, increase the levels. A number of major manufacturers, including TwinLab, Enzymatic Therapy and KAL, have inositol hexiacinate."

I give this prescription before the supportive research because it's long past time that this simple therapy became well-known to people. The evidence that supports this approach is compelling.

As noted earlier, the National Cholesterol Education Program has concluded that diet is the first therapeutic choice for high cholesterol. This study ranked niacin as the first "drug" to use.[3] It safely lowers cholesterol levels. It extends life. The Coronary Drug Project (CDP) affirmed this. Niacin was the only "drug" evaluated that demonstrated decreased mortality.[15] The long-term death rate was evaluated in a followup report from the CDP. Patients on niacin had an 11 percent decrease in mortality rates over those on placebos.[16]

One other piece of research fills out the picture. In Europe, for over thirty years, the form of niacin called inositol hexaniacinate has been used to improve blood flow and to lower cholesterol levels. This form of niacin is actually more effective than its parent product. More important, inositol hexaniacinate is much better tolerated than niacin.[17] No adverse reactions were reported in one study, from 153 patients who took doses that ranged between 600 and 1,800 milligrams per day.[18]

Standard niacin is known to have pronounced side effects in many people. At the therapeutic dose of 1,000 milligrams, three times daily, complaints ranging from flushing of the skin, fatigue, and stomach irritation, to serious problems like ulcers and liver damage, have been noted. Sustained-release preparations may not make you flush, but they are much harder on your liver.[19] For this reason, many physicians have stayed away from niacin. But the safer alternative is available at most health food stores.

Garlic

I have already recommended increased dietary consumption of garlic and onions. Each has sulfur-containing compounds that are thought to be responsible their cholesterol-lowering effects. The odor of these foods limits consumption for some, so for those who feel their relationships may be at risk, some relatively "odorless" garlic supplements are available.

Garlic supplements have been shown to be of general benefit to the cardiovascular system. Like vitamin E, they prevent the oxidation of cholesterol. Other effects include reduced platelet aggregation and lowering of blood pressure (see High Blood Pressure, page 269). These are what I call "positive side effects."[11]

When we look specifically at the effects of garlic preparations on cholesterol levels, a great deal of supportive research is found. The important HDL-to-LDL ratio is positively altered by garlic. For people with cholesterol levels above 200, LDL levels go down 15 percent. HDL levels usually rise by about 10 percent. Total blood cholesterol levels also tend to go down. The range is 10 to 12 percent. In addition, triglycerides will drop by roughly 15 percent.[10]

Garlic Supplements and Recommended Dosages

Product (Company Name)	Tablet Size	Allicin Yield	Daily Dosage
Kwai (Lichtwer Pharma)	100 mg	600 mcg	9 tablets
Garlicin (Nature's Way)	100 mg	1,800 mcg*	6 tablets
Beyond Garlic (Kal)	125 mg	2,000 mcg*	4 tablets
Garlinase (Enzymatic Therapy)	317 mg	4,850 mcg	1 tablet

*Allicin yield at time of printing.

Good garlic products are available from a number of companies. (See table for dosages I recommend to gain the maximum benefit.)

Elevated cholesterol levels frequently go hand-in-hand with other signs of a strained cardiovascular system. If the other signs are not yet visible, they will be soon. While garlic preparations can have a benefit on cholesterol alone, I particularly recommend it for its numerous benefits as an excellent part of a healthy cardiovascular program.

Gugulipid

If the Wise Men who were said to follow a star to Bethlehem 2,000 years ago came from as far away as India, the myrrh presented as a gift may have, taken internally, helped prevent signs of heart disease in the Christian Holy Family.

A myrrh tree of India, the mukul myrrh (*Commiphora mukul*), has a resin called *gugulipid*. This resin has been tested in a number of clinical studies ranging from four to twelve weeks.[20] It has been found to lower cholesterol from 14 to 27 percent. Triglyceride levels decreased from 22 to 30 percent.

Researchers have concluded that two compounds in this resin, called *Z-guggulsterone* and *E-guggulsterone*, are the most active agents in myrrh resin's cholesterol-lowering abilities. Look for a product which is standardized for guggulsterones. Several companies, including Doctor's Best, Enzymatic Therapy, and Nature's Herbs, offer gugulipids in a standardized form. This will help determine appropriate dosage. I recommend that you take enough of the extract to provide 25 milligrams of guggulsterone, three times a day.

Carnitine

If, after another month, cholesterol levels are still elevated, add 900 milligrams of carnitine daily to the program. (Carnitine was discussed earlier in the treatment of angina.) It has also been shown to be quite useful in lowering LDL cholesterol and triglyceride levels while raising HDL levels.[21] It is somewhat expensive, which is the reason I save it for last.

If Cholesterol Levels Won't Come Down

In the unlikely event that your cholesterol levels won't come down after taking all these steps, consider these additional guidelines.

1. Don't worry. Despite what your doctor might tell you, you are not a walking time bomb. Remember, the level of vitamin E was recently shown to be a more significant risk factor than cholesterol levels (see Chapter 2). As long as you follow the recommendations given in the Whitaker Wellness Program, you are protecting yourself from heart disease and stroke.

2. Follow the recommendations in Chapter 4. Since the liver is the major site of cholesterol manufacture, elevated cholesterol levels reflect liver dysfunction. I have seen patients with high cholesterol levels that were unresponsive to typical measures see dramatic reductions by simply supporting the liver with silymarin.

3. I also recommend my book *Reversing Heart Disease* (Warner Books, 1985) or Dr. Peter Kwiterovich's book, *The Johns Hopkins Complete Guide for Preventing and Reversing Heart Disease* (Prima Publishing, 1993).

Chronic Fatigue Syndrome

Dr. Whitaker's Prescription for Chronic Fatigue Syndrome:

1. Follow the Whitaker Wellness Program.
2. Follow the recommendations in Chapter 7 on enhancing immune function.
3. Follow the recommendations in Chapter 6 on enhancing adrenal function.

Description

Undoubtedly you have heard of the chronic fatigue syndrome. It is the catch-all diagnosis of the 1990s. But what exactly is this syndrome? It is associated with a varying combination of symptoms, including recurrent sore throats, low grade fever, lymph node swelling, headache, muscle and joint pain, intestinal discomfort, emotional distress

Frequency of Symptoms in Chronic Fatigue Syndrome

Symptom/Sign	Frequency (%)
Fatigue	100
Low-grade fever	60–95
Muscle pain	20–95
Sleep disorder	15–90
Impaired mental function	50–85
Depression	70–85
Headache	35–85
Allergies	55–80
Sore throat	50–75
Anxiety	50–70
Muscle weakness	40–70
Fatigue after exercise	50–60
Premenstrual syndrome (women)	50–60
Stiffness	50–60
Visual blurring	50–60
Nausea	50–60
Dizziness	30–50
Joint pain	40–50
Dry eyes and mouth	30–40
Diarrhea	30–40
Cough	30–40
Decreased appetite	30–40
Night sweats	30–40
Painful lymph nodes	30–40

and/or depression, and loss of concentration. (See table for a list of common symptoms and their frequency in patients with chronic fatigue syndrome.

In the past, chronic fatigue syndrome (CFS) has been known by a variety of names including chronic mononucleosis-like syndrome, chronic EBV syndrome, Yuppie flu, postviral fatigue syndrome, postinfectious neuromyasthenia, chronic fatigue and immune dysfunction syndrome (CFIDS), Iceland disease, Royal Free Hospital disease, and many more. In addition, symptoms of chronic fatigue syndrome mirror symptoms of neurasthenia, a condition first described in 1869.

In 1988, a consensus panel convened by the Centers for Disease Control (CDC) formally defined the chronic fatigue syndrome and established formal diagnostic criteria.[1] In order to fit the diagnosis, you must meet both major criteria. In addition, you must exhibit 8 of the 11 symptoms listed or present 6 of the 11 symptoms plus 2 of the 3 signs listed in the minor criteria category.

CDC Diagnostic Criteria for Chronic Fatigue Syndrome

Major Criteria

New onset of fatigue causing 50 percent reduction in activity for
at least six months
Exclusion of other illnesses that can cause fatigue

Minor Criteria

SYMPTOMS

1. Mild fever
2. Recurrent sore throat
3. Painful lymph nodes
4. Muscle weakness
5. Muscle pain
6. Prolonged fatigue after exercise
7. Recurrent headache
8. Migratory joint pain
9. Neurological or psychological complaints:
   Sensitivity to bright light
   Forgetfulness
   Confusion
   Inability to concentrate
   Excessive irritability
   Depression
10. Sleep disturbance (hypersomnia or insomnia)
11. Sudden onset of symptom complex

SIGNS

1. Low-grade fever
2. Nonexudative pharyngitis
3. Palpable or tender lymph nodes

Using the CDC criteria, the prevalence of the chronic fatigue syndrome in individuals suffering from chronic fatigue is thought to be
about 11.5 percent.[2] In other words, in about 90 percent of the cases of
chronic fatigue, the cause is something other than what these scientists
are calling the chronic fatigue syndrome. Here is a list of some of the
major causes of chronic fatigue:

CAUSES OF CHRONIC FATIGUE

Pre-existing Physical Condition
   Diabetes
   Heart disease

Lung disease
Rheumatoid arthritis
Chronic inflammation
Chronic pain
Cancer
Liver disease
Multiple sclerosis
Prescription Drugs
    Antihypertensives
    Anti-inflammatory agents
    Birth control pills
    Antihistamines
    Corticosteroids
    Tranquilizers and sedatives
Depression
Stress/low adrenal function
Impaired liver function and/or environmental illness
Impaired immune function
    Chronic fatigue syndrome
    Chronic candida infection
    Other chronic infections
Food allergies
Hypothyroidism
Hypoglycemia
Anemia and nutritional deficiencies
Sleep disturbance
Unknown cause

What causes chronic fatigue syndrome? Using the "germ theory," most of the research has focused on trying to identify a specific infectious organism, such as the Epstein-Barr virus (EBV). I prefer to focus on "host susceptibility." Two findings are consistent in CFS patients: (1) a disturbed immune system, and (2) impaired adrenal function.[3] In short, in sufferers of CFS, the host is susceptible to infiltration by disease.

What causes the general immune system failure and low adrenal function seen in CFS? Numerous factors work together to produce CFS; therefore, effective treatment must be comprehensive and address the underlying factors contributing to the weakened status of the immune system.

Comments on the Whitaker Prescription for Chronic Fatigue Syndrome

My approach to the complex problem of chronic fatigue syndrome is simple, straightforward, and, most important, effective. It is based on a simple truism of nondrug health care: a multifactorial problem is best addressed with a multifactorial solution.

The Whitaker Wellness Program, on its own, will often lead to complete recovery from chronic fatigue (see Chapter 2). The major factors that determine your energy levels and the status of your immune system are diet and lifestyle. Once you improve these factors, the rest is easier.

Obviously, enhancing immune function is a critical factor in treating CFS; the recommendations in Chapter 7 are extremely important to follow. It is also extremely important to support the adrenal glands. Individuals with CFS typically have low adrenal function, and following the recommendations in Chapter 6 will help.

Supplements

1. Take a high-potency multiple vitamin-mineral formula according to the guidelines in Chapter 2.
2. Take an additional 3,000 to 8,000 milligrams of vitamin C each day. Use at least two packets of E-mergen-C (from Alacer) daily, to provide 2,000 milligrams of the vitamin C and 400 milligrams of potassium.
3. Take an additional 1,200 IU of vitamin E.
4. Take 1,000 milligrams of elemental magnesium as magnesium aspartate.
5. Take one tablespoon of flax oil daily.
6. Take two tablets of ThymuPlex (see page 118), twice daily.
7. Take one or two capsules of Raw Adrenal (see page 106) with meals.
8. Take Siberian ginseng extract. Use products standardized for eleutheroside-E content (greater than 1 percent) at a dosage of 100 milligrams, three times daily. High-quality extracts are sold by Enzymatic Therapy, Nature's Herbs, Herbal Choice, and Sibergin.

Cold Sores

Dr. Whitaker's Prescription for Cold Sores:

1. Follow Dr. Whitaker's Prescription for Wellness.
2. Follow recommendations for herpes (see page 268).
3. Apply Herpilyn cream to affected areas two to four times daily.

Description

Cold sores are caused by the herpes virus. They are characterized by the appearance of single or multiple clusters of small blisters filled with a clear fluid on a reddened base.

Cold sores differ from genital herpes in that the strain of virus is different. Cold sores are usually caused by herpes simplex virus 1 (HSV1), while genital herpes is usually caused by the type 2 virus (HSV2). Most people, perhaps as high as 90 percent worldwide, are infected by HSV1. After the initial infection, the virus becomes dormant in the nerve cells, in most people; in others, however, it can be reactivated. This causes recurring outbreaks, usually following minor infections, trauma, stress, or sun exposure. The focus of my therapy is to create conditions in the host that limit the likelihood of recurrence.

Comments on Dr. Whitaker's Prescription for Cold Sores

Cold sores are a continual nuisance to many people, but they don't have to be. Follow the guidelines for herpes (see page 268). This will go a long way in preventing recurrences.

Use a special product that is simply phenomenal for healing and preventing cold sores, called Herpilyn. It is an all-natural medicated cream that is new to the United States, but has been used effectively for many years in Germany, under the product name Lomaherpan® Cream. The Lomaherpan company has licensed a U.S. version of this important product to Enzymatic Therapy. As a result, Americans now have access to a product that will give them the relief from cold sores that they desire.

The active component in the product is a special extract of *Melissa officinalis*, a member of the mint family. Melissa is endowed with powerful antiviral activity against the herpes virus.[1] The melissa extract in Herpilyn is a 70:1 concentrate, which means it takes 70 pounds of melissa to produce 1 pound of the extract. Rather than any single antiviral chemical, the melissa extract in the formula contains several components that work together to prevent the virus from infecting human cells.

When Lomaherpan® Cream was used in patients with the initial herpes infection, in comprehensive trials from three German hospitals and a dermatology clinic, there was not a single recurrence.[2] In other words, by using the cream not a single patient with a first herpes outbreak developed another cold sore.

Furthermore, these studies noted that Lomaherpan® Cream produced a rapid interruption of the infection and promoted healing of the herpes blisters much quicker than normal. The control group receiving other topical creams had a healing period of ten days, while patients receiving Lomaherpan® were completely healed within five days.

Lomaherpan® Cream was also studied in patients suffering from recurrent cold sores. If they used Lomaherpan® Cream regularly they either stopped having recurrences, or they experienced a tremendous reduction in the frequency of recurrences. This meant an average cold-sore free period of greater than 3 1/2 months.

Herpilyn, the United States version of Lomaherpan® Cream, should be applied to the lips two to four times a day during an active recurrence. You can apply it fairly thickly (1 to 2 millimeters). Detailed toxicology studies have demonstrated that it is extremely safe and suitable for long-term use.

Herpilyn is available at most health food stores. (If you can't find it, call Enzymatic Therapy (1-800-783-2286) for names of stores or mail-order companies in your area.)

Common Cold

Dr. Whitaker's Prescription for the Common Cold:

1. Rest!
2. Drink 8 ounces of water every hour that you are awake.
3. Take 1,000 milligrams of vitamin C with your water.
4. Take a zinc lozenge (such as those made by McZand Herbal, KAL, or Nature's Life) every two hours.
5. Take two tablets of Thymuplex (Enzymatic Therapy), three times daily.
6. Take one dropper of fresh-pressed juice echinacea, four times daily.
7. Avoid the use of over-the-counter cold remedies.

Description

The common cold is caused by a variety of viruses that infect the oral and nasal passages and the sinuses. We are constantly exposed to these viruses. So the onset of a cold is more likely caused by a breakdown in immune defenses than exposure to particular viruses.

The symptoms of a cold are indicative of the battle between the body and the invading viruses: fever, headache, nasal congestion, sore throat, or generalized malaise. The achy feeling is due largely to the release of interferon, a potent immune stimulator from the blood cells. These symptoms are, in fact, your friends. They may be unpleasant, but it is not reasonable or helpful to vigorously suppress them as most over-the-counter medications do, as this can prolong the time it takes the body to rid itself of the virus.

Comments on Dr. Whitaker's Prescription for the Common Cold

Prevention

The best treatment of a cold is to prevent it altogether. Since colds and flu are caused primarily by weakness in the immune system, a strong immune system can prevent them. Building a strong immune system requires the steps outlined in the Whitaker Prescription for Wellness (see Chapter 2), including special nutritional supplementation.

Chapter 7 discusses enhancing immune function by supplementing the diet with a multiple vitamin-mineral formula. Doing so can enhance the ability of the immune system to prevent colds. In *Lancet* (November 7, 1992), professor R.K. Chandra from Johns Hopkins University reported that a low-potency vitamin and mineral regimen over the course of one year dramatically reduced sick days in healthy 65-year-olds. Those taking the vitamin and mineral supplements had 23 sick days, compared to 48 for those on placebo. These elderly people had nearly an entire additional month each year without being sick.

The researchers concluded that elderly people using supplementation can experience "significant improvement in several indices of immunocompetence." They concluded that "the nutrients led to a striking reduction in illness, a finding that is of considerable clinical and public health importance."

Treatment

A healthy immune system can help prevent colds. But what if you do catch a cold? What can be done? There are a number of natural ways to enhance the immune system and thus speed up your recovery. Let's take a look at the seven recommendations in my prescription for the common cold.

1. Rest. This seems like good advice, but why? During periods of rest, relaxation, visualization, meditation, and sleep, potent immune-enhancing compounds are released and many immune functions are greatly increased.[1] The value of sleep and rest during a cold cannot be overemphasized.

2. Drink eight ounces of water every hour. The immune system works better when you are well hydrated. In addition, if you have a fever, the body can lose a lot of fluid and mucus membranes can dry up, which provides an excellent environment for viruses. Do not drink concentrated fruit juices, or any fluids that contain sugar; this depresses the ability of the white blood cells to destroy viruses.[1] Sugar and vitamin C are very similar in molecular structure, and sugar retards the transport of vitamin C into the white blood cells where it is

most needed. If you want to drink fruit juice, be sure it is diluted: one part fruit juice to three parts water.

3. Take 1,000 milligrams of vitamin C every hour with your water. As mentioned in Chapter 1, over twenty double-blind studies have shown that vitamin C is effective in reducing the severity of symptoms, as well as the duration, of the common cold.[2]

4. Take a zinc lozenge (such as those made by McZand Herbal, KAL, or Nature's Life), every two hours. In one study, zinc gluconate lozenges containing 23 milligrams of zinc taken every two hours reduced the average duration of the common cold by roughly seven days.[3] Use these lozenges only for one week—prolonged use of high doses of zinc can inhibit the immune system.

5. Take two tablets of Thymuplex (Enzymatic Therapy), three times daily. Each tablet of ThymuPlex contains 375 milligrams of active polypeptide fractions from calf thymus. It also includes nutrients essential to immune and thymus functions, L-lysine, and herbal extracts including echinacea, goldenseal, and blue flag. ThymuPlex is a great nutritional formula to enhance the immune system during any infectious process.

6. Take one dropper of fresh-pressed juice echinacea four times daily. (Echinacea was discussed in Chapter 7.) Although there is echinacea in ThymuPlex, I like to recommend the use of liquid echinacea products during a cold or sore throat because of the benefit of literally dousing the virus with echinacea. Two brands to choose from are EchinaFresh from Enzymatic Therapy and EchinaGuard from Nature's Way. Use the echinacea fluid extract only as long as you have symptoms.

7. I do not recommend any over-the-counter cold remedies. These remedies are geared primarily to alleviate the symptoms (such as fever or cough) that the body generates to fight the flu. Taking these medications can sometimes prolong the disease.[4] In addition, careful reading of the fine-print warnings on almost every cold remedy will mention a list of possible side effects.

Constipation

Dr. Whitaker's Prescription for Constipation:

1. Follow Dr. Whitaker's Prescription for Wellness.
2. Drink six to eight glasses of fluid per day, including two glasses of water mixed with powdered barley green juice. Use either Green Magma (Green Foods) or Kyo-Green (Wakunaga).
3. Dramatically increase your intake of vitamin C.
4. Increase intake of bran. Begin by eating 1/2 cup of bran cereal for breakfast, increasing to 1 1/2 cups over several weeks.

5. Eat four whole prunes or eight ounces of prune juice daily.
6. Drink aloe vera juice.
7. Use a fiber formula at night.
8. Retrain bowels if you have used stimulant laxatives for more than one month.

Description

Constipation affects over 4 million people in the United States on a regular basis.[1] This high rate of constipation translates to over $400 million in annual sales of laxatives in the U.S. There are a number of possible causes of constipation. One is that it is a side effect of many drugs. The most common cause of constipation is a low-fiber diet.

CAUSES OF CONSTIPATION

Dietary   highly refined and low-fiber foods, inadequate fluid intake

Physical inactivity   inadequate exercise, prolonged bed rest

Pregnancy

Advanced age

Drugs   anesthetics, antacids (aluminum and calcium salts), anticholinergics (bethanechol, carbachol, pilocarpine, physostigmine, ambenonium), anticonvulsants, antidepressants (tricyclics, monoamine oxidase inhibitors), antihypertensives, antiParkinsonism drugs, antipsychotics (phenothiazines), beta-adrenergic blocking agents (propanolol), bismuth salts, diuretics, iron salts, laxatives and cathartics (chronic use), muscle relaxants, opiates, toxic metals (arsenic, lead, mercury)

Metabolic abnormalities   low potassium stores, diabetes, kidney disease

Endocrine abnormalities   low thyroid function, elevated calcium levels, pituitary disorders

Structural abnormalities   abnormalities in the structure or anatomy of the bowel

Bowel diseases   diverticulosis, irritable bowel syndrome (alternating diarrhea and constipation), tumor

Neurogenic abnormalities   nerve disorders of the bowel (aganglionosis, autonomic neuropathy), spinal cord disorders (trauma, multiple sclerosis, *tabes dorsalis*), disorders of the splanchnic nerves (tumors, trauma), cerebral disorders (stroke, Parkinsonism, neoplasm)

Enemas   chronic use

Comments on Dr. Whitaker's Prescription for Constipation

Constipation will usually respond to a high-fiber diet, plentiful fluid consumption, and increased physical activity. Unfortunately, these changes appear to be too much to ask of many sufferers of chronic constipation. Instead of following this natural approach, it is easier for many people to rely on laxatives, which do not work over the long term.

One of the first questions I ask my patients who complain of constipation is how much water they are drinking. Consistently, I find out that they are simply not meeting their body's requirement for water. You must drink at least six to eight glasses per day. In two of those glasses, mix in one tablespoon of powdered barley green juice. Use either Green Magma (Green Foods) or Kyo-Green (Wakunaga).

Another simple recommendation is to boost vitamin C levels. In Germany, vitamin C is an approved laxative. If a person is not used to taking high doses of vitamin C, I recommend a daily dose of 5,000 milligrams. If your are already taking that much, increase it to 10,000 milligrams.

Eating more dietary fiber is another effective treatment of chronic constipation. High levels of dietary fiber increase both the frequency and quantity of bowel movements. Fiber decreases the transit time of stools, as well as the absorption of toxins from the stool. It also appears to be a preventive factor in several diseases.

Particularly effective in relieving constipation are bran and prunes. The typical recommendation for bran is 1/2 cup of bran cereal, increasing to 1 1/2 cups over several weeks. Corn bran is more effective than wheat bran, while oat bran is less irritating and a better absorber of fats. For best results, adequate amounts of fluids must also be consumed (at least 32 ounces per day). Whole prunes and prune juice possess good laxative effects; your grandmother was right. Eight ounces is usually an effective dose. A similar amount of aloe vera juice is also helpful.

If you need additional support, consider using fiber formulas, which act as bulking agents. They can be composed of natural plant fibers derived from psyllium seed, kelp, agar, pectin, and plant gums like karaya and guar. Alternatively, they can be purified semi-synthetic polysaccharides like methylcellulose and carboxymethyl cellulose sodium. Psyllium-containing laxatives are the most popular and usually the most effective. Fiber formulas are the laxatives that approximate most closely the natural mechanism that promotes a bowel movement.

If you have been using stimulant laxatives, even natural ones like cascara sagrada (*Rhamnus purshiana*) or senna (*Cassia senna*), you will need to "retrain" your bowels. Listed below are the recommended rules for re-establishing bowel regularity, as presented in the *Encyclopedia of Natural Medicine* (Murray MT and Pizzorno JE, Prima Publishing, Rocklin, CA, 1991). The recommended procedure will take four to six weeks.

Rules for Bowel Retraining

Find and eliminate known causes of constipation.

Never repress an urge to defecate.

Eat a high-fiber diet, particularly fruits and vegetables.

Drink six to eight glasses of fluid per day.

Sit on the toilet at the same time every day (even when the urge to defecate is not present), preferably immediately after breakfast or exercise.

Exercise at least twenty minutes, three times per week.

Stop using laxatives (except as discussed below to reestablish bowel activity) and enemas.

- Week One: Every night before bed take a stimulant laxative containing either cascara or senna. Take the lowest amount necessary to reliably ensure a bowel movement every morning.
- Weekly: Each week decrease laxative dosage by half. If constipation recurs, go back to the previous week's dosage. Decrease dosage if diarrhea occurs.

Crohn's Disease and Ulcerative Colitis

Dr. Whitaker's Prescription for Crohn's Disease and Ulcerative Colitis:

1. Eliminate food allergies.
2. Follow the Whitaker Wellness Program.
3. Drink 16 to 24 ounces of fresh vegetable juice per day or use powdered barley green juice. Mix one tablespoon of either Green Magma (Green Foods) or Kyo-Green (Wakunaga) with eight ounces of water, two to three times daily.
4. Take 3 to 5 grams of water-soluble fiber at bedtime.

Description

Crohn's disease and ulcerative colitis are the two major categories of inflammatory bowel disease (IBD). Crohn's disease most often affects the ileum or terminal portion of the small intestine. Ulcerative colitis affects the lining of the colon. Both diseases are characterized by intestinal pain, diarrhea, and malabsorption of nutrients. Ulcerative colitis is slightly more common than Crohn's disease.

Theories about the cause of IBD can be divided into several groups: (1) genetic predisposition; (2) infectious agent or agents; (3) immunologic abnormality; (4) dietary factors; and (5) an assortment of miscellaneous concepts implicating psychosomatic, vascular, traumatic, and other mechanisms.

The likely factor is hardly considered, in standard medical and gastroenterology texts. Yet several lines of evidence suggest that dietary choices may be the most important causative factor.

The incidence of Crohn's disease is increasing in cultures consuming the "Western" diet (high-refined sugar, high-fat diet). It is virtually nonexistent in cultures consuming a more primitive diet.

Food is the major factor in determining the intestinal environment. Common sense implicates food. In fact, the considerable change in dietary habits over the last century could explain the rising rates of Crohn's disease. The biggest culprit appears to be a diet high in refined sugar.[1]

Comments on Dr. Whitaker's Prescription for Crohn's Disease and Ulcerative Colitis

Diets that eliminate food allergies have proven to be extremely effective in the treatment of IBD.[2] These studies demonstrate that elimination of food allergies should be the primary therapy in the treatment of chronic IBD. (A complete discussion on how to identify and avoid food allergies appears on page 244.)

After eliminating food allergens, the next step is to correct any underlying nutritional deficiency. Nutrient deficiencies lead to altered gastrointestinal function and structure. The nature of the disease and the standard medical treatment cause nutritional deficiencies to be quite common.[3] This may lead the patient into a vicious cycle. Here is a list of common nutritional deficiencies in IBD patients.

NUTRITIONAL DEFICIENCY IN IBD PATIENTS

Deficiency	Prevalence (%)
Protein	25–80
Anemia	60–80
Iron deficiency	40
Low serum vitamin B12	48

Low serum folate	54–64
Low serum magnesium	14–33
Low serum potassium	6–20
Low serum retinol	21
Low serum ascorbate	12
Low serum vitamin D	25–65
Low serum zinc	40–50

The Whitaker Wellness Program in Chapter 2 provides a suitable guideline for nutritional therapy for IBD, including the optimum level of nutrients to supplement the diet. The dietary recommendations focus on providing a diet rich in plant foods, which is also a diet rich in dietary fiber. Treatment with a high-fiber, plant-based diet has been shown to have a favorable effect on the course of Crohn's disease.[4]

This recommendation is in direct contrast to one of the oldest medical treatments of IBD, which was to use a low-fiber diet. But dietary fiber has been shown to have a profound effect on the intestinal environment and is now thought to promote a more optimal intestinal flora composition.[5] Some foods may be too "rough" to handle; the individual will have to chose among many fiber options. But dietary treatment of IBD clearly should utilize an unrefined-carbohydrate, fiber-rich diet.

As in other inflammatory conditions, manipulation of dietary oils is indicated. Animal fats should be reduced considerably. The consumption of omega-3 oils (linolenic acid and eicosapentaenoic acid as found in flax oil and fish oils, respectively) should be encouraged. The omega-3 oils lead to significantly fewer inflammatory leukotrienes and have been shown to reduce inflammatory processes.

The effect of fish oil on the course of ulcerative colitis was recently investigated in a well-designed clinical trial.[6] Eighty-seven patients received supplements of 20 grams of fish oil (4.5 grams of EPA) or olive oil (placebo), daily, for one year. Treatment with the fish oil resulted in measurable improvements, with a trend towards achieving remission. Remission, in this case, meant being able to end treatment with corticosteroids (with its risks and side effects). Twenty grams is admittedly a lot of fish oil. But if you are on corticosteroids, it is certainly worth it to try to get off them. To offset the high cost of so much fish oil, I recommend taking ten capsules of fish oils per day and one tablespoon of less-expensive flax oil.

I also recommend buying a juicer and drinking 16 to 24 ounces of fresh vegetable juice each day. Cabbage juice, due to its ability to soothe irritated membranes and promote healing, is especially beneficial in IBD. If you don't want to buy a juicer, add powdered barley green juice to water to make your own "fresh juice." Mix one tablespoon of either

Green Magma (Green Foods) or Kyo-Green (Wakunaga) to eight ounces of water, two to three times daily.

Also, a gel-forming fiber supplement containing such fibers as psyllium seed husks, pectin, guar gum, or oat bran should be used at night. This will help regulate bowel function and bind toxins that may irritate the bowels. Take between 3 and 5 grams daily.

Depression

Dr. Whitaker's Prescription for Depression:

1. If you are depressed, particularly if you are severely depressed, seek medical or psychological counseling, and make sure to discuss with your physician the possibility of incorporating, even as a primary treatment, regular physical exercise.
2. Follow the Whitaker Wellness Program.
3. Take St. John's wort extract at recommended dosages.
4. Take 2,000 milligrams of L-tyrosine before meals.

Description

The official definition of "clinical" depression, as defined by the American Psychiatric Association in its *Diagnostic and Statistical Manual of Mental Disorders* (DSM-III), is based upon the following eight primary criteria:

1. Poor appetite with weight loss, or increased appetite with weight gain
2. Insomnia or hypersomnia
3. Physical hyperactivity or inactivity
4. Loss of interest or pleasure in usual activities, or decrease in sexual drive
5. Loss of energy and feelings of fatigue
6. Feelings of worthlessness, self-reproach, or inappropriate guilt
7. Diminished ability to think or concentrate
8. Recurrent thoughts of death or suicide

These specialists have concluded that the presence of five of the eight symptoms definitely indicates depression. The individual with four of these symptoms is probably also depressed. According to the DSM-III, the depressed state must be present for at least one month in order to be called depression. In many cases, depression is an appropriate response to a life event. In such cases, specific medical treatment is not needed.

Nearly one of every four individuals experience some degree of clinical depression or mood disorder at some time in their lives. The rates are slightly higher in women than men.

The most popular theoretical model of depression is based more on physiological matters than psychological factors. The main reason that this model is so popular is that it is a better fit for drug therapy. The "biogenic amine" hypothesizes biochemical derangement. These lead to imbalances of amino acids which form compounds called neurotransmitters that transmit information to and from nerve cells. Antidepressant drugs and amino acids like tryptophan are designed to correct or lessen suspected imbalances in the biogenic amines (serotonin, melatonin, dopamine, epinephrine, and norepinephrine). These compounds are also known as *monoamines.* The amino acid tryptophan serves as the precursor to serotonin and melatonin, while phenylalanine and tyrosine are precursors to dopamine, epinephrine, and norepinephrine.

Comments on Dr. Whitaker's Prescription for Depression

Prescription Antidepressants

Most physicians treating depression rely almost exclusively on prescription drugs. The most commonly prescribed drug for depression these days is Prozac, the new drug from Eli Lilly. If there was ever a drug that I am truly afraid to prescribe, it is Prozac. This drug has been successful in alleviating depression in many, but it causes a condition called *akathisia,* from the Greek word meaning "can't sit down." Akathisia is a drug-induced state of agitation. In some people, it may induce truly violent and destructive outbursts. The violent reactions experienced by some patients taking Prozac have been so common and well publicized that several citizens groups have formed to create awareness of the dangers of the drug. Adverse drug reactions to the FDA-approved drug Prozac are alarmingly high.

Also, the drug is merely treating symptoms. The causes of the problem are not being addressed.

New problems for the patient, however, may be unfolding. The Citizen's Commission on Human Rights, through the Freedom of Information Act, received the adverse drug reaction reports on all of the major antidepressant drugs from 1985 to June 1992. During that time, Prozac received 23,067 claims of adverse drug reactions

(ADRs) compared to Elavil, a commonly used standby antidepressant, which received only 2,032. Suicide attempts in the Elavil group were ten, compared to 1,436 attempts with Prozac. Death rates in the Prozac group were 1,313 compared to 159 for Elavil. (Of course, the greater frequency of prescribing Prozac could explain this increase.) But serious, violent behavior associated with Prozac has even entered the courtroom in several cases. Remember the "Twinkie Defense?" We're now talking about the "Prozac Defense."

Because of the negative publicity, the FDA convened a special committee to examine the growing concern with Prozac. This included ten psychiatrists. A lengthy and insightful report by Gary Null entitled "Prozac, Eli Lilly, and the FDA" appeared in the *Townsend Letter for Doctors* in February of 1993.[1] Null pointed out that when Dr. Martin Teicher, a Harvard researcher, began to present substantial evidence of the link between Prozac and violent, suicidal thoughts, the panel refused to allow him to present his slides. They said they were not interested in his findings. Instead, the panel allowed three slide presentations in defense of Prozac.

Nor was the panel interested in other points brought up by Dr. Teicher after he sat through the presentations that Eli Lilly sponsored. For example, Jan Fawcett, a psychiatrist sponsored by Eli Lilly, pointed out that the common risk factors associated with suicide are anxiety, insomnia, panic attacks, and poor concentration. Dr. Teicher pointed out that Eli Lilly's prescribing information for Prozac lists anxiety and insomnia as two of the most common side effects noted. During the drug's clinical trials, 9 percent of trial subjects receiving Prozac experienced anxiety and 13.8 percent experienced insomnia. These side effects were not noted in the subjects taking the placebo.

Dr. Teicher sought to make a point: If anxiety and insomnia are risk factors for suicide, and if Prozac causes anxiety and insomnia, there may be a link between Prozac and suicide.

The FDA panel, however, simply ignored Dr. Teicher when he pointed out the contradiction.

Several experts in this matter concluded that the FDA panel had received enough evidence linking Prozac and violence to take action against the drug. Why did the panel choose not to do so? Eight of the ten panelists were psychiatrists. Nine of the ten members had financial conflicts of interest. One psychiatrist on the panel, Jeffrey Lieberman, had received $20,000 in grants from Sandoz Pharmaceuticals at the time he served. Sandoz is the manufacturer of Pamelor, the second most widely prescribed antidepressant. Sandoz had its own side effects to worry about.

Another panelist, psychiatrist James Claghorn, received $170,000 worth of grants from makers of antidepressants. The FDA undoubtedly might argue that these grants are evidence of Claghorn's expertise. But

Dr. Claghorn gave positive reviews of two other antidepressant drugs in the 1980s, zimelidine and nomifensine. Within two years of his review, both drugs were pulled off the market due to serious side effects.

Psychiatrist David Dunner had conflicts of interest totaling half a million dollars from four manufacturers of antidepressants, including $200,000 worth of grants "pending" from Eli Lilly, Prozac's maker, when the hearing took place. The Citizen's Commission on Human Rights discovered that Dr. Dunner's conflict of interest waiver did not include several relevant items. The conflicts not disclosed in Dr. Dunner's waiver included two pending grants worth $250,000 from antidepressant drug makers, and an engagement to speak at a series of seminars funded by Eli Lilly. Dr. Dunner not only failed to mention these conflicts; in his waiver he stated that he had no current commitments to speak.

This omission violates federal laws. Dr. Jonathan Wright, who thought his patients should have access to tryptophan, a safer, less expensive alternative to Prozac, had his office raided and ransacked without any prior evidence of wrongdoing (see Chapter 1), yet Dr. Dunner was not prosecuted for his serious breach of federal disclosure laws.

Even without these oversights, Dr. Dunner certainly should not have been on the panel. He had received over $4 million worth of research grants from antidepressant manufacturers in an eight-year period prior to the hearings where he was supposed to serve the "public interest" and objectively discuss taking these very same drugs off the market.

Exercise

Perhaps the most natural, and certainly the safest, antidepressant is physical exercise. Prescription drugs for elevating the mood are prescribed to take once or twice a day. I recommend a prescription for brisk walking for half an hour once or twice a day instead of a drug.

Physical exercise enhances the most powerful mood elevators in the body, the endorphin system in the brain. There is a clear association between exercise and endorphin elevation. When endorphins go up, mood follows. Dr. Daniel Carr and other researchers studied seven women aged eighteen to thirty who had not engaged in any athletic training or dietary practices in the past. The study, published in the *New England Journal of Medicine,* showed that exercise training substantially increased the endorphins or the endogenous-produced opiates. The longer exercise training was continued, the more consistent and elevated was the response.[2]

Dennis Lobstein, Ph.D., a professor of exercise psychobiology at the University of New Mexico, compared the beta-endorphin levels and depression profiles of ten joggers versus ten sedentary middle-aged men.[3] The sedentary men tested out more depressed, perceived greater stress in their lives, and had more stress-circulating hormones and lower levels of beta-endorphins. Dr. Lobstein stated, this "reaffirms that depression is very sensitive to exercise and helps firm up a biochemical link between physical activity and depression."

Vitamin and Mineral Supplementation

There are many other natural approaches to depression. One is the use of vitamins and minerals. In several studies with elderly populations, those taking nutritional supplements and/or having higher levels of nutrients in their blood, had less depression. They also showed better cognitive function than those not taking supplements and/or with lower levels of the essential nutrients.[4]

St. John's Wort

One herb deserves special mention as a natural antidepressant. St. Johns wort (*Hypericum perforatum*) is a shrubby perennial plant native to many parts of the world, including Europe and the United States. Researchers in Germany have discovered that components in St. John's wort alter brain chemistry in a way that improves mood. In one study, six women with depressive symptoms, ages fifty-five to sixty-five, were given a standardized extract of St. John's wort (0.125 percent hypericin) as the only therapy.[5] There was a significant increase in urinary metabolites, indicating that there was greater dopamine production in the brain. This effect is consistent with antidepressant effects of many prescription drugs. In addition, these six patients and an additional nine cases were evaluated before and after with a series of surveys that measured anxiety, dysphoric mood, loss of interest, hypersomnia, anorexia, depression (usually worse in the morning), psychomotor retardation, and feelings of worthlessness. The rating was significantly lower after taking St. John's wort than the same ratings prior to taking the herb.

Other clinical studies with the standardized extract showed St. John's wort to be more effective in relieving depression than several standard drugs that are often used: amitriptyline (Elavil) and imipramine (Trofinil).[6] These drugs are associated with significant side effects, most often drowsiness, dry mouth, constipation, and impaired urination. St. John's wort extract is not associated with any significant side effects. In addition to improving mood, the extract has been shown to greatly improve sleep quality. It has been found effective in relieving both insomnia and hypersomnia.

The dosage of St. John's wort used in these German studies was typically 300 milligrams of the extract (0.125 percent hypericin content), three times daily. Enzymatic Therapy currently has the most potent St. John's wort extract in the United States. Each capsule provides 300 milligrams of an extract standardized to contain 0.3 percent hypericin. Take two to three capsules daily.

L-Tyrosine

Tyrosine is an amino acid that serves as the starting point in the manufacture of several important neurotransmitters. Studies of depressed individuals have indicated that many have low levels of tyrosine in the brain. Not surprisingly, many prescription drugs used in depression work by increasing tyrosine levels in the brain. Supplementing the diet with L-tyrosine has been shown to be as effective as antidepressant drugs, without the side effects.[4] Start out by taking 2,000 milligrams, three times per day before meals. After one month, drop the dosage by half.

Diabetes

Dr. Whitaker's Prescription for Diabetes:

Type I Diabetes
1. In newly diagnosed cases, take niacinamide. *For adults:* Take 25 milligrams per two pounds of body weight each day. *For children:* Take 100 mg to 200 milligrams per day.
2. Follow an intensified insulin program.
3. Follow the Whitaker Wellness Program.
4. Take 400 milligrams of *Gymnema sylvestre* extract daily.

Type II Diabetes
1. Achieve ideal body weight.
2. Exercise on a regular basis as described in Chapter 2 and Chapter 8.
3. Follow the Whitaker Wellness Program.
4. Take 400 milligrams of *Gymnema sylvestre* extract daily.

Special notes:
1. For diabetic retinopathy, see Macular Degeneration.
2. For conditions related to atherosclerosis, see Cholesterol and Peripheral Vascular Disease.

Description

Diabetes is one of the major killers of Americans. Greatly increased risk of heart disease, stroke, kidney disease, and loss of nerve function are all associated with this disease.

An estimated 10 million individuals have diabetes. Fewer than half, however, know this for a fact. They may be experiencing classic symptoms of the problem, such as frequent urination and excessive appetite and thirst. But they do not consult a physician so they are never given the diagnosis.

The major contributing factor in diabetes is obesity. While obesity is not considered a causal factor with type I diabetes, type I represents only about 10 percent of cases. Approximately 90 percent of those with Type II diabetes are obese. The obesity connection indicates a simple way for the layperson to distinguish the two major types of diabetes. Type II, which dominates, is clearly nutrition- and lifestyle-related. It generally occurs in individuals after age forty. Most type II diabetes can be controlled by diet alone. Discovery of clear, causal factors has thus far eluded type I researchers. Yet, although the two types have separate origins, diet is fundamental to the successful treatment of both.

Diabetes is a chronic disorder. One way it occurs is if the pancreas does not secrete enough of the hormone insulin. In type I diabetes, the beta cells of the pancreas (which manufacture insulin) are often found to be completely destroyed. In fact, they are destroyed by the person's own white blood cells.

What provokes this damaging activity of the body against itself? The probable explanation is that the white cells developed antibodies in response to cell destruction from other mechanisms. These mechanisms could include such things as chemical, viral, food allergy, or free radical attacks. Unfortunately, in diabetes, as in some other diseases, antibodies created for a beneficial purpose end up attacking the body's own tissues. These diseases are called "autoimmune diseases."

In diabetes, the insulin-producing beta cells are targeted. Some 75 percent of individuals with type I diabetes show evidence of antibodies to beta cells. These antibodies are evident in only 0.5 to 2 percent of the rest of the population. Normal individuals either do not experience a severe antibody reaction, or they repair the damage more efficiently.

The destruction of the beta cells in type I creates the need for the insulin injections that most people associate with diabetes. (See table of differences between type I and type II diabetes.) The full medical term for type I is Insulin-Dependent Diabetes Mellitus (IDDM). Type I diabetics must supply insulin externally all of their lives. This can be a long time, since type I usually occurs in children and adolescents.

Type I versus Type II Diabetes

Features	Type I	Type II
Age at onset	Usually under 40	Usually over 40
Proportion of diabetics	Less than 10%	Greater than 90%
Seasonal trend	Fall and winter	None
Family history	Uncommon	Common
Appearance of symptoms	Rapid	Slow
Obesity at onset	Uncommon	Common
Insulin levels	Decreased	Usually elevated
Insulin resistance	Occasional	Often
Treatment with insulin	Always	Usually not required
Ketoacidosis	Frequent	Rare
Complications	Frequent	Frequent

These individuals must continuously modify doses and types of insulin in response to regular blood sugar testing.

Type II diabetes is called Non-Insulin-Dependent Diabetes Mellitus (NIDDM). In most cases, there is plenty of insulin, but the cells of the body have become resistant to insulin's effect. With such resistance, the blood sugar can't get into the cells. As a result, there are simultaneous elevations of both blood sugar and insulin. This dual elevation is responsible for some rather serious long-term complications.

There are other, less frequently encountered types of diabetes. *Secondary diabetes* is a form of diabetes that follows after certain conditions and syndromes. These include pancreatic disease, hormone disturbances, drugs, and malnutrition. *Gestational diabetes* refers to glucose intolerance occurring during pregnancy.

In addition, *impaired glucose tolerance* is a condition that includes prediabetic, chemical, latent, borderline, subclinical, and silent diabetes. Individuals with impaired glucose tolerance have blood glucose levels and GTT that are intermediate. Their levels are between normal and those that are clearly abnormal. Many practitioners consider *reactive hypoglycemia* as a prediabetic condition.

If you suspect that you may have a problem with blood sugar control, it is vital that you see a physician for proper diagnosis. The standard method of diagnosing hypoglycemia and diabetes involves the measurement of blood glucose levels. The normal fasting blood glucose level is between 70 and 105 milligrams/deciliters. If a person has a fasting blood glucose measurement greater than 140 milligrams/deciliters on two separate occasions, the diagnosis is diabetes.

A more functional test of blood sugar control is the oral glucose tolerance test (GTT). It is used in the diagnosis of both reactive hypoglycemia and diabetes, although it is rarely required for the latter.

After fasting for at least twelve hours, a baseline blood glucose measurement is made. Then the subject drinks a very sweet liquid containing glucose. Blood sugar levels are rechecked at thirty minutes, one hour, and then hourly for up to six hours. If blood sugar levels rise to a level greater than 200 milligrams/deciliters, diabetes is indicated.

Comments on Dr. Whitaker's Prescription for Diabetes

Diabetes is a very serious disorder. It needs to be treated effectively. Current medical treatment has certainly helped many diabetics to live healthier and longer lives. This is especially true with that 10 percent of diabetes sufferers who have the type I insulin-dependent variety. Researchers and technicians have developed new understanding of insulin therapy. They have created new techniques for measuring blood glucose and administering insulin. These breakthroughs have definitely left many people thankful.

With that said, however, consider a 1978 report provocatively called a "Off Diabetes Pills: A Diabetic's Guide to Longer Life," written by Rebecca Warmer, Sydney Wol, M.D., and Rebecca Rich, in cooperation with the Public Citizens' Health Group in Washington, D.C.

Warning: Antidiabetic Pills Are Dangerous to Your Health

Are you taking tolbutamide (Orinase), tolazamide (Tolinase), chlorpropamide (Diabinese), or acetohexamide (Dymelor)? These pills could cost you your life. This booklet is written for you, to explain why you must do three things:

- Stop taking these antidiabetic pills as soon as you can;
- Change your diet and lose weight;
- Stop seeing your present doctor unless he or she agrees to help you lose weight.
- Switch to insulin if you still have diabetic symptoms once you are at or below your ideal weight.

These steps could mean the difference between life and death.

The drugs in question are all used in treatment of type II diabetes, which is 90 percent of all diabetics. These are sulfa drugs (sulfonylureas); other drugs in this group not mentioned by Public Citizens' Health Group but which are frequently used are glyburide (DiaBeta, Micronase) and glipizide (Glucotrol). Drugs in this class appear to do two things: They enhance the sensitivity of tissues to insulin. And they stimulate the pancreas to secrete more insulin. This would appear to be an excellent solution. So why would this consumer education group make such bold statements against these drugs? My clinical experience and understanding of diabetes research suggest that it is because they are right.

. Nearly two decades after their report was published, most of these drugs are still being used. The track record for effectiveness is passable, except when you measure it against the health costs of the side effects.

In terms of effectiveness, in 40 percent of cases, blood sugar levels can no longer be controlled by these drugs after three months of continual treatment at an adequate dosage. Diabetes is a lifelong disease. Sulfonylureas generally lose their effectiveness over time. The overall success rate of adequate control over long-term use of these drugs is no more than 20 to 30 percent.

There is tremendous evidence that these drugs produce harmful long-term side effects. The evidence also suggests that these drugs can contribute to your death. The University Group Diabetes Program (UDGP) conducted a study on the long-term effects of tolbutamide, and concluded that the rate of death due to a heart attack or stroke was 250 percent greater for users of tolbutamide than for the group controlling their type II diabetes by diet alone.[1] The drug had magnified the heart disease risk that diabetes sufferers already face.

Other side effects noted with these drugs are hypoglycemia, allergic skin reactions, headache, fatigue, indigestion, nausea and vomiting, and liver damage.

The damaging potential of sulfonylurea drugs indicates that there are times when these drugs should not be used. These drugs have to be used with extreme caution. They should not be used during pregnancy, in persons with a known allergy to sulfa drugs, during infection, injury, or surgery, or during long-term corticosteroid use. They must be used with extreme caution in treating the very old, alcoholics, those taking multiple drugs, and those with impaired liver or kidney function.

Multiple drug interactions are a major problem in many arenas of the disease-management system that prevails today. Because of the range of health problems associated with obesity, the likelihood of multiple prescriptions from chronic problems is quite high in the population being treated with sulfonylurea drugs.

Roughly one of every five patients may have long-term benefits, but 100 percent of these patients face potentially serious risks. The cost-benefit picture doesn't look good. So are there alternatives to drug therapy for patients with type II diabetes?

This question is best answered by Dr. Michael Berger, M.S., Professor of Medicine at Dusseldorf University, Germany. In the book *Oral Agents in the Treatment of Diabetes Mellitus* (Davidson JK (ed). Thieme Inc., New York, 1986, p. 268), Dr. Berger writes:

Unfortunately the use of sulfonylurea drugs has become entrenched as the "treatment of laziness," both on the part of the physician and the patient. How much easier it is to prescribe or swallow a pill than to explain or observe a weight-reducing diet in combination with an increase in caloric expenditure [exercise].

Dr. Berger focuses on the obesity issue associated with the onset of type II diabetes:

The central problem of the syndrome for which Sims has coined the term *diabesity* (representing more than 90 percent of the patients with NIDDM in the industrialized world) is insulin resistance due to hyperinsulinemia [excessive insulin secretion by the pancreas] associated with obesity/hyperphagia [overeating] and immobilization. Any rational attempt to treat this disorder should be based upon attempts to decrease, rather than increase, insulinemia in order to improve sensitivity to endogenous insulin.

Dr. Berger's recommendation reflects my own:

Thus, hypocaloric dieting and increased physical activity must remain the basis for therapy for overweight patients with non-insulin-dependent diabetes mellitus. Only if patients are still hyperglycemic despite significant weight loss of several weeks, or if they are already of normal weight and reasonably physically active, is the use of sulfonylurea drugs justified."

In short, except in a very few cases, drug therapy should be the option of last resort. The first line of defense is not the "treatment of laziness" but the "treatment of empowerment." Most diabetics can learn through the strategy I prescribe that they hold their health in their own hands. The side effects of Dr. Whitaker's program? How about a healthier, longer life?

Dietary Treatment of Diabetes

Diet is fundamental to the successful treatment of diabetes, whether it is type I or type II. This has been recognized (to an extent) for many years. But the conventional dietary recommendations for diabetics reflect the general lack of nutritional awareness in conventional medicine.

Prior to 1955, the main dietary advice to diabetics was to derive a majority of their calories from fat. The recommendation seemed to follow from evidence of short-term glucose control. Over the long run, however, (we know now) such a diet is extremely detrimental and can be fatal. Similarities to the data on sulfonylurea drugs should be noted:

possible short-term benefits, significant long-term damage. In fact, the link between a high-fat diet and diabetes is almost as strong as the link between refined sugar intake and diabetes. Such a diet leads to insulin insensitivity. It also greatly increases the risk of atherosclerosis.[2]

The American Diabetes Association (ADA) no longer promotes a high-fat diet. However, the association still has not endorsed the optimal diet suggested by available research. The evidence of the shortcomings of the ADA diet was found in a study that put type I diabetics on "the best diet" and then had them switch to the ADA diet. The result was that these individuals, once back on the ADA diet, had to increase their insulin requirements to prior levels.[3]

The other shortcoming of the diet recommended by the ADA is that it does not recognize the need for dietary supplementation.

The diet that I have found to be "the best" for diabetics, whether type I or type II, was popularized by Dr. James Anderson.[3] This diet features cereal grains, legumes, and root vegetables. Simple sugar and fat intake are restricted. In short, it is a specialized version of the basic diet recommended in the Whitaker Wellness Program—a high-complex-carbohydrate, high-fiber diet (HCF).

The HCF diet has substantial support in the literature. Tissues show increased sensitivity to insulin. The cholesterol ratio moves in the positive direction: HDL goes up and LDL goes down. Weight goes down. Blood sugar levels are reduced after meals. The benefits of the lowfat intake have been noted.

A star player in this diet is the legume family. These foods are full of fiber-rich compounds. Fiber is an important dietary strategy with obesity. (See Chapter 8.) But in the bloodstream of the diabetic, legume fibers have particular value. They help control blood glucose levels. My recommendation is actually for a "HCLRHF Diet": high-complex-carbohydrate, legume-rich, high-fiber. This combination helps to improve all aspects of diabetic control.[4]

Maintenance HCF Diet for Diabetics—Caloric Intake and Sources

55% TO 60% FROM COMPLEX CARBOHYDRATES

> 50% grain products
> 48% fruits and vegetables
> 2% skim milk

20% FROM PROTEIN

> 50% fruits and vegetables
> 36% grain products
> 14% skim milk and lean meat

20 TO 25% FROM FAT

60% grain products
20% fruits and vegetables
12% skim milk and lean meat

FIBER

Nearly 100 grams per day

Dr. Anderson recommends a slightly varied form of this diet for individuals who are hospitalized with diabetes. Here, the complex carbohydrate portion of calories is up to 70 to 75 percent, and that from fat is down to 5 to 10 percent. Protein stays roughly the same at 15 to 20 percent.

Note how closely this diet approximates the diets of our nearest primate cousins (see Chapter 2).

Insulin Treatment

Many doctors follow the "treatment of laziness" with type II diabetics. Diet and exercise suggestions may be made, but if such a change of habits is perceived as difficult, the core treatment is usually that with which the physician is most familiar and asks less of the patient.

Using a typical disease-management strategy, insulin is the treatment of choice following sulfonylurea drugs. Healthy individuals generally produce in the range of 31 units per day of insulin. No problems exist in the tissue uptake of insulin for these people, and these pancreatic secretions are efficiently utilized. The obese type II diabetic, on the other hand, secretes nearly 400 percent more insulin than a healthy person, roughly 114 units daily. Lean type II individuals secrete only about 14 units per day, and type I insulin-dependent diabetics secrete just 4 units per day. Clearly the lean type II and the type I diabetic needs insulin support.

But in the obese type II individual, the cells of the body have become insulin-resistant. This tissue failure is associated with the loss of nerve function in diabetics, which can lead in turn to the amputations often seen in end-stage diabetes. The pancreas only gets a message that the body needs more insulin; it doesn't know that the problem is not with insulin production. The problem is on the receiving end.

In short, the problem is not with the quarterback. The problem is that the "receivers" can't catch. In fact, the cells may be batting down the passes. The conventional insulin strategy sends in a new quarterback, more insulin, when it would be better to focus on the receiver, not flood the body with more insulin. Recall that one outcome of the

HCF diet promoted by Dr. Anderson (and which I recommend) is that it increases tissue sensitivity to insulin.

Unfortunately, the advice of Dr. Berger and other nutrition-oriented doctors like Dr. Anderson, has had little effect on conventional diabetes care.

There is no question that an established type I diabetic requires insulin. Here the strengths of conventional medicine shine. Important breakthroughs have been made with patented devices that help the insulin-dependent diabetic monitor blood sugar levels and administer insulin at home. First, to take a blood sample, the diabetic uses a simple, spring-triggered device equipped with a disposable lancet. Usually the sample is taken from the lateral sides of the distal fingers, then placed on a reagent strip. Some of these strips give satisfactory values on mere visual inspection. A colored scale indicates blood sugar levels. Others need to be inserted into a small, commercially available machine known as a glucometer. This machine displays the blood glucose levels.

Another method has been developed to assess the degree of blood sugar control over a longer period of time. This is the hemoglobin A_{1c} (HgbA$_{1c}$) assay. The assay takes advantage of the 120-day average life span of a red blood cell. In healthy individuals, between 5 and 7 percent of the hemoglobin A in red blood cells is combined with glucose. A measurement of 8 to 10 percent marks mild glucose elevations. Concentrations of up to 20 percent signal severe imbalances. The HbgA$_{1c}$ is believed to represent time-averaged values for blood glucose over the life of the red blood cell, or two to four months.

These tests establish an individual's potential need for insulin. In doing so, they also help monitor the effectiveness of dietary measures. With type II diabetics, insulin need can ebb and flow, based partly on the dietary and lifestyle choices the individual makes.

Insulin cannot be absorbed orally, and must be injected. Conventional insulin therapy involves administering crystalline insulin. The preparations come in concentrations of 100 units per milliliter (U-100) and 500 units per milliliter (U-500). Human synthetic insulin is gaining increasing acceptance as the preferred source, but insulin can also come from beef or pork. The injections are further distinguished by the duration of action. Some are short, some intermediate, and some long-acting. A soluble, noncrystalline type is sometimes used.

With conventional treatment, the diabetic receives one or two injections per day, usually a mixture of intermediate and long-acting varieties. Research has shown, however, that the chronic complications of insulin therapy are promoted by this relatively crude approach. A new method has been developed which has been shown to limit complications.[5]

The goal with the new approach is to mimic, as closely as possible, the way a healthy pancreas continuously varies plasma insulin levels. The approach is called "intensified insulin therapy." One intensified method involves increasing the number of injections daily, to three or five. A second option comes closer yet to the body's own process. It also requires more motivation and involvement on the part of the individual.

The patient wears a small pump device next to the abdomen. The pump is basically a small syringe filled with soluble insulin. From the bottom of the pump, a flexible tube leads directly into a needle which remains inserted into a site in the abdomen. The patient merely presses the plunger on the syringe to release insulin, fifteen minutes prior to meals, or at other times that are appropriate.

The pump method has its drawbacks. It must be worn twenty-four hours per day. There is some evidence that the risk of hypoglycemia is somewhat higher. In addition, not all physicians are yet aware of this method.

Clearly, most of the choices are difficult with this very serious disease. The bottom line, for type I or type II, is a good diet and regular physical activity.

Recent research from Europe casts a potentially hopeful light for some type I individuals who have just been initially diagnosed. Like many medical breakthroughs, this new strategy had accidental roots. European researchers were looking at the effects of a form of niacin on animals. We know that niacin is necessary for proper energy production and for fat, carbohydrate, and cholesterol metabolism. While investigating other questions, the researchers observed that this form of niacin, called *niacinamide* or *nicotinamide,* was preventing diabetes in the animals that they were studying.

The researchers then set up some pilot studies with human subjects.[6] The results are exciting. Niacinamide seems to prevent diabetes from developing in humans as well as animals. In fact, if administered early enough after the onset, niacinamide can help restore the activity of insulin-manufacturing beta cells. In other individuals, results suggest that the niacinamide may not actually restore beta cell activity but does slow down beta cell destruction. Some newly diagnosed type I diabetics have had complete resolution with niacinamide.

This preliminary research has provoked a major follow-up project. Eighteen European nations, plus Israel and Canada, are involved in a multicenter study that commenced in 1992. Other studies are also underway. The dose of niacinamide required is based on body weight. Studies on children used 100 to 200 milligrams each day. For adults, use 25 milligrams per two pounds of body weight.

Preventing the Complications of Diabetes

At this time, a diagnosis of diabetes is lifelong. The therapeutic goal is to hold the development of diabetes in check, reverse it where possible, and to prevent complications.

The list of complications can be frightening to a newly diagnosed diabetic. Some are acute. Diabetic ketoacidosis primarily inflicts type I individuals. Nonketogenic hyperosmolar syndrome primarily afflicts type II individuals. Hypoglycemia can be a complication for both types.

Over the long run, many major complications can occur, including atherosclerosis, diabetic retinopathy, diabetic neuropathy, diabetic nephropathy, and diabetic foot ulcers.

All of these complications reflect the level of blood sugar control the diabetic can achieve. A great deal of evidence shows that better control reduces the incidence of complications of all kinds. My program for type I and type II individuals helps stabilize blood sugar. It also takes advantage of research which shows that supplementing special nutritional compounds can both prevent and improve these complications. I have found this approach to be extremely effective in preventing complications of diabetes.

Follow the Whitaker Wellness Program in Chapter 2. Begin by making the dietary recommendations, paying particular attention to the modifications by Dr. Anderson described in this section. Follow the prescription for supplementation. Diabetics have great need for nutrients.

Gymnema Sylvestre

One way to support the body in countering the effects of diabetes is to administer substances that assist the pancreas in producing insulin. A fascinating finding about an herb called *Gymnema sylvestre* suggests that this is exactly what this plant does.

The herb, used for many years in India in the Ayurvedic medical tradition, has been found by modern researchers to enhance glucose control in rabbits and dogs. To understand the mechanism of this helpful action, the researchers removed the pancreas in some animals and re-administered *Gymnema sylvestre*. In the group with no pancreas, they found no effect from the herb. The herb's value seemed to be associated directly with the pancreas. Did *Gymnema sylvestre* actually enhance pancreatic activity by helping regenerate insulin-producing beta cells?

In studies in humans, a pattern emerged which seems to confirm this speculation. In a study of twenty-seven type I individuals, an extract of the leaves of *Gymnema sylvestre* was administered. All were on insulin therapy. Fasting blood sugar levels dropped. Insulin requirements dropped. Blood sugar control improved.[5] Similar results have been found with type II diabetics. Of twenty-two patients who were already on oral hypoglycemic drugs, all showed better blood sugar control. All but one able to reduce drug dosages considerably, therefore reducing the probability of drug side effects. In fact, five of the patients were able to maintain their blood sugar control with the extract alone. They were able to stop taking drugs altogether.[7]

Excellent result. The intriguing role of this herb when healthy individuals are given *Gymnema* is that nothing happens! No lowering of blood sugar. No hypoglycemia. The herb's powerful assistance is invoked only if the pancreas needs it. And when administered to the diabetic individuals studied, *Gymnema* administration showed no side effects.

The dose for *Gymnema sylvestre* extract is 400 milligrams per day for either type of diabetic. A number of companies, such as Nature's Herbs (Gymnesyl) and Enzymatic Therapy (Dia-Comp), market these extracts in the United States.

Recent scientific studies of *Gymnema sylvestre* did not "discover" the plant's power. As noted, doctors practicing in India's Ayurvedic tradition have long used it for the symptom complex that Western doctors call diabetes. These health problems needed treatment before the advent of insulin. In 1980, recognizing that many such valuable herbal agents are used by indigenous peoples around the world, the World Health Organization called upon researchers to investigate them further. Those who heeded this call have discovered many different herbal preparations for diabetes in the past decade. *Gymnema sylvestre* happens to be the standout. Compare the character of its activity to that of the insulin-control drugs favored by Western doctors: Side effects are nonexistent; the body's natural activity is supported; the need for potentially damaging intervention is diminished; serious complications may be avoided; short- and long-term costs of care are lower.

Nutrient Support

The most important vitamins and minerals for diabetics of both types are vitamin C, vitamin E, vitamin B6, chromium, and magnesium. The amounts recommended in Chapter 2 are sufficient, except vitamin B6 should be elevated somewhat.

Some of these nutrients are directly involved with the pancreas in its "quarterbacking" of insulin or, alternatively, the activity of the cells of the body as "receivers." Vitamin E is known to improve the action of insulin. High doses (400 to 600 IU per day) may reduce insulin requirements. Chromium works closely with insulin in facilitating the reception of glucose by the cells. Chromium deficiency will block insulin's action. The "ball is dropped." Glucose levels elevate. And if the receiving cells aren't doing their job, the transport of vitamin C into cells of the body is hindered, because this transport is facilitated by insulin. Studies have shown that a relative vitamin C deficiency exists even in those diabetics with adequate dietary vitamin C.[8]

The role of chromium supplementation has been widely studied. Trials have shown mixed results.[9] In some clinical studies, supplemental chromium has been shown to decrease fasting glucose levels. Insulin levels have been lowered. Glucose tolerance has improved. With the vital role of chromium in blood sugar control, it is a key component of the "glucose tolerance factor." Studies have also found decreased total cholesterol and triglyceride levels, with elevations of HDL cholesterol.[8] Other researchers have reported no effect from chromium supplementation in improving the glucose tolerance in diabetics. All researchers agree, however, that this mineral, the nutritional importance of which was discovered in 1957, is important to blood sugar metabolism.

Deficiencies of vitamin B6, vitamin C, and magnesium are found in most diabetics. These deficiencies can promote complications. Diabetics with neuropathy have been shown to be deficient in Vitamin B6 and have benefited from supplementation.[11] The neuropathy produced by deficiency of vitamin B6 is actually indistinguishable from diabetic neuropathy. Peripheral nerve abnormalities are a good indication that supplemental B6 is definitely in order. The dosage should be 150 milligrams, a little higher than that recommended in the Whitaker Wellness Program. Supplementation of vitamin B6 as a preventive measure is also indicated for those with long-standing diabetes.

Magnesium levels are usually low in diabetics, particularly those who have developed the complication of retinopathy. Supplementation may prevent some of this, as well as complications that appear as heart disease.[12] (More information on this role of magnesium may be found in Chapter 2. Follow the overall recommendations in that chapter.)

Vitamin E may help prevent many long-term complications of diabetes.[10] The recommended amount is 400 to 800 IU per day. Since trace mineral selenium functions very closely with vitamin E, I also recommend supplementing with selenium (200 to 400 micrograms) any time you are supplementing with high doses of vitamin E.

A chronic, latent deficiency of vitamin C will lead to a number of problems for diabetics. Wounds heal poorly. Immune function will be depressed. Cholesterol levels will climb. The increased permeability of capillaries will show up as a tendency to bleed. Supplementing vitamin

C at one to two grams a day has reduced the accumulation of factors that can lead to diabetic complications of the eyes and nerves.[13] The 5,000 milligrams per day recommended in Chapter 2 is appropriate.

Diet, Supplementation, and Drug Therapy

A natural approach to diabetes can alter the need for both insulin and the insulin-control drugs a physician may administer. For this reason it is imperative that a diabetic have a good working relationship with his or her physician before engaging the therapeutic approaches I recommend. Diabetes is a very serious disease. Careful attention to symptoms, home glucose monitoring and the HgbA$_{1c}$ tests should be used. The need to work closely with a physician is particularly important for those individuals with type I diabetes.

Ear Infection

Dr. Whitaker's Prescription for Ear Infection:

1. Avoid cigarette smoke, even if passive.
2. Eliminate food allergies.
3. Strengthen the immune system by avoiding overconsumption of sugar and by taking a multiple vitamin-mineral formula.
4. For acute ear infections in children, use a topical herbal-oil combination such as Ear Drops from Eclectic Institute.
5. Use measures to assist drainage from the Eustachian tube.

Description

Chronic ear infections affect 20 to 40 percent of children under the age of six. They account for over 50 percent of all visits to pediatricians.

Ear infections help keep pediatric practices humming. A conservative estimate suggests that approximately $8 billion are spent annually on medical and surgical treatment of ear infections in the United States. Unfortunately, this money is not being wisely spent.

There are basically two types of ear infections: chronic and acute. An acute middle ear infection (otitis media) is characterized by a sharp, stabbing, dull, or throbbing pain in the ear. The pain is due to inflammation, swelling, or infection of the middle ear. Acute ear infections are usually preceded by an upper respiratory infection or allergy. The organisms most commonly cultured from middle-ear fluid during acute otitis media include *Streptococcus pneumoniae* (40 percent) and *Haemophilus influenzae* (25 percent).

Chronic ear infections are known in medical terms as serous, secretory, or nonsuppurative otitis media with effusion. A more descriptive name is *glue ear*. Chronic infection refers to a constant swelling of the middle ear.

Abnormal Eustachian tube function is the underlying cause in virtually all cases of otitis media. The Eustachian tube regulates gas pressure in the middle ear. It also protects the middle ear from nose and throat secretions and bacteria, and clears fluids from the middle ear. Swallowing causes active opening of the Eustachian tube due to the action of the surrounding muscles. Because this tube is smaller in diameter and more horizontal in infants and small children, they are particularly susceptible to Eustachian tube problems.

Obstruction of the Eustachian tube leads to buildup of fluid. If bacteria start to grow, this leads to bacterial infection. Obstruction results from a variety of causes. The tube can collapse due to weak tissues holding the tube in place and/or an abnormal opening mechanism. Or the collapse can occur due to allergic blockage with mucous, or infection.

Comments on Dr. Whitaker's Prescription for Ear Infection

The standard medical approach to ear infections in children begins with antibiotics and/or antihistamines. If the first administration fails, a second will be tried, frequently with a different drug. Often the infection will subside under attack from the antibiotic, then rebound. This is because the cause of the problem is not addressed by the antibiotic.

If the ear infection is ultimately unresponsive to the drugs, surgery is performed. The surgery involves the placement of a tiny plastic tube through the eardrum. The tube assists drainage of fluid into the throat via the eustachian tube. This procedure is known as a *myringotomy*. Like antibiotics, this medical procedure does not address the possible causes of the problem. It relieves the pressure, the symptom that something is wrong.

Myringotomy is not a curative procedure; this is evident from the outcome. Children with tubes in their ears are in fact more likely to have further problems with ear infections.

Myringotomies are currently being performed on nearly 1 million American children each year. The most common unnecessary surgery of the past, the tonsillectomy, has been replaced in numbers by this new procedure. The decline of the tonsillectomy was followed by a rise in the myringotomy. Over 2 million myringotomy tubes are inserted into children's ears each year, along with 600,000 tonsillectomies and adenoidectomies.

Are all these surgeries necessary? Are any of these surgeries effective? Is current standard medical treatment successful? A number of well-designed studies have demonstrated that there are no significant differences in the clinical course of acute otitis media when conventional treatments were compared with placebos. Specifically, no differences were found between nonantibiotic treatment, ear tubes, ear tubes with antibiotics, and antibiotics alone.[1] Children not receiving antibiotics, however, had fewer recurrences than those who did. This reduced recurrence rate is undoubtedly a reflection of the suppressive effects that antibiotics have on the immune system. Antibiotics, because they are systemic, can also kill the biota in the gut which are necessary for healthy digestion. In short, administration of antibiotics, repeat administration in particular, can be very harmful.

The studies clearly suggest that conservative treatment alone would reduce the rate and decrease the yearly financial costs of otitis media. By conservative, I mean nonantibiotic and nonsurgical. By conservative I also mean conserving and working with the body's own ability to heal. By conservative, I mean saving measures like antibiotics and surgery for the very last—after all else has been tried.

Doctors often scare patients into believing that drugs and ear tubes are necessary to reduce the risk of the infection spreading to the mastoid and brain. The rate of such infection is 0.2 to 2 percent. This is of major concern, but there is no documented evidence that the rate is any different with or without antibiotics, or with or without myringotomy.

The results of these studies, when coupled with the high rate of recurrent ear infections following insertion of ear tubes, lead to an awful conclusion. Studies show that the typical basic care for ear infections provided by most pediatricians (which represents 50 percent of pediatric practice) is harmful to our children.

Overuse of antibiotics is stimulating a rapid evolution of more virulent strains of bacteria. Pharmaceutical firms and government-funded researchers are already struggling to stay a step ahead of the game with some of these agents. We are in a vicious circle with this bacteria. We could be facing a very serious, community-wide problem.

Cigarette Smoke

Parents who smoke cigarettes are much more likely to have children with chronic ear or respiratory tract infections. Several case-controlled studies found that elementary school children who underwent myringotomy tube placement were more likely to have lived in a households where cigarettes were smoked.[2] In a recent study, children with higher serum conitine levels were found to have a 38 percent higher rate of ear infections. Conitine is a nicotine metabolite that indicates exposure to cigarette smoke.[3] All of this evidence indicates that children should not be exposed to passive cigarette smoke.

Breast-Feeding and Infant Care

The best thing a mother can do to prevent ear infections in her children is to breast-feed them, if possible. Just four months of breast-feeding has been shown to have a protective effect.[4] Human milk has a high antibody content, which can help inhibit infectious agents.[5] It diminishes the "host susceptibility" of the infant until its immune system is fully up and running. With breast-feeding, the potential harmful activity of the causative agents is inhibited. The benefit is there whether the agent is bacterial or viral.

One reason that antibiotics are so overprescribed is that doctors often administer them before testing to see whether the problem agent is bacterial or viral. Breast milk can help protect against either, but an antibiotic facing a virus will merely pass it by in the bloodstream, and seek and destroy the gut biota one needs for healthy digestion.

The breast-feeding mother can further safeguard the child by altering her own food habits. By avoiding the foods to which she may be allergic, the child won't be exposed. Optimally, allergic foods will also be avoided during pregnancy.

Breast-feeding a baby helps prevent ear infections in a couple of other, indirect ways. The child won't have the problems typically associated with bottle-feeding. For example, if a baby bottle-feeds while lying on his or her back, the contents are easily regurgitated into the middle ear. For the same reason, bottle-propping should be avoided.

A baby who gets its primary nourishment from a mother has less contact with foods that may be problematic, such as cow's milk. It is not known conclusively whether it is the protective effect of mother's milk or allergy to cow's milk that is the primary factor in ear infections. Most likely, both are factors. Other foods to which many children are allergic are wheat, eggs, fowl, and dairy products. Good eating habits during the infant's first nine months are important.

Infants have high permeability of the digestive tract, especially during the first three months. To reduce and prevent allergic problems, it is best to carefully control the baby's food intake. Don't repeat the same foods all the time. Introduce new foods one at a time and watch for reactions. Note which foods are problematic.

Diet and Inhalants

Between eight and nine out of every ten children with chronic ear infections have them because of allergies. This connection is well established through published research. Most studies put the number between 85 and 93 percent.[5] With statistics like these, we are getting pretty close to naming the problem, and no one has said bacteria or virus.

The primary culprits are inhalants and food, or some combination of both. One study of children found 14 percent of allergies were only to foods, 16 percent only to inhalants, and 70 percent to a combination of both allergens. Try removing these agents. One study that used this therapy produced a 92 percent success rate.[6] The 119 children involved were put on elimination diets for their food allergies and desensitized from inhalant-related problems. The study compared this group with controls who used conventional, surgical ear treatment. Only 52 percent in that group responded positively; even so, they came out of conventional care with tubes in their ears, and often without either tonsils or adenoids.

Some simple but stringent dietary recommendations will bring relief to most children in a matter of days. Since it is just about impossible to determine an exact allergen during an acute attack, the best strategy is to remove all of the most common allergic foods: milk and dairy products, eggs, wheat, corn, oranges, and peanut butter. Foods known to inhibit immune function should also be removed: simple carbohydrates such as sugar, honey, dried fruit, and concentrated fruit juices. The microscopic lens that focuses attention only on microbial causative agents will miss placing blame where it belongs, on environmental and dietary factors such as food or inhalant allergies.

Many positive side effects can come if a child eats right starting early in life. The parent and child get an early understanding about food allergies and many problems can be avoided if these food sensitivities are known and dealt with. The risks of surgery and the side effects of antibiotics are not mandatory parts of childhood.

Other Measures

Frequent ear infections may represent a weak immune system. Measures should be taken to enhance the immune system by supplementing the diet with a good children's multiple vitamin-mineral formula. A deficiency of any of a number of essential nutrients increases the likelihood of ear infections, particularly the trace minerals zinc, selenium, and manganese. Vitamin C and the B vitamins are also critically important.

In addition to preventive measures like avoiding allergens and enhancing the immune system, locally applied heat is often very helpful in reducing discomfort. It can be applied as a hot pack or by blowing hot air into the ear with the aid of a straw and a hair dryer.

Hygroscopic anhydrous glycerine (available at most pharmacies) or commercial preparations of mullein oil, such as Ear Oil from Eclectic Institute (available at most health food stores), may be put directly into the ear. These earache preparations generally include soothing oils as well as herbs that combat the infection, such as garlic or goldenseal. A child will often demonstrate the presence of an ear infection by tugging or pulling at the ear. Use the oil at the earliest sign. These measures help reduce the pressure in the middle ear and promote fluid drainage.

Eczema

Dr. Whitaker's Prescription for Eczema:

1. Eliminate food allergies.
2. Follow the Whitaker Wellness Program.
3. Apply CamoCare (Abkit) or Simicort (Enzymatic Therapy) to affected areas twice daily.

Description

Eczema, also known as *atopic dermatitis,* is an intensely itchy, inflammatory disease of the skin. It is commonly found on the face, wrists, and insides of the elbows and knees. Although it may occur at any age, it is most common in infants. It completely clears in half the cases by 18 months of age. Eczema affects 2.4 to 7 percent of the population and is often associated with asthma.

Comments on Dr. Whitaker's Prescription for Eczema

As is the case with ear infections, eczema exemplifies the importance of diet and food in health from the earliest stages of an individual's life. One recent study of eczema in children took place at Middlesex Hospital in London.[1] The researcher concluded that perhaps 75 percent of cases of childhood eczema could be resolved merely by shifting some dietary factors. Cow's milk, as in ear infections, is a major culprit. Removing this substance to treat ear infections may serve to limit the likelihood of developing eczema. Other key foods these researchers removed were eggs and tomatoes, and agents which are added to foods in processing, such as food preservatives and food coloring.

    The causal role of food allergies in childhood eczema is well established in the scientific literature. If eliminating those foods which the researchers in the Middlesex study removed does not work, it is still possible that other foods are the problem. The best way to discover what the offending food might be is through an elimination diet (see page 245).

Here is an illustrative case: Francesca T. first developed eczema when she was four years old. She would scratch until the skin on her arms and legs was almost raw. After careful evaluation, through trial and error, a link was observed between her eczema and certain foods: peanuts, nuts, seeds, and chocolate. When Francesca avoided these foods, her skin cleared up dramatically. While some may view keeping a child off peanut butter and chocolate as a challenge, the rewards are worth it. Francesca had no new episodes of eczema.

Essential Fatty Acid Deficiency

A deficiency of essential fatty acids is associated with decreased synthesis of anti-inflamatory prostaglandins. My basic recommendation is to increase the dietary intake of fatty acids (as described in Chapter 2). Research has shown that using evening primrose oil can relieve the symptoms of eczema in many patients.[2] Fatty acid imbalances are normalized through this strategy. This requires a substantial dose of at least 10 grams per day if you want to see a benefit. Gamma-linolenic acid (GLA) supplements like borage and black currant provide similar benefits. However, I have found flax oil to produce good results, and it is less expensive than these much higher priced oils.

Topical Creams

A number of excellent all-natural creams can be used in place of cortisone creams in the topical relief of eczema. Preparations containing extracts of licorice and German chamomile are the most active. Creams with these ingredients have demonstrated an effect that is equal to or better than cortisone when applied topically. CamoCare (Abkit) uses chamomile extract. Simicort (Enzymatic Therapy) includes chamomile, licorice, and allantoin. These creams have been demonstrated to be effective, and they do not have the side effects associated with cortisone.

For example, the licorice compound (glycyrrhetinic acid) contained in Simicort has been shown to be superior to topical cortisone, especially in chronic cases of eczema. In one study of patients with eczema, 93 percent of the patients applying glycyrrhetinic acid demonstrated improvement, compared to 83 percent using cortisone.[3] The anti-inflammatory action of glycyrrhetinic acid (as well as chamomile) is largely due to its ability to inhibit the formation and secretion of inflammatory compounds.[4] This is an extremely important feature when the skin is irritated and inflamed, as commonly occurs in eczema.

Fibrocystic Breast Disease

Dr. Whitaker's Prescription for Fibrocystic Breast Disease:

1. Follow the Whitaker Wellness Program.
2. Eliminate sources of caffeine and other methylxanthins from the diet.

Description

Fibrocystic breast disease (FBD), also known as cystic mastitis, is a mildly uncomfortable to severely painful benign cystic swelling of the breasts. Fibrocystic breast disease is very common. It affects 20 to 40 ·percent of premenopausal women. It is usually a component of the premenstrual syndrome (PMS) and is considered a minor risk factor for breast cancer. It is not as significant a factor as the classical breast cancer risk factors such as family history, early menarche, and late or no first pregnancy.

The development of fibrocystic breast disease is apparently due to an increased estrogen-to-progesterone ratio. With each menstrual cycle, there is a recurring hormonal stimulation of the breast. As the hormone levels fall after a few days, the breasts normally return to their prestimulation size and function. In many women these changes are so slight that clinical signs or symptoms do not appear. In others, however, significant inflammatory processes occur.

Comments on Dr. Whitaker's Prescription for Fibrocystic Breast Disease

Following the Whitaker Wellness Program is often all that is needed to significantly improve or eliminate the problem of fibrocystic breast disease. The key point is the focus on plant foods and the recommendation for vitamin E supplementation. (If other PMS symptoms are present, the recommendations for Premenstrual Syndrome are also appropriate).

Why is a diet rich in plant foods important? (1) It will relieve constipation, and (2) it reduces circulating estrogen levels. Women having fewer than three bowel movements per week have a risk of fibrocystic breast disease 4.5 times greater than women having at least one a day.[1] This association is probably due to the bacterial flora in the large intestine transforming colon contents into a variety of toxic metabolites. Some of these toxic products are carcinogens and mutagens.[2]

In addition, fecal microorganisms are capable of resynthesizing estrogen from previously excreted and detoxified estrogen. Women on a vegetarian diet excrete two to three times more detoxified estrogens than women on an omnivorous diet. More estrogens are also re-absorbed by women not on vegetarian diets.[3] Furthermore, omnivorous women have 50 percent higher mean levels of undetoxified estrogens.

Vitamin E supplementation is very effective in relieving fibrocystic breast disease, in some cases. Several double-blind clinical studies have shown vitamin E (alpha-tocopherol) to relieve many premenstrual symptoms, including fibrocystic breast disease.[4] The mode of action appears to be that vitamin E normalizes altered levels of circulating hormones in women with PMS.[5]

There is also very strong evidence supporting an association between fibrocystic breast disease and the consumption of caffeine, theophylline, and theobromine, as found in coffee, tea, cola, chocolate, and caffeinated medications.[6] Caffeine, theophylline, and theobromine are all known to stimulate overproduction of cellular products, such as fibrous tissue and cyst fluid.

In one study, limiting methylxanthines (caffeine, theophylline, and theobromine) in the diet resulted in improvement in 97.5 percent of the 45 women who completely abstained. Improvement was also found in 75 percent of the 28 who limited their consumption of coffee, tea, cola, chocolate, and caffeinated medications.[7] Those who continued with little change in their methylxanthine consumption showed little improvement.[4] According to this study, women may have varying thresholds of response to methylxanthines.

Food Allergy

Dr. Whitaker's Prescription for Food Allergy:

1. Identify food allergies with the aid of an elimination diet or food allergy testing.
2. Eliminate fixed-food allergens from the diet.
3. Use the rotary diversified diet.
4. Follow recommendations on enhancing digestion in Chapter 3.

Description

Food sensitivity. Food idiosyncrasy. Pharmacologic (druglike) reaction to food. Food intolerance. Metabolic reaction to food. Food anaphylaxis.

The diverse names given to the problem of food allergy signifies both the prevalence of the problem and the diverse ways of viewing it. At least 60 percent of Americans suffer from negative reactions to food, according to some physicians. The number has increased dramatically in the past fifteen years. The total number is not well known because many food allergy problems are diagnosed as "psychosomatic" or "in the head" of the patients. Many food allergy problems go undiagnosed. As physician awareness of the problem of food sensitivities goes up, problems without a diagnosis will go down.

Food allergies have been tabbed as important causes in a wide range of conditions.[1]

Symptoms and Diseases Commonly Associated with Food Allergy

SYSTEM	SYMPTOMS AND DISEASES
Gastrointestinal	Canker sores, celiac disease, chronic diarrhea, stomach ulcer, gas, gastritis, irritable colon, malabsorption, ulcerative colitis
Genitourinary	Bedwetting, chronic bladder infections, kidney disease
Immune	Chronic infections, frequent ear infections
Brain	Anxiety, depression, hyperactivity, inability to concentrate, insomnia, irritability, mental confusion, personality change, seizures
Musculoskeletal	Bursitis, joint pain, low back pain
Respiratory	Asthma, chronic bronchitis, wheezing
Skin Acne	Eczema, hives, itching, skin rash
Miscellaneous	Irregular heartbeat, edema, fainting, fatigue, headache, hypoglycemia, itchy nose or throat, migraine, sinusitis

There is hardly an aspect of impaired functioning that is not tied to food allergies. Where and how an individual's allergic response will appear is not well established. Research is not clear whether adverse reactions are mediated by the immune system. The location of symptoms in the body may be linked to the place in the body where the immune system is activated. Another factor may be the mediators of the inflammation involved. Tissue sensitivity to these mediators in different parts of the body may also be a factor.

We do know that the allergic reaction may be caused by a food protein, a starch, some other food component, or even contaminants in the food. By contaminants I mean the additives, preservatives, and colorings which food manufacturers use to prevent spoilage, enhance flavor, or make a food look better.

Between 10 and 15 percent of food allergies are *IgE-mediated allergies*. In such cases, a food molecule acts inside the body as an antigen. Antigens are substances that can be bound by an antibody. IGE is one such allergy-related antibody. Once the IGE has picked up its cargo, it hops freight on a special white blood cell called a *mast cell* or *basophil*. These special cells respond to this added load by releasing histamines and other substances that cause swelling. It's about this time that the individual in which this little drama is being carried out begins to realize he or she may have a problem.

Comments on Dr. Whitaker's Prescription for Food Allergies

I recall a news account about a group of neighbors who were suffering a range of odd health problems. They concluded that the problem must be in the community well from which they all took their water. The county health department came out and tested the water. The community was shocked when the report came back that the water was fine. They took the report to another scientist. He noticed that the county's test only looked at organic pollutants like bacteria. It didn't check for inorganic pollutants like industrial chemicals. A later, more thorough, test uncovered twenty separate carcinogenic inorganic compounds in the water.

The story is analogous to the skin prick or scratch tests most conventional allergy doctors use, which will only find IGE-mediated food allergies. As noted, these represent only 10 to 15 percent of all allergies. The results of this allergy test can come back negative and the doctor will conclude that food allergy is not a problem. The message to the patient: "It's in your head."

Better tests exist. I strongly recommend an elimination diet and a food challenge approach; it asks a lot of the patient, but returns exceptional rewards. In fact, in the act of diagnosis, a person can begin to discover the new habits and choices that will resolve the symptoms. The understanding an individual gains is not the same as a page of laboratory results shouting: "Don't eat this! Don't eat that." Instead, an individual directly experiences specific negative associations between food consumed and adverse responses. Your body, not a lab report, presents the results.

Elimination Diet

First, try an elimination diet or a short fast. The idea is to clear your system, to create a "blank slate" on which the outcome of your home research can be clearly written. (A fasting protocol is provided in Chapter 4.) A standard elimination diet consists of lamb, chicken, rice, banana, apple, and a vegetable from the cabbage family. This diet is also called an *oligoantigenic* diet. You may also choose to substitute a hypoallergenic meal replacement formula during this elimination period. Ultraclear (Metagenics) is one such formula (see Chapter 5).

Now, reintroduce certain foods. To prepare for this step, set up a daily record book and keep a detailed journal of the dates when new foods are introduced, and any adverse responses in your body.

Every other day, reintroduce a food to the diet. If the food is one to which you are sensitive, the symptoms of the adverse response will be stronger than before. Your body has had a chance to rest from fighting the food and so responds with more vitality. Note the response in your journal. Is it stiffness? Pain? If so, where? Itchy throat? Insomnia? Congestion? A two-day wait before reintroducing the next food allows a period of up to forty-eight hours where such symptoms will likely be an adverse response to the reintroduced food.

Once a sensitivity is felt from a food, omit it from the diet for a week. Then try reintroducing it a second time. Adverse reactions a second time probably mean that this food is one that should be cut out of your diet altogether. To do so effectively requires educating yourself to the variety of ways in which a specific food may show up in the diet. For instance, a problem with eggs may mean also cutting out breads made with eggs. Look closely at ingredient lists on processed foods. In fact, closely related foods with similar characteristics may also be problematic. One such example is rice and millet.

Lab Tests

A number of laboratory tests can be used by physicians to check for food allergies. The best one is the radio-allergo-sorbent (RAST) test, and the enzyme-linked immunosorbent assay (ELISA). The physician sends off a blood sample for these tests.

Multiple Food Allergies

The going gets tricky when an individual discovers multiple food allergies. The body is hypersensitive and responds adversely to any number of foods which may or may not be a problem. The good news is that tolerance for eliminated foods can return; these foods can eventually be added back into the diet without reactivating the allergic

Edible Plants and Animal Kingdom Taxonomic List

Vegetables

Legume	Mustard	Parsley	Potato	Grass	Lily
Bean	Broccoli	Anise	Chili	Barley	Asparagus
Cocoa bean	Brussels sprouts	Caraway	Eggplant	Corn	Chives
Lentil	Cabbage	Carrot	Pepper	Oat	Garlic
Licorice	Cauliflower	Celery	Potato	Rice	Leek
Peanut	Mustard	Coriander	Tomato	Rye	Onion
Pea	Radish	Cumin	Tobacco	Wheat	
Soybean	Turnip	Parsley			
Tamarind	Watercress				

Laurel	Sunflower	Beet	Buckwheat
Avocado	Artichoke	Beet	Buckwheat
Camphor	Lettuce	Chard	Rhubarb
Cinnamon	Sunflower	Spinach	

Fruits

Gourd	Plum	Citrus	Cashews	Nuts	Beech
Cantalope	Almond	Grapefruit	Cashews	Brazil nut	Beechnut
Cucumber	Apricot	Lemon	Mango	Pecan	Chestnut
Honeydew	Cherry	Lime	Pistachio	Walnut	Chinquapin nut
Melons	Peach	Mandarin			
Pumpkin	Plum	Orange			
Squash	Persimmon	Tangerine			
Zucchini					

Banana	Palm	Grape	Pineapple	Rose	Birch
Arrowroot	Coconut	Grape	Pineapple	Blackberry	Filbert
Banana	Date	Raisin		Loganberry	Hazelnut
Plantain	Date sugar			Raspberry	
				Rosehips	
				Strawberry	

Apple	Blueberry	Pawpaws
Apple	Blueberry	Papaya
Pear	Cranberry	Pawpaw
Quince	Huckleberry	

Animals

Mammals (Meat/Milk)	Birds (Meat/Egg)	Fish		Crustacean	Mollusk
Cow	Chicken	Catfish	Salmon	Crab	Abalone
Goat	Duck	Cod	Sardine	Crayfish	Clam
Pig	Goose	Flounder	Snapper	Lobster	Mussel
Rabbit	Hen	Halibut	Trout	Prawn	Oyster
Sheep	Turkey	Mackerel	Tuna	Shrimp	Scallop

Four-Day Rotation Diet

Food Family	Food
Day 1	
Citrus	Lemon, orange, grapefruit, lime, tangerine, kumquat, citron
Banana	Banana, plantain, arrowroot (musa)
Palm	Coconut, date, date sugar
Parsley	Carrot, parsnip, celery, celery seed, celeriac, anise, dill, fennel, cumin, parsley, coriander, caraway
Spices	Black and white pepper, peppercorn, nutmeg, mace
Subucaya	Brazil nut
Bird	All fowl and game birds, including chicken, turkey, duck, goose, guinea, pigeon, quail, pheasant, eggs
Juices	Juices (preferably fresh) may be made and used from any fruits and vegetables listed above, in any combination desired, without adding sweeteners
Day 2	
Grape	All varieties of grapes, raisins
Pineapple	Juice-pack, water-pack, or fresh
Rose	Strawberry, raspberry, blackberry, loganberry, rose hips
Gourd	Watermelon, cucumber, cantalope, pumpkin, squash, other melons, zucchini, pumpkin or squash seeds
Beet	Beet, spinach, chard
Legume	Pea, black-eyed pea, dry beans, green beans, carob, soybeans, lentil, licorice, peanut, alfalfa
Cashew	Cashew, pistachio, mango
Birch	Filbert, hazelnut
Flaxseed	Flaxseed
Swine	All pork products
Mollusks	Abalone, snail, squid, clam, mussel, oyster, scallop
Crustaceans	Crab, crayfish, lobster, prawn, shrimp
Juices	Juices (preferably fresh) may be made and used without added sweeteners from any fruits, berries, or vegetables listed above, in any combination desired, including fresh alfalfa and some legumes
Day 3	
Apple	Apple, pear, quince
Gooseberry	Currant, gooseberry
Buckwheat	Buckwheat, rhubarb
Aster	Lettuce, chicory, endive, escarole, globe artichoke, dandelion, sunflower seed, tarragon
Potato	Potato, tomato, eggplant, pepper (red and green), chili pepper, paprika, cayenne, ground cherries
Lily (onion)	Onion, garlic, asparagus, chive, leek
Spurge	Tapioca
Herb	Basil, savory, sage, oregano, horehound, catnip, spearmint, peppermint, thyme, marjoram, lemon balm

Four-Day Rotation Diet (*continued*)

Food Family	Food
Walnut	English walnut, black walnut, pecan, hickory nut, butternut
Pedalium	Sesame
Beech	Chestnut
Saltwater fish	Herring, anchovy, cod, sea bass, sea trout, mackerel, tuna, swordfish, flounder, sole
Freshwater fish	Sturgeon, salmon, whitefish, bass, perch
Juices	Juices (preferably fresh) may be made and used without added sweeteners from any fruits and vegetables listed above, in any combination.
Day 4	
Plum	Plum, cherry, peach, apricot, nectarine, almond, wild cherry
Blueberry	Blueberry, huckleberry, cranberry, wintergreen
Pawpaw	Pawpaw, papaya, papain
Mustard	Mustard, turnip, radish, horseradish, watercress, cabbage, Chinese cabbage, broccoli, cauliflower, Brussels sprouts, kale, kohlrabi, rutabaga
Laurel	Avocado, cinnamon, bay leaf, sassafras, cassia buds or bark
Sweet potato or yam	
Grass	Wheat, corn, rice, oats, barley, rye, wild rice, cane, millet, sorghum, bamboo sprouts
Orchid	Vanilla
Protea	Macadamia nut
Conifer	Pine nut
Fungus	Mushrooms and yeast (brewer's yeast, etc.)
Bovid	Milk products—butter, cheese, yogurt, beef and milk products, oleomargarine, lamb
Juices	Juices (preferably fresh) may be made and used without added sweeteners from any fruits and vegetables listed above, in any combination desired.

response. You might not have to swear off a favorite food forever! In fact, some favorite foods to which one has cyclic, rather than fixed, allergic responses can gradually be reintroduced, in moderation, and enjoyed without fear of problems.

If multiple allergies are discovered, try a *rotary diversified diet*. A highly varied assortment of foods is eaten in a fixed, rotating schedule. Tolerated foods are eaten at regularly spaced intervals of four to seven days. The idea is that infrequent eating of tolerated foods is less likely to produce new allergies. Nor will it stimulate mild allergic responses and make them more severe.

Successful use of the rotary diversified diet requires knowledge of the various food families (see figure, "Edible Plants and Animal Kingdom Taxonomic List"). If one food in a food family can "cross-react" with an allergy-inducing food, another food from the same family might also. The rotation plan prevents too much food from any one family being eaten at a time. A usual recommendation is not to eat foods from the same family two days in a row. This rotation of food families need not be as strict as rotation of individual foods (see figure, "Four-Day Rotation Diet").

Food Additives

The various agents that processors use in foods, such as additives, preservatives, acidifiers, artificial flavors, and artificial colors, often produce an allergic response, and are especially problematic for children. Hyperactivity and learning disabilities have been linked to these substances, which are also associated with depression, asthma, and migraine headaches.[2]

Gallstones

Dr. Whitaker's Prescription for Gallstones:

1. Follow the Whitaker Wellness Program.
2. Drink six 8-ounce glasses of pure water each day.
2. Eliminate food allergies or foods which aggravate the condition.
3. Take a lipotropic formula.
4. Take one or two capsules of Super Milk Thistle (Enzymatic Therapy) with meals, three times daily.

Description

Water, cholesterol, bile acids, and lecithin (phosphatidylcholine), mixed together in the gallbladder, determine solubility of the bile. If these concentrations shift too dramatically, gallstones can form. The solubility of the bile is the most important factor in the formation of gallstones.

Once gallstones have formed, measures can be taken to alter the solubility of the bile. Foods that aggravate the condition can be avoided. Sometimes the gallstones remain and symptoms don't die down. Persistence or worsening of symptoms usually leads to surgical removal of the gallbladder. As with most diseases, gallstones are easier to prevent than to reverse.

The ratio of the substances determining bile solubility is unbalanced in many Americans. Each year, an estimated 1 million gallstones develop; some 300,000 gallbladders are removed.

Comments on Dr. Whitaker's Prescription for Gallstones

Gallstones are associated with the Western diet.[1] Such a diet, high in refined carbohydrates and fat, and low in fiber, leads to a reduction in the synthesis of bile acids by the liver and a lower bile acid concentration in the gallbladder.

A diet high in water-soluble fibers, such as those found in vegetables and fruits, pectin, oat bran, and guar gum, is extremely important in the prevention as well as the reversal of most gallstones.

A vegetarian diet has been shown to be protective against gallstone formation. A study performed in England compared a large group of healthy nonvegetarian women to a group of vegetarian women. Ultrasound diagnosis showed that gallstones occurred significantly less frequently in the vegetarian group.[2]

While this may simply be a result of the increased fiber content of the vegetarian diet, other factors may be equally important. Animal proteins, such as casein from dairy products, have been shown to increase the formation of gallstones in animals. Vegetable proteins, such as soy, have been shown to be preventive against gallstone formation.

Another important dietary recommendation in the treatment of gallstones is to make sure that you drink enough water. Drink at least six 8-ounce glasses of pure water each day. This simple recommendation can go a long way in preventing gallstones from forming.

One of the leading experts in food allergy, Dr. J.C. Breneman, has been telling us since 1948 that allergy elimination diets are successful in preventing attacks of gallstones. A 1968 study put a group of patients on a basic allergy elimination diet of beef, rye, soybeans, rice, cherries, peaches, apricots, beets, and spinach.[3] All of the patients (100 percent) remained symptom-free while on the diet.

Foods that induced gallbladder symptoms, in order of their effect (with the most pronounced first), were eggs, pork, onions, fowl, milk, coffee, citrus, corn, beans, and nuts. Adding eggs to the diet caused gallbladder attacks in 93 percent of the patients.

Several mechanisms have been proposed to explain the association of food allergy and gallbladder attacks. Dr. Breneman believes the ingestion of allergy-causing substances causes swelling of the bile ducts, which impairs bile flow from the gallbladder.

Other recommendations for patients with gallstones may be found in Chapter 4. A lipotropic formula and silymarin (described in Chapter 4) are the best supplements to take. Silymarin has been shown in human studies to dramatically improve the solubility of bile.[4,5] A special form of silymarin deserves special mention, Super Milk Thistle from Enzymatic Therapy. This formula provides silymarin bound to phosphatidylcholine, the main component of soy lecithin. This combination leads to improved absorption of silymarin and to greater therapeutic effect (see Hepatitis, page 265). Take two capsules of this formula with meals.

Glaucoma

Dr. Whitaker's Prescription for Chronic (Open-Angle) Glaucoma:

1. Follow the Whitaker Wellness Program.
2. Take 1 gram of mixed bioflavonoids daily.

Description

Glaucoma refers to increased pressure within the eye due to an imbalance between the production and outflow of fluid in the eye. Obstruction of outflow is the main cause of this imbalance in acute glaucoma. A number of physiological abnormalities have been observed in glaucomatous eyes, such as unusual tissues at the back of the eye through which the optic nerve fibers and blood vessels pass. Abnormalities have also been seen in the connective tissue network that eye fluid must pass through to leave the eye. Blood vessels in the eye may be problematic, resulting in elevated inner eye pressure or progressive loss of peripheral vision.

Glaucoma can be acute or chronic. Chronic glaucoma is much more common. In the United States, there are approximately 2 million people with glaucoma, 25 percent undetected. Ten percent have the acute closed-angle type; 90 percent suffer from the chronic open-angle type. In chronic glaucoma, there will usually be no symptoms until significant elevations in pressure readings occur. When the pressure of fluids in the eye reaches high levels, the individual will experience a gradual loss of peripheral vision, or "tunnel vision." Extreme pain, blurring of vision, and severely reddened eyes may also be associated with the acute phase of the chronic condition.

Acute closed-angle glaucoma is a very serious condition, a medical emergency. Usually a person will experience severe throbbing pain in the eye. Vision will markedly blur. Nausea and vomiting are often associated with its onset. A person who suspects this condition should go immediately to an ophthalmologist or hospital emergency room. Effective therapy must be started within twelve to forty-eight hours or permanent loss of vision will occur within three to five days.

Comments on Dr. Whitaker's Prescription for Chronic Glaucoma

High doses of vitamin C have been shown to lower pressure levels on the inner eye in many clinical studies.[1] A daily dose of 500 milligrams per kilogram (2.2 pounds) of body weight, whether in single or divided doses, reduces inner eye pressure by an average of 16 millimeters/hydrargyrums. Almost-normal tension levels have been achieved in some patients who were unresponsive to standard drug therapies (acetazolamide and pilocarpine).

This pressure-lowering action of vitamin C is long-lasting if supplementation is continued. In an emergency, intravenous administration results in an even greater initial reduction.[2] I also recommend bioflavonoids (at least 1 gram of mixed flavonoids daily) along with the vitamin C. Rutin, a common bioflavonoid, has been shown to be of benefit even at very low dosages (20 milligrams, three times daily).[3]

Another way to lower eye pressure is to avoid food and environmental allergens.[4] One study challenged 113 patients with the appropriate allergen. The allergens employed were both food and environmental, depending on what was problematic for the individual. Many demonstrated an immediate rise in intraocular pressure of up to 20 millimeters, in addition to other typical allergic symptoms.

Gout

Dr. Whitaker's Prescription for Gout:

1. Follow the Whitaker Wellness Program.
2. Do not drink alcohol.
3. Do not eat foods high in purines (organ meats, other meats, shellfish, brewer's and baker's yeast, herring, sardines, mackerel, and anchovies).
4. Achieve ideal body weight.
5. Drink six 8-ounce glasses of water daily.
6. Eat the equivalent of one-half pound of cherries daily.
7. Use high-dose folic acid therapy, if necessary.

Description

In old novels and histories, gout is often a recurring bit player. The bit player arrives in the middle of the night, generally to the great consternation of a wealthy man. This man likes his rich foods and his drink. He overconsumes and is on the rotund side. The man is successful in the world, yet we find him awake at night, one painful foot resting on an ottoman. Gout, like a messenger in a moral tale, has arrived to take the rich man down a notch. This condition is associated with affluence and is often called "the rich man's disease."

This picture reflects in many particulars the typical portrait of an individual with gout. Over 95 percent of sufferers are men over thirty years of age. A rich diet, high in consumption of alcohol and meats, is associated with the development of gout. The initial gout attack generally comes at night. Some specific event, such as eating or drinking too much, can provoke a gout attack. An attack can also be provoked by trauma, by certain drugs, or surgeries. The attack zone is likely to be the foot.

Here is how gout develops from a biochemical perspective. A substance called *purines* is manufactured in the body, or ingested in foods. Meats, particularly organ meats, are high-purine foods. As purines are metabolized, uric acid is formed. Uric acid is the final breakdown product of purines. Excess uric acid needs to be secreted. This is the kidney's job. Unfortunately for the man who likes his meat and likes his drink, alcohol inhibits the kidney's secretion of uric acid. The uric acid stays in the body.

Gout is caused by increased concentration of uric acid in biological fluids. The uric acid crystals end up migrating in the blood until they eventually find a nest in the body. Joints, tendons, kidneys, and other tissues are favored home sites. The neighborhood of one of these uric acid "homes" can go downhill quickly. Considerable damage and inflammation can result. Gout is a common type of arthritis.

For nearly half of those afflicted, the damaging interaction of these factors will appear initially in the first joint of the big toe. The pain is usually intense. In fact, 90 percent of those with gout will at some time feel the pain in this joint. An attack will lead to fever and chills if it progresses. Although uric acid levels are elevated in 10 to 20 percent of the American population with its high meat and alcohol diet, only a small fraction, of 1 percent (.15 percent) will get gout.

There are basically two types of gout medications: drugs used to treat acute attacks of gout and drugs which reduce the level of uric acid in the body. In the treatment of acute attacks, colchicine or nonsteroidal anti-inflammatory drugs (NSAIDs) such as indomethacin, phenylbutazone, naproxen, and fenoprofen are used.

In the treatment of chronic gout, physicians often measure the amount of uric acid in a twenty-four hour collection of urine. This identifies whether a patient is an overproducer of uric acid (greater than 800 milligrams) or an underexcretor (less than 800 milligrams). The overproducer is usually prescribed allopurinol while the underexcretor is given probenecid or sulfinpyrazone.

Comments on Dr. Whitaker's Prescription for Gout

It is a well-accepted fact that most cases of gout can be treated effectively with diet alone. However, with the advent of modern drug therapy, many physicians do not stress the value of diet therapy to their patients. It is far easier to simply prescribe a pill than it is to educate the patient on healthier food choices and to assist them in making the necessary changes. Given the side effects of the drugs, and the safety and effectiveness of dietary therapy, the failure of physicians to discuss dietary therapy with their patients is a great disservice.

The dietary treatment of gout involves the following guidelines:

Elimination of alcohol intake
Low-purine diet (elimination of organ meats, meats, shellfish,
    brewer's and baker's yeast, herring, sardines, mackerel, and
    anchovies)
Achievement of ideal body weight
Liberal consumption of complex carbohydrates
Low fat intake
Low protein intake
Liberal fluid intake
Increased consumption of flavonoids

All of these factors are equally important. They are designed either to limit the production of uric acid and/or promote uric acid excretion in the urine.

Another useful dietary prescription for gout is to increase the intake of fruits like cherries, blackberries, blueberries, and raspberries. Consuming the equivalent of one-half pound of fresh cherries per day has been shown to be very effective in lowering uric acid levels and preventing attacks of gout.[1] These fruit are rich sources of flavonoid compounds, which give them their deep red-blue color. In addition to lowering uric acid levels, these flavonoids also prevent destruction of joint structures.

When these fruits are out of season (or if you have diabetes or hypoglycemia), consider using cherry extracts instead, to gain the benefits of the flavonoids without stressing control of blood sugar levels.

Folic Acid

If additional support is necessary, ask your physician to prescribe high doses of folic acid therapy. Folic acid has been shown to inhibit xanthine oxidase, the enzyme responsible for producing uric acid.[2] In fact, research has demonstrated that a derivative of folic acid is an even greater inhibitor of xanthine oxidase than the drug allopurinol. This suggests that folic acid at pharmacological doses may be an effective treatment for gout. Positive results have been reported, but the data is incomplete and uncontrolled.[3] The dosage of folic acid required is in the range of 10 to 40 milligrams per day.

Folic acid has been used at these high dosages with no reported toxicity and is certainly safer than current drugs used in gout. However, there have been reports of high-dose folic acid interfering with some drugs used to treat epilepsy. High doses of folic acid may also mask the symptoms of a vitamin B12 deficiency. Because of these concerns, folic acid therapy should only be utilized under the supervision of a physician.

Hayfever

Dr. Whitaker's Prescription for Hayfever:

1. Follow the recommendations asthma (see page 163).
2. Avoid relying on over-the-counter and prescription antihistamines.

Description

Beautiful springtime. For some, the season of renewal means only one thing: Trees will be reproducing and creating pollen. The playtime of summer comes next, when grasses and weeds set free their pollens into the air. The pollens are carried on the spring and summer winds to their destinations.

In the nasal passages and airwaves of some individuals, the poetry of the warm seasons induces just one sensation: hayfever. During spring and summer, trees, weeds, and grasses produce the most significant hayfever-inducing pollens. Ragweed pollens account for nearly three-quarters of the hayfever in the United States.

If this allergic reaction is indeed seasonal, it is called *seasonal allergic rhinitis*. If hayfever symptoms persist year-around (as they do in some individuals), pollens and the poetry of new life may not be the major cause of the symptoms. This is called *perennial allergic rhinitis*.

Comments on Dr. Whitaker's Prescription for Hayfever

The underlying mechanisms responsible for hayfever are similar to those which produce asthma. An individual with hayfever should therefore follow my recommendations for asthma (see page 163).

Conventional hayfever therapies feature antihistamine drugs, all of which have significant side effects. I strongly encourage you to avoid the use of antihistamine drugs like chlorpheniramine (Allerest, Chlor-Trimeton, Coricidin, Triaminic Allergy) and astemizole (Hismanal). These drugs do not block the release of histamine. Instead, they block the action of histamine at receptor sites. This can cause real problems.

Some of the histamine receptor sites are in the brain. Histamines help the brain maintain alertness. For the brain, anti-histamine means anti-alert. So a side effect of most antihistamines is drowsiness. Now "drowsy" has a meaning rather different than "drunk driving" in our minds. But as little as 50 milligrams of the antihistamine diphenhydramine (Benadryl) may produce as much driving impairment as a 0.1 percent blood alcohol content. This blood alcohol level will get you arrested for driving while intoxicated.[1]

Antihistamine drugs have additional possible side effects: allergic reactions, headache, nausea, and drying of the nose, mouth, and throat.

Seldane (terfenadine) and Hismanal (astemizole) are two antihistamine drugs that do not cause drowsiness. Developers of these drugs managed to remove this side effect; unfortunately, in the process, they created other problems. These problems are so significant that the FDA now requires Marion Dow, the maker of Seldane, and Hismanal's manufacturer, Janssen, to issue special warnings to physicians.

The FDA's unusually stern action grew out of a pattern of serious cardiovascular side effects. As of May 1992, fifteen deaths were reported caused by Seldane or Hismanal.[2] Records show that another 110 additional serious cadiovascular events have been suffered by individuals taking these drugs to control hayfever.

The manufacturers of these drugs must warn physicians about the range of situations in which severe adverse reactions are likely to occur, such as when individuals take more of the product than the manufacturer recommends. Patients with significant liver dysfunction are at risk with these drugs. In addition, serious side effects can be produced in patients who are also on the drugs ketoconazole or erythromycin. These warnings must be printed inside a heavy black frame on advertisements for the drugs. This is called the FDA's "black box" designation.

Despite these problems, many medical doctors choose to skirt the drowsiness side effect by prescribing Seldane or Hismanal instead. The list of adverse reactions to these drugs is long. Both Seldane and Hismanal dry out the mucous membranes, bothering or harming activity in the nose, mouth, and throat. Other possible side effects include allergic reactions, nausea, indigestion, vomiting, increased appetite, weight gain, headache, nervousness, and fatigue.

These side effects of commonly prescribed hayfever medications can present a dark conclusion to the poetry of spring's reawakening and summer's abundance. Take the Whitaker Prescription for Asthma or Hayfever to ensure that the next time the season of new life rolls around, you can enjoy it without restriction.

Headache

Dr. Whitaker's Prescription for Headache:

1. Eliminate factors, such as food allergies, which can precipitate a headache.
2. Follow the Whitaker Wellness Program.
3. For migraines, take feverfew for prevention, and higher doses to diminish acute attacks.
4. Consider seeing a chiropractor, acupuncturist, or a practitioner of a relaxation technique.

Description

"This project is a real headache."

"Working with (insert name of choice) can be a real headache."

Sometimes when we use phrases like these, or hear them, the actual aching in the head doesn't exist. But we know what is meant by it. Stress. A constant aggravation.

This is the classic *tension headache* that most of us suffer from at one time or another. Tension headaches are usually caused by a tightening of the muscles of the face, neck, or scalp. Nerves may get pinched. Blood supply may get hindered due to this constriction. These physiologic changes become known to us as a steady, constant pain that starts at the forehead or back of the head. The pain spreads over the entire head. The sensation is of having a vice grip applied to the skull.

"He's not a headache. He's a migraine!"

This piece of the dialect begins to distinguish the two types of headaches based on the strength of the pain. The migraine tends to be a throbbing pain, which pounds sharply in the head of the sufferer. The immediate physiological cause is excessive expansion of a blood vessel in the head.

Sometimes migraines hit without warning. Many who suffer migraines get unusual symptoms called *auras* before the pain hits. The aura may be a tingling or numbness in the body. Alternatively, the individual's vision may become blurred or show bright spots. Thinking may become disturbed. Anxiety or fatigue may suddenly set in.

A surprisingly high percentage of Americans suffer from migraines. The percentage is higher for women (25 to 30 percent) than for men (14 to 20 percent). A family history of the illness is discovered with more than half of the sufferers.

Comments on Dr. Whitaker's Prescription for Headaches

A good place to start dealing with a headache is to determine whether you have a tension headache or a migraine. Those who have migraines may say, almost bragging: "You'll know you have a migraine if that's what you have."

Think about the factors that precipitated your headache. What was going on? Some of the more common factors are food allergies, eyestrain, muscle tension, poor posture, too little sleep, or, alternatively, too much sleep. Headache onset can be associated with hormonal changes, such as menstruation, ovulation, and the use of birth control pills. Another major immediate promoter of headaches is emotional change. In particular, the letdown after stress or anger can produce a headache. Headaches can also result from withdrawing from caffeine or other drugs which constrict blood vessels.

The best strategy to ending headaches is more easy to prescribe than it is to carry it out. That is: Remove the cause. Here are some tips.

Food Allergies

The major factor for most people with chronic headaches, particularly chronic migraine, is food allergy. The top of the watch-list for migraine sufferers includes milk, wheat, chocolate, tomatoes, and fish. Food additives and artificial sweeteners, like aspartame (Nutrasweet) are also known to be problematic. Studies have determined causal relationships between food allergens and migraines. Research has also shown that removal of the foods to which a person is sensitive can diminish or eliminate symptoms of the migraine.[1]

Some foods actually have a double-whammy effect in promoting migraines. These foods have compounds called *vasoactive amines*. One of their effects is to cause blood vessels to expand, triggering migraine in some individuals. Examples of these foods are chocolate, cheese, beer, and wine.

Magnesium and Feverfew

Research has discovered that magnesium has a special relationship with headache development, whether the headache is the tension or migraine type. Individuals with frequent headaches have been found to have low brain and tissue magnesium.[2] The tone of the blood vessels and nerves, however, is dependent on the availability of adequate levels of this mineral. Low levels of magnesium can set the stage for migraine attacks. Supplementing magnesium at the levels recommended the Whitaker Wellness Program in Chapter 2 should offer sufficient protection.

The herb feverfew (*Tanacetum parthenium*) has recently gained some deserved notoriety for its value with migraines. Clinical research in England has given it this boost. The research didn't, however, "discover" feverfew's value. Many accounts of scientific examination of plants tend to make this suggestion. In truth, feverfew has been used for centuries to relieve migraines, and against fevers and arthritis. Some old crone was gathering feverfew in a field long before a white-coated researcher ever blessed it with statistics. We do now have better understanding of the specific biochemical activity of feverfew. And we can be more certain of the level of certain active constituents which are needed to produce an effect.

The scientific resurrection of feverfew began with popular interest in the 1970s. The value of the herb spread by word of mouth and informal channels. A survey project in 1983 contacted 270 individuals who had chosen to eat feverfew daily to combat migraines. Nearly three-quarters (70 percent) believed that feverfew diminished the intensity of their attacks or decreased the frequency. Many of these were individuals who came to this nonconventional treatment after failing to respond to usual medicines.

Some researchers decided to test these claims through controlled clinical trials. The first study took place at the London Migraine Clinic.[3] The researchers decided to focus on the individuals who said they were being helped by feverfew. Some were kept on a dose of feverfew; others were taken off the herb and given a placebo. Those who continued with feverfew saw no change in the frequency or severity of symptoms. But those on the placebo began to see a range of negative effects during the six months of the study. Headaches came back. Some felt nausea. Others vomited. The difficulty was so intense for two of the subjects that they guessed they were taking the placebo. They left the study and began taking feverfew again. With self-treatment, their incapacitating migraines subsided into remission again. A followup study at the University of Nottingham confirmed the London Migraine Clinic study.[4]

Since that time, more attention has focused on determining the specific mechanisms of feverfew's activity. The herb appears to slow blood vessel dilation by inhibiting the release of substances from the platelets which promote this effect. The tone of blood vessels is enhanced by feverfew, as it is by magnesium.[5] The production of various inflammatory substances is also inhibited, perhaps suggesting a reason for its traditional use against arthritis.

Researchers have determined that one substance in feverfew, called *parthenolide*, is the herb's "active principle." The scientific use of the herb is based on ensuring that high enough levels of this agent are in a given dose. In the clinical trials noted above, the parthenolide content was between 0.4 and 0.6 percent. The London study used a dose of 25 milligrams of freeze-dried, pulverized leaves twice a day. The Nottingham study took a different dosage attack. One capsule with 82 milligrams of dried, powdered leaves was given, but only once a day.

I recommend that individuals with acute migraines take a substantially higher dose of 1 to 2 grams. The herb has no serious side effects and has been shown to be well-tolerated.[6] The lower dose may be effective for ongoing administration, to ward off the onset of migraines.

Stress and Tension Reduction

If it is indeed a work situation, a person, or a project that seems to be giving you a headache, the option of leaving your job or your relationship is always worth considering. Often this isn't an option and good coping strategies are in order. Try a relaxation technique (see Chapter 6). Consider treating yourself to a regular massage, cranial-sacral therapy, or some other physical therapy to help release tension. For a tension headache, a warm bath or shower can sometimes make a world of difference.

If your headaches, whether migraine or tension, are chronic, see a professional with expertise in this area. Both chiropractic and acupuncture have been shown to be effective in assisting with headache relief. Biofeedback and transcutaneous electrical nerve stimulation (TENS) may also help. Psychological counseling is a good choice if the cause is an ongoing emotional situation.

Heart Disease

Dr. Whitaker's Prescription for Heart Disease:

1. Follow the Whitaker Wellness Program.
2. Take 500 milligrams of carnitine, twice daily.
3. Take 30 to 100 milligrams of coenzyme Q10, three times daily.
4. Take two tablets Rogenic (Enzymatic Therapy), three times daily, with meals.
5. Read *Reversing Heart Disease* (Warner Books, 1985) to learn more.
6. See sections on Angina (page 145), Cholesterol (page 191), and High Blood Pressure (page 269), if applicable.

Description

Heart disease is a term that is often used to describe a disease of the heart's blood vessels. These blood vessels, the coronary arteries, supply the heart muscle with vital oxygen and nutrients. If the blood flow through these arteries is restricted or blocked, angina (see page 145), severe damage, or death to the heart muscle often occurs. This is known as a *heart attack*. In most cases, the condition which blocks the blood and oxygen supply is *atherosclerosis* or hardening of the artery walls. The mortar that hardens the arteries is a plaque-containing cholesterol, fatty material, and cellular debris.

Heart disease can also be used to describe other conditions of the heart. These include congestive heart failure, disturbances in heart rate and rhythm (arrhythmias), and various disorders of the heart muscles (cardiomyopathies).

Comments on Dr. Whitaker's Prescription for Heart Disease

If you have any heart disease, read the section on angina, which reviews the data on conventional care choices (see page 145). Many of the same natural therapeutic suggestions and principles apply here. As in angina, my approach utilizes nutritional measures designed to improve the blood supply to the heart and improve energy metabolism within the heart. The program assists in the movement of ingredients essential for health to the heart. Then it helps the heart utilize them. These goals are interrelated. An increased blood flow means improved energy metabolism and vice versa. Both will produce improved heart function.

Diet and Supplements

Dietary intervention as detailed in the Whitaker Wellness Program (see Chapter 2) is the first step. The second step involves special nutritional and herbal factors. If you have heart disease, you definitely need to be taking carnitine and coenzyme Q10. A deficiency of carnitine or coenzyme Q10 (CoQ10) in the heart is like trying to run an automobile without a fuel pump. There may be plenty of fuel, but there is no way to get it to the engine. The supplements help restore proper levels of these important substances to heart tissue. The dosage of carnitine is 500 milligrams, twice daily, and the dosage of CoQ10 is 30 to 100 milligrams, three times daily.

Coenzyme Q10   Coenzyme Q10 is particularly beneficial. Numerous studies have shown the benefit of CoQ10 supplementation for both congestive heart failure (CHF) and cardiomyopathy. In one study, twenty patients with congestive heart failure were treated with coenzyme Q10, 30 milligrams per day for one to two months.[1] Fifty-five percent of the patients reported subjective improvement. They felt better. According to standard methods of disease classification, 50 percent showed a decrease and a full 30 percent showed a "remarkable" decrease in chest congestion as seen on chest X-rays.

One interesting outcome is that patients with mild disease tended to improve more often than those with more severe disease. The subjective improvements in CHF have been confirmed by various objective tests, including increased cardiac output, stroke volume, cardiac index, and ejection farction.[2]

Another study looked at eighty patients with cardiomyopathy. They received daily doses of 100 milligrams of CoQ10 for twelve weeks. This supplement alone significantly increased the amount of blood pumped by the heart, called the *cardiac ejection fraction.* CoQ10 also reduced shortness of breath and increased muscle strength in 89 percent of the subjects. These improvements lasted as long as the patients were continuously treated. In this study, that was a full three years. However, cardiac function deteriorated as soon as CoQ10 was discontinued.

Note that in this study CoQ10, alone, clearly has a disease-management value. It does not help the body to restore its healthy function. It plays a role. But function falls off if administration is discontinued.

In a third clinical trial, thirty-four patients with severe cardiomyopathy were given 100 milligrams of CoQ10 daily.[3] Eighty-two percent of the patients improved. Mean ejection fraction increased from about 25 to about 40 percent. A more graphic benefit of CoQ10 was that a two-year survival rate was 62 percent, as compared to 25 percent for a similar series of patients treated by conventional drugs.[4] In short, 2.5 times as many patients on conventional drugs might still be alive after two years had they been taking CoQ10 instead; this is a powerful tool.

Rogenic   I recommend Rogenic (Enzymatic Therapy) to my patients with any heart disease. Rogenic provides essential vitamins and minerals for the heart and vascular system, along with some special herbal extracts. While the Whitaker Wellness Program recommends 1,000 milligrams of magnesium daily, a person with heart disease requires more. Two tablets of Rogenic, three times daily, will provide an additional 450 milligrams of magnesium, in the form of magnesium aspartate.

The Rogenic formula also provides a dose of a special hawthorn extract. (This herb is discussed under Angina, page 145.) Hawthorn extracts are widely used by physicians in Europe. They can be beneficial therapeutically for angina, minor forms of congestive heart failure, and cardiac arrhythmia. Double-blind studies have shown effectiveness in all of these applications.[5] Improvements in heart function were shown in all standard measures of evaluation. In severe congestive heart failure, hawthorn extracts can be safely used in combination with digitalis.

If you take two tablets of Rogenic three times daily you will be getting 150 milligrams of a hawthorn extract standardized to contain 1.8 percent vitexin-4'-rhamnoside. If you simply want to take a hawthorn product, be sure that you use the standardized extracts. The dosage for extracts standardized to contain 1.8 percent vitexin-4'-rhamnoside or 10 percent procyanidins is 120 to 240 milligrams three times daily. For extracts standardized to contain 18 percent procyanidolic oligomers, the dosage is 240 to 480 milligrams daily.

Coleus Forskohlii   Another herb which may be useful in mild to moderate congestive heart failure is *Coleus forskohlii.* The root of this plant has long been used in Ayurvedic medicine in the treatment of asthma, high blood pressure, and heart disorders. It contains a diterpene molecule known as *forskolin* which is a powerful activator of adenylate cyclase in various tissues, resulting in elevations of cyclic adenosine monophosphate (cAMP)—one of the key regulators of cellular function. In the heart, an elevation of cAMP leads to an increased force of contraction. This may be useful in congestive heart failure and various cardiomyopathies.[6]

The effectiveness of coleus root is dependent upon the level of forskolin. Because the forskolin content of coleus root is typically 0.2 to 0.3 percent, using crude preparations may not supply sufficient levels of forskolin to produce a beneficial effect. I prefer the standardized extracts which have concentrated forskolin content. Enzymatic Therapy's Coleus Extract, for example, contains 18 percent forskolin, or roughly 100 times the amount in the crude plant. Each 50-milligram capsule provides 9 milligrams of forskolin. Take one capsule two to three times daily. The only other standardized coleus extract being marketed in the United States (that I am aware of) provides only 1 milligram of forskolin per capsule. You would have to take 18 to 27 capsules per day for the same effect.

Hemorrhoids

Dr. Whitaker's Prescription for Hemorrhoids:

1. Avoid activities that increase intra-abdominal pressure.
2. Increase the intake of high-fiber foods.
3. Use a bulk-forming fiber formula.
4. Use topical preparations to relieve symptoms.
5. Follow recommendations for varicose veins (see page 354).

Description

If a low-fiber, highly refined diet needed approval as a medicine, one side effect would be "increased straining during defecation." A result of such increased straining is that blood congests in the rectum. Because no valves exist in the venous system of the rectum to relieve such pressure, a varicose vein effect occurs, known to us as *hemorrhoids.*

In fact, hemorrhoids are personally known to a lot of us. Symptomatic hemorrhoidal disease has been estimated to afflict nearly one in every three Americans. For those over age fifty, the percentage approaches nearly one in two. Hemorrhoids are most common in Western, industrial nations where a low-fiber, highly refined diet is most often the fare.

However, diet is not the only causal factor with hemorrhoids. Other activities also push venous pressure in the rectum beyond its design limits. Among these are pregnancy, coughing, sneezing, vomiting, physical exertion, and portal hypertension due to cirrhosis. In fact, standing or sitting for long periods of time can be causal factors.

If the hemorrhoids appear near the beginning of the anal canal, they are known as *internal hemorrhoids.* At the end of the canal, they are called *external hemorrhoids.*

There is a general misconception that links anal itching to hemorrhoids. This is generally not the case unless a prolapsed internal hemorrhoid is producing a mucous discharge. In fact, usually anal itching is associated with coarse toilet paper, allergies, candida albicans, or parasitic infection.

However, swelling, bleeding, seepage, burning, inflammation, irritation, and pain are all among the unpleasant symptoms of of hemorrhoids.

Comments on Dr. Whitaker's Prescription for Hemorrhoids

Unlike in the United States and England, hemorrhoids are rarely seen in parts of the world where high-fiber, unrefined diets are consumed.[1] Individuals consuming a low-fiber diet tend to strain more during bowel movements. Their smaller and harder stools are more difficult to pass. This straining increases the pressure in the abdomen, which obstructs venous return. The increased pressure promotes pelvic congestion and may significantly weaken the veins, causing hemorrhoids to form.

A high-fiber diet is perhaps the most important component in the prevention of hemorrhoids. A diet rich in vegetables, fruits, legumes, and grains promotes peristalsis. Many fiber components attract water and form a gelatinous mass that keeps the stools soft, bulky, and easy to pass. The net effect of a high-fiber diet is significantly less straining during defecation.

Natural bulking agents, particularly powdered psyllium seed husks, can also be used to reduce fecal straining and relieve hemorrhoids.[2] Take 3 to 5 grams of psyllium fiber per day.

The warm sitz bath is an effective noninvasive treatment for uncomplicated hemorrhoids. A sitz bath is a partial immersion bath for the pelvic region. The temperature of the water in the warm sitz bath should be between 100 and 105ºF.

The use of medicated creams, pads, suppositories, and ointments can provide temporary relief. Many over-the-counter products for hemorrhoids, as well as products in health food stores, contain natural ingredients. These may be witch hazel (*Hamamelis* water), shark liver oil, cod liver oil, cocoa butter, Peruvian balsam, vitamin E, zinc oxide, live yeast cell derivative, and allantoin. Use these products according to the directions on the label.

Hepatitis

Dr. Whitaker's Prescription for Hepatitis:

1. Follow the Whitaker Wellness Program.
2. High-dose intravenous vitamin C (40 to 100 grams), or oral administration to bowel tolerance.
3. Take 210 milligrams of silymarin, three times daily, or two capsules of Super Milk Thistle (Enzymatic Therapy) three times daily.
4. Take two tablets of ThymuPlex (Enzymatic Therapy) three times daily.

Description

Hepatitis in most instances is caused by a virus. Viral types A, B, and C are the most common. Hepatitis A occurs sporadically or in epidemics, and is transmitted primarily through fecal contamination. Its incubation period is two to six weeks; carrier states are unknown. The death rate from hepatitis A is low (0 to 0.2 percent).

The rate of hepatitis A in the general population of the United States is surprisingly high. Antibodies to the hepatitis A virus are detected in 10 to 20 percent of children below ten years of age. Detection increases to 50 to 60 percent of adults by age 50. Yet only 3 to 5 percent of adults are aware that they have had hepatitis A, indicating that the majority of cases are mild or without symptoms.[3]

Hepatitis B is transmitted through infected blood or blood products. It is occasionally transmitted through saliva and sexual secretions. It is found most often in intravenous drug users and homosexuals, about 5 to 10 percent of whom become carriers. Its incubation period is six weeks to six months and fatality rate is moderate (0.3 to 1.5 percent).

Hepatitis C (formerly known as hepatitis non-A, non-B), is less common. Unfortunately, we are beginning to see more of it. Its primary route of transmission is blood transfusion. In fact, about 10 percent of people receiving blood transfusions develop hepatitis C. Its incubation period is two to twenty weeks; its mortality rate is unclear, but higher than for the other forms (1 to 12 percent).[1,2]

Hepatitis can also be caused by other viruses, including the type D virus, Epstein-Barr virus, and cytomegalovirus.[2]

For as yet unknown reasons, 10 percent of hepatitis B and 10 to 40 percent of hepatitis C cases develop into chronic viral hepatitis forms. The symptomatology varies. The symptoms can be latent, and they can lead to chronic fatigue, serious liver damage, and even death.[1]

Acute viral hepatitis is characterized by loss of appetite, nausea, vomiting, fatigue, and other flu-like symptoms; fever; enlarged, tender liver; jaundice (yellowing of skin due to increased levels of bilirubin in the blood); dark urine; and elevated liver enzymes in the blood.

Comments on Dr. Whitaker's Prescription for Hepatitis

The recommendations given here are useful in all forms of hepatitis, whether in an acute or chronic phase. In severe cases, I recommend large, intravenous doses of vitamin C (40 to 100 grams). According to Robert Cathcart, M.D., hepatitis is "one of the easiest diseases for ascorbic acid to cure." Dr. Cathcart demonstrated that vitamin C in these high doses was able to greatly improve acute viral hepatitis in two to four days. He showed clearing of jaundice within six days.[1] Other studies demonstrated similar benefits.[2] The doses could be given either orally or intravenously.

Given the safety of vitamin C and the potential benefit, it is certainly a good idea. If you cannot find a physician to administer the vitamin C intravenously, call the American College of Advancement in Medicine (1-800-532-3688) or take vitamin C to bowel tolerance (see page 41).

If you are planning to have surgery or be hospitalized for any reason, your risk for contracting hepatitis B is greatly enhanced. To reduce your odds of contracting hepatitis, take the high dosage of vitamin C given in the Whitaker Wellness Program. This recommendation is simple and effective. In one well-designed study it was shown that 2 grams or more of vitamin C per day was able to dramatically prevent hepatitis B in hospitalized patients.[3] While 7 percent of the control patients (receiving less that 1.5 grams of vitamin C per day) developed hepatitis, none of the patients taking more than 1.5 grams per day developed hepatitis.[5]

Silymarin, an extract from the common milk thistle (discussed in Chapter 4) is an herbal extract that can work as a preventive measure to protect the liver from damage and enhance liver function. In addition, studies have shown silymarin to be quite useful therapeutically in both chronic and acute hepatitis. Take 210 milligrams of silymarin three times daily, or two capsules of Super Milk Thistle (Enzymatic Therapy). Super Milk Thistle contains silymarin bound to phosphatidylcholine (the main component of soy lecithin). By binding the silymarin with this component, the result is improved absorption of silymarin and greater therapeutic effect.[4] So far, two studies in patients with chronic viral hepatitis have produced better results with the phosphatidylcholine-bound silymarin in comparison to studies with unbound silymarin.[5]

In one study, eight patients with chronic viral hepatitis (three with hepatitis B, three with both hepatitis B and hepatitis C, and two with hepatitis C) were given one capsule of phosphatidylcholine-bound silymarin between meals for two months. After treatment, serum malondialdehyde levels (an indicator of lipid peroxidation) decreased by 36 percent, and the quantitative liver function showed an increase of 15 percent. Elevated liver enzymes decreased by at least 16 percent.

The value of thymus extracts in chronic viral conditions, including hepatitis, is discussed in Chapter 7. Thymus extracts have been shown to be effective in several double-blind studies, in both acute and chronic cases. In these studies, therapeutic effect was noted by accelerated decreases of liver enzymes (transaminases), and elimination of the virus.[6]

These results prompted Carson Burgstiner, M.D., a prominent surgeon in Savannah, Georgia, to try a thymus extract product for his own hepatitis.[7] As past president of the Medical Association of Georgia, Dr. Burgstiner was well aware of the risks of chronic hepatitis, like cirrhosis of the liver and an increased risk of cancer. After agonizing over his medical condition for nine years, Dr. Burgstiner began taking ThymuPlex from Enzymatic Therapy. Six weeks later, blood studies showed that his body had finally rid itself of the virus.

Herpes

Dr. Whitaker's Prescription for Herpes:

Prevention
1. Follow the Whitaker Wellness Program.
2. Follow the recommendations for enhancing immune function in Chapter 7.
3. Eat a diet low in arginine and rich in lysine.
4. Take 1,000 milligrams of L-lysine, three times daily, with meals.

During an active infection
1. As above.
2. Apply Herpilyn cream to affected areas two to four times daily.

Description

Herpes is often the term used to describe a sexually transmitted disease that produces a painful rash on the genitals. However, the herpes simplex virus (HSV) can produce a recurrent viral infection on virtually any area of skin or mucous membranes. The most common sites are around the mouth (cold sores) and the genitals. Cold sores are usually caused by herpes simplex virus 1 (HSV1), while genital herpes is usually caused by the type 2 virus (HSV2). (See Cold Sores, page 206.)

The rash in genital herpes is characterized by the appearance of single or multiple clusters of small blisters filled with a clear fluid on a reddened base. The blisters eventually burst. When they do, they leave small, painful ulcers which heal within ten to twenty-one days.

After the initial infection, the virus becomes dormant in the nerve root near the spine. It's as if herpes has a hidden guerrilla compound where it retreats. From time to time it strikes, usually when the host is compromised in some ways. In short, it likes to strike when your guard is down. Herpes tends to become reactivated following minor infections, trauma, and stress. The stress can be emotional, dietary, or environmental. While about 40 percent of people never have a second outbreak, others may suffer four or five attacks a year for several years. For these people, the herpes virus can almost be viewed as a barometer of their "stress pressure" in their lives. Gradually, however, the attacks become less severe and the intervals between recurrences become longer.

Comments on Dr. Whitaker's Prescription for Herpes

Herpes tends to strike when the immune system is compromised. By following the Whitaker Wellness Program and the recommendations in Chapter 7, you are going a long way toward strengthening your immune system.

I also recommend that you take advantage of the amino acid L-lysine, a therapy which fools the virus. In order for the herpes virus to reproduce, it needs an amino acid called arginine. Lysine and arginine look similar to the virus. So the virus incorporates L-lysine instead of arginine. This blocks the steps in the development of the herpes virus which requires arginine. The result is that the virus will not become reactivated.[1]

Our goal in preventing herpes recurrences is clearly to keep lysine levels high and arginine levels low. First, avoid foods high in arginine. These are chocolate, peanuts, almonds and other nuts, and seeds. Foods that are high in lysine are most vegetables, legumes, fish, turkey, and chicken. Along with these dietary recommendations, I recommend that you supplement each meal with 1,000 milligrams of L-lysine.

Several double-blind, placebo-controlled studies have shown that lysine supplementation, along with avoidance of foods high in arginine, can be very effective in preventing recurrences in many cases. In one study, the group receiving L-lysine rated it 74 percent effective.[2] In contrast, the group receiving the placebo noted a success rate of 28 percent.

During an active infection, use Herpilyn cream on genital lesions in the way you would use it for a cold sore. (See Cold Sores, page 206.)

High Blood Pressure

Dr. Whitaker's Prescription for High Blood Pressure:

For Borderline to Mild Hypertension (140–160/90–104)
1. Do not take blood pressure lowering drugs.
2. Reduce weight if you are overweight.
3. Follow the Whitaker Wellness Program.

For Moderate Hypertension (140–180/105–114)
1. As above.
2. Take two tablets of Rogenic (Enzymatic Therapy) three times daily.
3. Take 30 to 100 milligrams of Coenzyme Q10 three times daily.

4. Take an odor-free garlic preparation at a high enough dosage to provide 8 milligrams of allicin or an allicin yield of 4,000 micrograms per day.
5. Follow these guidelines for three months. If blood pressure has not dropped below 140/105, you will need to work with a physician to select the most appropriate medication. If a prescription drug is necessary, calcium channel blockers or ACE inhibitors appear to be the safest.

For Severe Hypertension (160+/115+)
1. Consult a physician immediately.
2. Employ all the measures above.
3. A prescription drug may be necessary to achieve initial control.
4. When satisfactory control over the high blood pressure has been achieved, work with the physician to taper off the medication.
5. Consider intravenous EDTA chelation therapy (see page 145).

Description

When the doctor takes your blood pressure, he or she gets two readings, a high one and a low one. The first number is the systolic or contraction reading. The second is the diastolic or expanding one. A normal blood pressure reading is 120 over 80 (120/80). High blood pressure or hypertension refers to a reading of greater than 140/90. Over 60 million Americans have high blood pressure. An elevated blood pressure is one of the major risk factors for a heart attack or stroke. High blood pressure is divided into different levels: Borderline (120–160/90–94), Mild (140–160/95–104), Moderate (140–180/105–114) and Severe (160+/115+). Over 80 percent of patients with high blood pressure are in the borderline to moderate range.

Comments on Dr. Whitaker's Prescription for High Blood Pressure

My first recommendation in the treatment of high blood pressure is to avoid taking blood pressure lowering drugs. It is for a very good reason: Taking these drugs could be more dangerous to your health than high blood pressure.

Several well-designed, long-term clinical studies have looked at people taking the blood pressure-lowering drugs, typically diuretics and beta-blockers. The conclusion of these studies is that people suffer from a range of unnecessary side effects, among them an increased risk for heart disease.[1]

The side effects of the drugs must be examined in close detail. Diuretics cause the loss of potassium, magnesium, and calcium from the body. All of these minerals have been shown to exert blood pressure lowering effects and prevent heart attacks. The drugs also increase cholesterol and triglyceride levels. They increase the viscosity of the blood, raise uric acid levels, and increase the stickiness of the platelets, which makes them more likely to aggregate and form clots. All of these factors may explain why diuretics may actually increase the risk of dying from a heart attack or stroke.

Thiazide diuretics worsen blood sugar control, so they cannot be used safely in diabetics. Beta-blockers, on the other hand, actually reduce heart function as well as elevate triglyceride and cholesterol levels. Furthermore, long-term use of beta-blockers can lead to heart failure.

Virtually every medical authority (textbook, organization, or journal), including the Joint National Committee on Detection, Evaluation, and Treatment of High Blood Pressure, has recommended that nondrug therapies be used in the treatment of borderline to mild hypertension. At this stage of the disease, the drugs carry with them no benefit, yet possess significant risks. An article examining drug treatment in hypertension appeared in the *American Journal of Cardiology,* and is consistent with current medical opinion: "Few patients with uncomplicated marginal hypertension require drug treatment . . . there is little evidence that these patients (with marginal hypertension) will achieve enough benefit to justify the costs and adverse effects of antihypertensive drug treatment."[2]

The two most definitive trials are the Australian and Medical Research Council trials. Five other large trials also support this conclusion, including the famous Multiple Risk Factor Intervention Trial (MRFIT). In short, drugs offer no benefit in protecting against heart disease in borderline to moderate hypertension.[1,3]

These studies compared drug treatment to no treatment (placebo), and the drugs came off looking very bad. If a third group were kept off drugs and were also given the natural, nondrug therapies I am recommending, this group would probably have outlived those using drug therapy by a significant amount.

There are no negative side effects with the natural approach. There are many positive benefits. The diet that protects against high blood pressure will help ward off many other health problems, from gout to hemorrhoids to cancer.

In contrast, the drugs commonly used to lower blood pressure are associated with a whole host of side effects. Typical side effects of diuretics are light-headedness, increased blood sugar levels, and muscle weakness and cramps caused by low potassium levels. Decreased libido and impotence are also reported. Less frequent side effects include allergic reactions, headache, blurred vision, nausea, vomiting, and diarrhea. Beta-blockers and other blood pressure-lowering drugs make it difficult to get enough blood and oxygen to the hands, feet, and brain. This failure results in cold hands and feet, nerve tingling, impaired mental function, fatigue, dizziness, depression, lethargy, reduced libido, and impotence.

These side effects are not necessary. Most cases of high blood pressure can be brought under control through changes in diet and lifestyle. In fact, in head-to-head comparisons, many nondrug therapies, such as diet, exercise, and relation therapies, have proved superior to drugs in cases of borderline to mild hypertension.[4]

Despite this substantial evidence and medical opinion, blood pressure lowering drugs are still among the most widely prescribed. According to an article in the *Journal of the American Medical Association*, "Treatment of hypertension has become the leading reason for visits to physicians as well as for drug prescriptions."[5] Yearly sales of blood pressure medications are estimated to be greater than $10 billion.

It is estimated that approximately 80 percent of patients with high blood pressure are in the borderline to mild range. If doctors began prescribing the nondrug protocols that have been recommended by the authorities, it would mean a loss of $8 billion in sales to the drug companies each year.

The Natural Approach

Attaining ideal body weight is perhaps the single most important recommendation to lower blood pressure. Specific dietary factors include a high sodium-to-potassium ratio; low-fiber, high-sugar diet; high saturated fat and low essential fatty acids intake; and a diet low in omega-3 fatty acids, calcium, magnesium, and vitamin C. Some of the other important lifestyle factors that may lead to high blood pressure include coffee consumption, alcohol intake, lack of exercise, stress, and smoking.

Following the Whitaker Wellness Program provides the ideal dietary, lifestyle, and nutritional supplementation program to lower blood pressure. In fact, in most cases this is all that is needed to help you reach normal blood pressure.

Hives

Dr. Whitaker's Prescription for Hives:

1. Eliminate food allergies.
2. Eliminate food additives from the diet.
3. Eliminate dairy products from the diet.

Description

Hives or urticaria are localized swellings of the skin. Hives usually itch intensely. Hives are caused by the release of histamine within the skin. About 50 percent of patients with hives develop *angioedema,* a deeper, less-defined swelling involving tissues beneath the skin.

Hives and angioedema are relatively common conditions. It is estimated that 15 to 20 percent of the general population has had hives at some time. Although persons in any age group may experience acute or chronic hives or angioedema, young adults (post-adolescence through the third decade of life) are most often affected. Medications are the leading cause of hives in adults. In children, hives are usually due to foods, food additives, or infections.[1]

Comments on Dr. Whitaker's Prescription for Hives

An elimination or low-antigenic diet is of upmost importance in the treatment of most cases of hives, particularly in children. The diet should not only eliminate suspected allergens, but also all food additives. The strictest elimination diets allow only water, lamb, rice, pears, and vegetables. Those foods most commonly associated with inducing urticaria (milk, eggs, chicken, fruits, nuts, and additives) should definitely be avoided.[2] Foods containing vasoactive amines should also be eliminated, even if no direct allergy to them is noted. The primary foods to eliminate are cured meats, alcohol, cheese, chocolate, citrus fruits, and shellfish.

Food additives also appear to be a major factor in hives. Colorings (azo dyes), flavorings (salicylates, aspartame), preservatives (benzoates, nitrites, sorbic acid), antioxidants (hydroxytoluene, sulfite, gallate), and emulsifiers/stabilizers (polysorbates, vegetable gums) have all been shown to produce hives in sensitive individuals.[3]

The most common cause of hives in adults are the antibiotic drugs taken intentionally as prescriptions, or unintentionally, when the antibiotics administered to animals are passed through to humans in the food chain. Because it cannot be destroyed by boiling or steam distillation, penicillin and related compounds can exist undetected in foods.

Researchers are not yet clear on the extent to which unintended consumption of antibiotics, including penicillin and related compounds, contributes to hives. One suggestive study looked at 245 individuals with chronic uticaria.[5] Of these, over a third showed allergic sensitivity to penicillin. It is important to note that skin tests revealed this sensitivity in roughly 25 percent of those in the trial, while another 12 percent showed penicillin sensitivity through other allergy testing. Because penicillin administered to dairy cows is a major contributor to the penicillin in the food supply, the individuals were placed on a dairy-free diet. Over 50 percent improved clinically. Yet only 5 percent of those with negative skin tests improved on the same dairy-free diet. The study suggests that penicillin in the food supply can be a factor in hives. Allergic symptoms have also been traced to penicillin in soft drinks and frozen dinners.[4] This suggests that a chronic sufferer of hives who wishes to create an environment most conducive to ending these symptoms would be smart to limit or end dairy consumption.

Allergy to penicillin is very high in the population. The exact percentage is estimated to be roughly 10 percent. Studies suggest that nearly 25 percent of these allergic individuals will experience urticaria, angioedema, or severe reactions.[1] Thus, some 2.5 percent of all individuals may have hives or a related symptom in response to penicillin.

Hyperactivity and Learning Disorders

Dr. Whitaker's Prescription for Hyperactivity and Learning Disorders:

1. Eliminate food additives and food allergies from the diet.
2. Have a hair mineral analysis performed to rule out heavy metal toxicity.
3. Follow the Whitaker Wellness Program.

Description

Attention deficit disorder is the term currently used to describe a condition that has had multiple labels in the past, such as *hyperactivity* and *learning disability*. This condition describes three separate disorders: (1) attention deficit disorder without hyperactivity; (2) attention deficit disorder with hyperactivity; and (3) attention deficit disorder—residual type. Residual attention deficit disorder (individuals 18 years or older) is viewed primarily as a continuation of the process.

Attention deficit disorder with hyperactivity is the most common. About 3 percent of all school-age children carry this diagnosis. Boys are more likely to be given this diagnosis. In fact, ten boys will have it for every one girl.

The characteristics of this disorder, in order of their frequency, are (1) hyperactivity; (2) perceptual motor impairment; (3) emotional instability; (4) general coordination deficit; (5) disorders of attention (short attention span, distractibility, lack of perseverance, failure to finish things off, not listening, poor concentration); (6) impulsiveness (action before thought, abrupt shifts in activity, poor organizing, jumping up in class); (7) disorders of memory and thinking; (8) specific learning disabilities; (9) disorders of speech and hearing; and (10) neurological signs and electroencephalograph (EEG) irregularities.

Comments on Dr. Whitaker's Prescription for Hyperactivity and Learning Disorders

The treatment of attention deficit disorders is basically threefold: (1) eliminate food additives and food allergies from the diet; (2) rule out heavy metal toxicity; and (3) provide optimal nutrition.

The belief that food additives can cause hyperactivity in children stemmed from the research of Benjamin Feingold, M.D. It is commonly referred to as the Feingold Hypothesis. According to Feingold, perhaps 40 to 50 percent of hyperactive children are sensitive to artificial food colors, flavors, and preservatives. They may also be sensitive to naturally occurring salicylates and phenolic compounds in foods.[1]

Feingold's assertion that food additives are a problem in learning disorders has been subject to great debate over the past two decades. Practices that are profitable carry on and major economic interests have responded by hiring their own researchers to combat the results. Questions are asked in ways that will produce answers that undercut the challenging work and please the funding interests. The media publishes "conflicting reports." Politicians and regulators cite this conflict as their reason for inaction. Habits do not change easily. Feingold's work has stimulated a classic example of such debate, because the American food supply and American agribusiness is profitably enmeshed in the use of food additives.

Dr. Feingold made his original presentation to the American Medical Association in 1973. His strong claims were based on experience with 1,200 individuals in whom behavior disorders were linked to consumption of food additives. Followup research in Australia and Canada has tended to support Feingold's thesis.[2] In fact, in these and other countries outside the United States, such research has led to public policy changes. Fear of possible harmful effects has led to significant restrictions on artificial food additives.[3]

The story has been different in the United States. Most of the research published here suggests that the additives are just fine.[4] This research, Feingold points out, has mainly been funded by an entity called the Nutrition Foundation, an organization that is largely supported by major financial contributions from Coca Cola, Nabisco, General Foods, and other interests that make a profit on food additives. The results of the double-blind research associated with the Nutrition Foundation have been essentially negative on the Feingold Hypothesis.[5] Their research, however, has focused almost entirely on just ten food dyes. Feingold's research, on the other hand, looked at the 3,000 additives which in fact are part of the diets of our children.

The bottom line is that if your child is suffering from hyperactivity or an attention deficit disorder, the Feingold Hypothesis may help guide you to an answer to the riddle of your "difficult child."

Learning Disabilities

As discussed in Chapter 5, a deficiency of virtually any nutrient can result in impaired brain function. Numerous studies have shown that nutrient deficiency, particularly iron deficiency, exists in a significant number of children with learning disabilities.[6] Correcting any underlying nutritional deficiency will result in an almost immediate improvement in mental function. Even when there is no true nutrient deficiency, taking vitamins and minerals may help improve mental function. Also mentioned in Chapter 5, a recent study published in the respected medical journal *The Lancet* demonstrated that a multiple vitamin-mineral supplement increased intelligence in children, even when the children were not malnourished.[7]

There is a strong relationship between childhood learning disabilities (and other disorders including criminal behavior) and body stores of heavy metals.[8] Lead is particularly implicated. Numerous studies have shown children with learning disabilities and hyperactivity often have high body stores of heavy metals.[9] Poor nutrition and elevation of heavy metals usually go hand in hand. This is due to decreased consumption, in poor diets, of food factors which chelate heavy metals or decrease their absorption (see Chapter 4). If you have a child with learning difficulties, have your doctor perform a hair mineral analysis for heavy metals. If they are elevated, follow the recommendations on page 76.

Hypoglycemia

Dr. Whitaker's Prescription for Hypoglycemia:

1. Follow the Whitaker Wellness Program.
2. Avoid foods with a high glycemic index.
3. Take 200 to 400 micrograms of chromium each day.

Description

Hypoglycemia refers to a condition of low blood sugar. Because glucose is the primary fuel for the brain, when levels are too low, the brain feels the effects first. The brain responds to this sugar deficiency in a multitude of ways. Symptoms of hypoglycemia can range from mild to severe. They include such things as headache; depression, anxiety, irritability and other psychological disturbances; blurred vision; excessive sweating; mental confusion; incoherent speech; bizarre behavior; and convulsions.

CONDITIONS LINKED TO HYPOGLYCEMIA

Depression[1]
Aggressive and criminal behavior[2]
Premenstrual syndrome[3]
Migraine headaches[4]
Leg cramps[5]
Angina[6]

Hypoglycemia is divided into two main categories, reactive hypoglycemia and fasting hypoglycemia. Reactive hypoglycemia is the more common type. It is characterized by the development of symptoms of hypoglycemia two to four hours after a meal. Reactive hypoglycemia may also result from the use of certain drugs.

Fasting hypoglycemia is extremely rare. It usually only appears in severe disease states such as pancreatic tumors, extensive liver damage, prolonged starvation, and various cancers.

The diagnosis of hypoglycemia can be made with the help of the oral glucose tolerance test (GTT). After fasting for at least twelve hours, a baseline blood glucose measurement is made. Then the subject drinks a very sweet liquid containing glucose. Blood sugar levels are rechecked at thirty minutes, one hour, and then hourly for up to six hours. Basically, if blood sugar levels rise to a level greater than 200 milligrams per deciliter, diabetes is indicated. If levels fall below 50 milligrams per deciliter, the results indicate reactive hypoglycemia.

Hypoglycemia Questionnaire

No = 0   Mild = 1   Moderate = 2   Severe = 3

Crave sweets	0	1	2	3
Irritable if a meal is missed	0	1	2	3
Feel tired or weak if a meal is missed	0	1	2	3
Dizziness when standing suddenly	0	1	2	3
Frequent headaches	0	1	2	3
Poor memory (forgetful) or concentration	0	1	2	3
Feel tired an hour or so after eating	0	1	2	3
Heart palpitations	0	1	2	3
Feel shaky at times	0	1	2	3
Afternoon fatigue	0	1	2	3
Vision blurs on occasion	0	1	2	3
Depression or mood swings	0	1	2	3
Overweight	0	1	2	3
Frequently anxious or nervous	0	1	2	3

Total: _____

Scoring:

Less than 5: hypoglycemia is not likely a factor
6–15: hypoglycemia is a likely factor
Greater than 15: hypoglycemia is extremely likely

However, relying on blood sugar levels alone is often not enough in diagnosing hypoglycemia and blood sugar disorders. It is now widely recognized that signs and symptoms of hypoglycemia can occur in individuals having blood glucose levels well above 50 milligrams per deciliter.[2] Many of the symptoms linked to hypoglycemia appear to be a result of increases in insulin or epinephrine. Therefore, it has been recommended that insulin or epinephrine (adrenaline) be measured at the same time as glucose levels. Symptoms often correlate better with elevations in these hormones than with glucose levels.[7]

In most cases, all of this laboratory data is simply a waste of money. When all is considered (especially cost), the most useful measure of diagnosing hypoglycemia is often a more old-fashioned method: assessing symptoms. The questionnaire on page 278 is an excellent screening method for hypoglycemia.

Comments on Dr. Whitaker's Prescription for Hypoglycemia

You decide to indulge yourself with a refined carbohydrate treat. A sugar donut. "Just a little something." Unfortunately, your body responds to your little indulgence as though it were an act of war.

Refined carbohydrates are quickly absorbed into the bloodstream. The pancreas gets the message and begins to produce more insulin. Excessive secretion of insulin drives blood sugar levels down. The message that something is amiss with blood sugar reaches the adrenal glands. The adrenals give your body the ability to make a "fight or flight" decision. They send a rush of adrenaline (epinephrine) into your system to jack the blood glucose level back up again and keep you on your toes. In short, it's war time.

The body and the adrenals will survive the irregular treat without much problem. They are built for that. But if a diet rich in refined carbohydrates continuously sets off this cascade of events, the adrenals wear down. They become exhausted. The blood sugar control mechanisms are thrown out of balance. This produces reactive hypoglycemia.

This condition can be viewed as "pre-diabetes." For hypoglycemia to become this more serious diagnosis, the body's sugar control mechanisms take the next step out of balance. The pancreas gets tired of responding to the constant demand for insulin. It too becomes exhausted and slows or stops production. At the same time, the tissues of the body may develop insensitivity to the continuous insulin assaults. They won't respond as rapidly, the pancreas works to send out more, the negative spiral tightens. The condition now has the characteristics of diabetes, with all the potentially grave complications.

In 1981, David Jenkins developed a tool that can help guide an individual with reactive hypoglycemia away from further complications and toward health. Before Jenkins developed his tool, it was generally accepted that the basic dietary treatment plan meant avoiding refined sugars. But what of other foods? Which are most likely to provoke the cascade of detrimental blood sugar responses? If ingesting straight glucose is considered the worst choice, how do others compare?

Jenkins gave a value of 100 to describe the rise in blood sugar after consuming pure glucose. The values of other foods were then established in reference to this standard value. This scale gives a good indication of the body's insulin response to carbohydrate-containing foods, since this response is similar to the rise in blood sugar levels. Jenkins called this scale the *Glycemic Index.*[8]

There are some surprises here. The highest value is a baked potato (98). Puffed rice and corn flakes are very high, at 95 and 80, respectively. On the low end are ice cream (36) and sausage (28). The basic recommendation for a hypoglycemic person is to avoid foods with high values.

Does this mean that eating ice cream instead of a potato is the best way to go? How about some sizzling sausage?

Nice try! The reason for the low rating of these foods on the Glycemic Index is that diets high in fat impair glucose tolerance. This provides at best a short-term benefit based on a very limited perspective. This reductive perspective on ice cream and sausage led conventional doctors, until 1955, to wrongly promote a high fat diet for diabetics (see Diabetes, page 226). We now know that such a diet is harmful in many ways. One such harmful effect is its role in the development of obesity which in turn has a very high association with the onset of type II diabetes.

In short, use of the Glycemic Index should be moderated by common sense.

GLYCEMIC INDEX OF SOME COMMON FOODS[9]

Sugars		Grains	
Glucose	100	Rice, puffed	95
Maltose	105	Corn flakes	80
Honey	75	Bread, whole grain	72
Sucrose	60	Rice	70
Fructose	20	Bread, white	69
		Wheat cereal	67
		Corn	59
Fruits		Bran cereal	51
Raisins	64	Oatmeal	49
Bananas	62	Pasta	45
Orange juice	46		
Oranges	40	Legumes	
Apples	39	Peas	39
		Beans	31
		Lentils	29
Vegetables			
Potato, baked	98	Other foods	
Potato (new), boiled	70	Ice cream	36
Beets	64	Milk	34
Carrot, cooked	36	Sausages	28
Carrot, raw	31	Nuts	13

Chromium

Chromium has been mentioned earlier for its role in the *glucose toler-ance factor*. Chromium works closely with insulin in facilitating the up-take of glucose into cells. Without chromium, insulin's action is blocked and glucose levels are elevated. Obviously, chromium is a critical nutrient in diabetes, but it is also very important in hypo-glycemia. In one study, eight female patients with hypoglycemia were given 200 micrograms a day for three months and demonstrated alle-viation of their symptoms of hypoglycemia.[10] In addition, glucose tol-erance test results were improved and the number of insulin receptors on red blood cells were increased.

Although there is no RDA for chromium, it appears that we need at least 200 micrograms each day in our diet. Chromium levels can be depleted by refined sugars, white flour products, and lack of exercise. I believe the individual with hypothyroid should supplement the diet with 200 to 400 micrograms of chromium each day. Chromium poly-nicotinate, chromium picolinate, and chromium-enriched yeast are the best forms.

Hypothyroidism

Dr. Whitaker's Prescription for Hypothyroidism:

1. Follow the Whitaker Wellness Program.
2. Try a health food store thyroid preparation. If your basal body tem-perature does not rise to normal levels after two months, you may require a prescription for thyroid hormone from your doctor.

Description

Hypothyroidism is a condition in which an individual's metabolic processes slow down. They often feel cold in their hands and feet. The sluggish metabolism can appear as fatigue, lethargy, and depression. Weight is no longer "burned off" as it was in the past. Individuals ex-perience difficulty in losing weight. Some experience moderate weight gain. In addition, infections tend to recur, perhaps because the body struggles to mount the energy required to fight off infections.

Other signs and symptoms linked to hypothyroidism are dry skin, elevated cholesterol, constipation, muscle and joint stiffness, and headaches.

The immediate biochemical cause of hypothyroidism is that the cells of the body are receiving poor regulatory oversight from the thyroid. Thyroid hormones regulate metabolism in every cell. Without the biochemical direction provided by these hormones, the individual's altered metabolism hits him or her as chronic fatigue or depression. These are the two most common features of hypothyroidism.

Sometimes the cause of this regulatory problem is that the pituitary gland is not telling the thyroid to synthesize enough hormone. This is called secondary hypothyroidism. To see if the fault lies in the pituitary, levels of the pituitary's thyroid-stimulating hormone (TSH) are compared to levels of thyroid hormone. If TSH levels are high and thyroid hormone levels are low, then the thyroid should be getting the message from the pituitary, but it is just not responding. The problem is in the thyroid's ability to follow the pituitary's direction. It is not synthesizing enough thyroid hormone. This is called *primary hypothyroidism.*

Laboratory blood tests will definitely pick up on severe thyroid-deficiency states. These can in fact be life-threatening (myxedema). It is paradoxical that while these tests are quite sophisticated, they are also crude. The mild hypothyroidism that many people experience does not register on these sophisticated tests. These mild conditions, which account for the majority of cases, are frequently undiagnosed.[1] We are in the gray area known to most physicians as subclinical. Hypothyroidism is a condition which, because it is invisible to most laboratory tests, leads many physicians to believe the symptoms are merely "in the head" of the patient.

However, hypothyroidism is a condition for which older, more primitive tests are more functional instruments, when you are evaluating whether or not the thyroid is involved in producing the patient's symptoms. One test is the *Achilles tendon reflex time,* otherwise known as "rubber hammer diagnostics." The test is useful because reflex time slows down with hypothyroidism.

Basal Body Temperature

The other, more telling diagnostic tool is measurement of the temperature of the body while at rest, or the *basal body temperature.* Your body temperature reflects your metabolic rate. This rate is largely determined by hormones secreted by the thyroid gland. The only piece of medical technology required for this test is a thermometer. Basal body temperature is perhaps the most sensitive functional test of thyroid function.

Procedure

1. Shake down the thermometer to below 95ºF and place it by your bed before going to sleep at night.

2. On waking, place the thermometer in your armpit for a full ten minutes. It is important to make as little movement as possible.

Lying and resting with your eyes closed is best. Do not get up until the ten-minute test is completed.

3. After ten minutes, read and record the temperature and date.

4. Record the temperature for at least three mornings (preferably at the same time) and give the information to your physician. Menstruating women must perform the test on the second, third, and fourth days of menstruation. Men and postmenopausal women can perform the test at any time.

Interpretation   Your basal body temperature should be between 97.6 and 98.2º. It is below the "normal" of 98.6 because you are taking your temperature under the arm rather than orally or anally. Temperature registers roughly a point lower in this spot, and low basal body temperatures are quite common. They do not prove hypothyroidism. The likelihood that a thyroid problem is behind your low temperature is higher only if you also have some of the symptoms noted earlier.

High basal body temperatures (above 98.6) are less common. They may be evidence of *hyperthyroidism.* Common signs and symptoms of hyperthyroidism include bulging eyeballs, fast pulse, hyperactivity, inability to gain weight, insomnia, irritability, menstrual problems, and nervousness. In short, the symptoms of hyperthyroidism tend to be what would reasonably be associated with heating up or speeding up the body.

Comments on Dr. Whitaker's Prescription for Hypothyroidism

Severe hypothyroidism must be treated by a physician. This is a "do not pass go, go directly to" directive. The treatment is thyroid hormone replacement therapy. The physician will generally prescribe a synthetic thyroid hormone to stabilize the body's metabolic activity. I recommend the desiccated natural thyroid in these instances. The whole desiccated thyroid contains a range of thyroid hormones, whereas the synthetic thyroid is more limited.

Discovering hypothyroidism in the "pre-clinical" stage provides other options. The first is to make sure the thyroid has all the necessary building blocks to synthesize its hormones. Many vitamins and minerals are involved. The most critical is iodine. In fact, at this time the only known function of iodine in the body is in thyroid hormone synthesis. Interestingly enough, both a deficiency of iodine and an excess of iodine are associated with limiting synthesis of thyroid hormone.

Nature's best sources of iodine are from the sea. Seaweeds such as kelp are one source. Hypothyroidism will give many people an opportunity to explore a new section of the health food store! Clams, oysters, lobsters, sardines, and other saltwater fish are others. Surprisingly, given that most of these sources come from the sea, sea salt itself has very little iodine.

Our main source of iodine is the iodized salt which is used in food processing, cooking, and as a condiment. Roughly 45 percent of salt intake is from the processing of food, 45 percent from the cooking of food, 5 percent as a table condiment and 5 percent that is naturally occurring in foods. The excess salt in the American diet has put iodine in the unusual category of being 400 percent above the FDA's recommended dietary allowance. The RDA is 150 micrograms and the average intake is roughly 600 micrograms per day. The problems associated with excess iodine in thyroid function suggest that supplementation should not exceed 1,000 micrograms for any length of time.

Individuals with mild hypothyroidism may be helped by thyroid preparations sold in health food stores. While the FDA prohibits any thyroxine in these products, it is actually virtually impossible for a manufacturer to entirely remove thyroxine. In a sense, the health food store thyroid formulas are mild forms of desiccated natural thyroid. Manufacturers will usually enhance these formulas with additional thyroid support, such as iodine, zinc, and tyrosine.

To check the effectiveness of a health food store product, keep tabs on your basal body temperature. Try modulating the dose a bit, based on effectiveness. For health food products, optimal dosage varies depending on the potency of the supportive nutrients. I am familiar with Enzymatic Therapy's Thyroid and L-Tyrosine Complex. For this formula, I recommend a dosage of one capsule, three times a day.

If your basal body temperature does not come back to normal in two months, see your doctor for a desiccated natural thyroid.

Impotence

Dr. Whitaker's Prescription for Impotence:

1. Follow the Whitaker Wellness Program.
2. Exercise.
3. If your cholesterol levels are high, follow the recommendations on page 191.
4. If you have diabetes, follow the recommendations on page 221.
5. Take one or two capsules of Masculex (Enzymatic Therapy) three times daily.
6. If there is no improvement after three months, give yohimbine a try.

Description

The most effective public health campaign the United States government could engage to promote positive diet and lifestyle choices in American men might be a little crude, but it would take advantage of a condition that horrifies most men: impotence.

"A highly refined, high-fat diet can be hazardous to your sex life," the health warning would say. Picture a man saying "I'm sorry," next to a partner in bed.

"Smoking and drinking can make you impotent." Picture a man in a robe standing sadly by the window at night.

"Can't get an erection? Take a look at your diet and lifestyle, man. Take a look at the beer and chips in your hands." These public service announcements would be well-placed during breaks in professional sports coverage on television.

The smaller print text of the public service message would give the supportive details: One out of every four men over the age of fifty will suffer from the inability to attain or maintain an erection long enough to permit satisfactory sexual intercourse.[1] An estimated 10 million to 20 million men suffer from impotence.

One factor linked to impotence is long-term alcohol consumption. Another is long-term tobacco use.

The biggest causal factors in impotence are health conditions that are strongly linked to diet and lifestyle decisions. For half of the men over fifty suffering from impotence, atherosclerosis of the penile artery is the primary cause. Diabetes, another disorder related to diet and lifestyle, is also considered an organic cause of impotence.

The major "inorganic causes" of impotence are also closely, but indirectly, tied to diet and lifestyle. These are the many prescription drugs that have erectile dysfunction as a possible side effect. The most common of these drugs are those designed to lower blood pressure, a health concern also closely tied to dietary and lifestyle decisions. These antihypertensive drugs include beta blockers, calcium channel blockers, angiotensin-converting enzyme inhibitors, and diuretics.

Maybe such a campaign would get the attention of those men who haven't yet started to work toward a healthier diet and lifestyle.

Meantime, the drugs that have sexual dysfunction as a side effect are probably not necessary. Virtually every medical authority recommends against these drugs (and their side effects) for individuals with moderate hypertension. Instead, nondrug therapies are recommended for individuals with blood pressure less than 140/105. (See High Blood Pressure, page 269, for ideas on how to avoid the risk of sexual dysfunction.)

Many other prescription medications can interfere with sexual function. Take a look at the small print on the bottle. Ask your physician whether any prescription drugs you are taking have impotence as a side effect. Usually, natural alternatives to these drugs will produce safer and better clinical results. Work with your physician. If your physician will not work with you to make the change, try finding one who will.

Other causal factors thought to be associated with impotence are hypothyroidism, excess prolactin, and low levels of testosterone.

Comments on Dr. Whitaker's Prescription for Impotence

The frequency of impotence increases with age. But aging itself is not a cause of impotence. This is an important distinction. It is the customary diets and lifestyles of our aging population that has helped create these high statistics on impotence.

Nutrition clearly plays a role in determining sexual impotence. Optimal sexual function requires optimal nutrition. The Whitaker Wellness Program recommendations in Chapter 2 should be sufficient. Vegetables, fruits, whole grains, and legumes are key food groups. For proteins, fish, chicken, turkey, and lean cuts of hormone-free beef are preferred sources. Nutrients such as zinc, essential fatty acids, vitamin A, vitamin B6, and vitamin E are important for healthy sexual function. If you have diabetes, look at that section on page 221; if you have elevated cholesterol, see my recommendations on page 191.

Zinc deserves particular consideration. Because it is concentrated in the semen, frequent ejaculation can deplete zinc stores. Zinc is required for more enzyme activity than any other mineral. There is some evidence that the body responds to deficiency of this precious mineral by decreasing sexual drive. Many of the foods which are said to enhance virility have zinc as a common denominator. These include nuts, seeds, legumes, and liver.

Exercise

Exercise is a must for good health. Will regular exercise improve a man's sexual performance? Yes. This answer is not just based on common sense, but on clinical research as well.

Let's look at just one study of this relationship. Seventy-eight sedentary but healthy men (mean age 48 years) were observed for nine months. Aerobic work capacity (physical fitness), coronary heart disease risk factors, and sexuality were studied.[2] The men exercised in supervised groups 60 minutes per day for 3.5 days per week. A control group of seventeen men (mean age, 44 years) participated in organized walking at a moderate pace 60 minutes per day, 4.1 days per week on average. Each subject maintained a daily diary of exercise, diet, smoking, and sexuality during the first and last months of the program.

This study, like many others, showed the beneficial effects of regular exercise on fitness and coronary heart disease risk factors. The diary entries were analyzed to measure the effects on sexual function. Analysis revealed significantly greater sexuality in the exercise group. This was measured in frequency of various intimate activities, reliability of adequate functioning during sex, and percentage of satisfying orgasms. Moreover, the degree of enhanced sexuality among exercisers correlated with the degree of their individual improvement in fitness. The better physical fitness the men were able to attain, the better their sexuality.

Ginseng

Perhaps the most popular herb in use for sexual enhancement is Chinese or Korean ginseng (Panax ginseng). Unfortunately, at this time there are no human studies available to support the claim that this herb is a sexual rejuvenator. However, the herb's reputation was not fabricated out of thin air. In studies with animals, sperm formation and testosterone levels increased with ginseng administration. Testes grew. And increased sexual activity and mating behavior was observed.[3]

The animal studies are suggestive enough that if an individual's common sense is provoked by desire, such a person might decide to allow himself to be the exception that has thus far proved the rule in human studies.

Yohimbine

Another popular herb in use for enhancing sexual function comes from the bark of a tree that is native to tropical West Africa, the yohimbe tree (Pausinystalia johimbe). There is a popular belief that an alkaloid isolated from this bark will actually increase testosterone levels. Studies have shown no such increase.

Yet this herb and its isolated alkaloid clearly have some potent effects on sexual function. The primary action of yohimbine hydrocholoride is to increase blood flow into erectile tissue. It increases libido. Used alone, yohimbine is successful in 34 to 43 percent of cases.[4] But if combined in formula with testosterone and strychnine, effectiveness increases further.

The problem with this potent medicine is its side effects. Individuals have been known to get anxious. Others have suffered panic attacks and hallucinations. Yohimbine can have an effect on the cardiovascular system. Blood pressure can rise. So can the heart rate. Dizziness, skin flushing, and headache have also been noted. Certain individuals should definitely not take yohimbine: those with psychological disturbances, women, and people with kidney disease.

Yohimbine is the one drug approved by the FDA for treating impotence. But because side effects can exist both with yohimbine and the extract from the bark, the FDA considers yohimbine to be an unsafe herb. The current status of commercial preparations does not help the consumer with this difficulty. None of the yohimbe products of which I am aware give the consumer a label specification of the amount of yohimbine per dosage. So it is difficult to prescribe and particularly difficult to prescribe safely. I support the FDA's caution with this herb. At the least, any patient using either of these powerful agents should be under the supervision of a physician.

Muira Puama

Muira puama (*Ptychopetalum olacoides*), an herb that is little known, but which boasts its own exotic origins, was shown in a recent French study to have clinical effectiveness in improving sexual function in some patients. This herb is from a shrub that is native to Brazil. A common name is "potency wood," which suggests that the locals didn't need to hear from the French researchers before giving it value in this arena.

The French study was carried out under the supervision of Dr. Jacques Waynberg, one of the world's premier authorities on sexual function.[5] It took place at the Institute of Sexology in Paris. The study looked at 262 men. Some were complaining of lack of sexual desire. Others had an inability to attain or maintain an erection. The subjects were given 1 to 1.5 grams of a muira extract each day. Of those in the first category, three out of five (62 percent) felt a positive dynamic effect within two weeks. Of those with concerns about erections, one in two felt the muira puama extract to be beneficial. No negative side effects were felt by either group.

The researchers have yet to put a finger on the biochemical mechanism or mechanisms by which these positive results were achieved. The speculation is that muira puama actually influences both the psychological and the physical.

Ginkgo Biloba

The atherosclerotic basis of sexual dysfunction in a high percentage of those suffering from impotence suggests that *Ginkgo biloba* extract may be useful. A battery of clinical studies have shown ginkgo's value in increasing both blood flow and oxygen to many tissues.

Stimulated by the clinical research on ginkgo, some researchers decided to look directly at the value of *Ginkgo biloba* in cases of impotence caused by lack of blood flow.[6] A group of sixty men with impotence were observed from twelve to eighteen months. They were given 60 milligrams per day of *Ginkgo biloba* extract. A high-tech measurement called duplex sonography was used to measure penile blood flow every four weeks. None of these subjects had reacted positively to injections of the drug papaverine at up to 50 milligrams in a previous study.

The results of this preliminary study on ginkgo were exceptional. Fully one-half (51 percent) regained potency within six months. In fact, within six to eight weeks, the sonograms began to show signs of increased penile blood supply. Those who did not respond to the ginkgo were then readministered the injected papaverine. One group, which represented 20 percent of the original sample, regained potency with the new papaverine trial. For a second group, representing 25 percent of the original, improved blood flow was noted after the second papaverine injection. Potency, however, was not regained. Only 5 percent remained unaffected.

What is particularly remarkable in this study is the size of the ginkgo dose. Other studies have shown that the optimal ginkgo dose for long-term administration to enhance blood supply is a full 250 percent above the 60-milligram dose of *Ginkgo biloba* in the trial. How might the results have come out if a dose of 120 milligrams per day had been given?

Some Practical Advice

The optimal clinical approach to enhancing sexual function in men would combine the attributes of all of these agents. Sexual dysfunction can be handled in a number of ways. Blood supply to erectile tissue can be enhanced. The brain's transmission of nervous signals can be stimulated. And the male glandular system's activity is targeted.

Because of the potential side effects of yohimbine, I do not recommend it until all else has failed. Give my program at least three months of conscientious administration first. Then make sure you see a physician before using any product derived from the yohimbe tree.

The herbal formula I use in my clinical practice is a formula called Masculex (Enzymatic Therapy). The formula includes extracts of Muira puama, *Ginkgo biloba* and *Panax ginseng*. Key nutrients for male sexual health are also included, such as zinc, liver extract, beta-sitosterol and a concentrate of wheat germ oil. In addition, the formula has an extract of saw palmetto. (See section on benign prostatic hyperplasia, page 324.) Take one to two capsules, three times a day. Though we do not have clinical information to prove this, these agents in combination may have more value than each of them taken individually.

Insomnia

Dr. Whitaker's Prescription for Insomnia:

1. Eliminate substances known to interfere with sleep, such as caffeine and alcohol.
2. If depression is the cause, follow the recommendations on page 216.
3. If anxiety is a problem, follow the recommendations on page 158.
4. Follow the Whitaker Wellness Program.
5. Take 150 to 300 milligrams of valerian root extract (0.8 percent valerenic acid content) 30 to 45 minutes before retiring.

Description

"Get a good night's sleep." This simple therapeutic recommendation is closely associated with the image of the old-style country doctor. The recommendation recognizes that healing requires sleep. Sleep is the most basic of "natural medicines."

If ever a nation needed this prescription, it is the United States as the turn of the century approaches. Various forces in our lives are stealing this most basic of natural medicines from us. Nearly one out of every three Americans experiences insomnia on a regular basis. Over 50 percent have some difficulty falling asleep.

But these days, the kind suggestion of the doctor or a loving family member no longer does the trick. Instead, drug stores do a brisk business in over-the-counter insomnia medications. Even these drugs don't bring sleep for many. For 10 million people each year, the desire for the balm of sleep leads them to physicians for prescription medications. The modern physician is more likely to say: "Take this drug and get a good night's sleep." Unfortunately, there are serious questions about how "good" such a drug-induced sleep is.

Tranquilizers (benzodiazepines) like Halcion, Librium, and Valium, have recently been receiving a great deal of negative attention in the media. More people are "waking up" to the fact that these drugs can be quite dangerous. These drugs are not designed to be used long-term; they are addictive, associated with numerous side effects, and cause abnormal sleep patterns.

These drugs can create a vicious cycle in the patient's life. The patient takes the drug to induce sleep. This causes further disruption of normal sleep by suppressing REM (rapid eye movement) sleep. It is during REM sleep that repair and rejuvenative processes take place. REM sleep is also when we dream. Because patients do not experience adequate REM sleep while on a benzodiazepine, they will typically wake up with a "hangover." They may feel more tired than when they went to sleep. So they turn to a stimulant, such as coffee, to get them going. This is the stimulant phase of the vicious cycle. The drug's role in maintaining this cycle does not end here. When a patient tries to withdraw from long-term use of benzodiazepines, REM sleep increases. Nightmares and further sleep disturbances are added to the other withdrawal symptoms.

An individual summons his or her willpower and commitment to break the vicious cycle. But waiting inside reintroduced REM sleep, like mythic beasts at the exit gate, are nightmares to scare the person back into drug sleep again. It can require the fortitude of a hero or heroine to get off these pills.

This mythic picture of the ordeal of release from the imprisoning cycle of benzodiazepines has an interesting reflection in their biochemical activity. These drugs work directly on brain chemistry. The most serious side effects are experienced by patients as minor to major personal transformations.

One person becomes extremely irritable and aggressive. Another becomes nervous and confused. Another begins to experience hallucinations. Others engage in bizarre behavior. Still others, instead of "acting out," turn inward. Feelings of depression increase. Greater suicidal thinking is observed. The serious side effects hit not only behavior, but memory. Some report severe memory impairment and even amnesia while on benzodiazepines.

A wide array of additional side effects are often experienced by patients on these drugs. One cluster of side effects alters a person's relationship to food: nauseau, indigestion, diarrhea, and constipation. Another cluster is linked to alertness: dizziness, drowsiness, impaired coordination. Others are allergic reactions, headache, and blurred vision. For these reasons, an individual taking these drugs should not drive or engage in any potentially dangerous activities. Alcohol should not be consumed while on "sleeping pills."

Comments on Dr. Whitaker's Prescription for Insomnia

Insomnia can have many causes. The most common reasons are depression, anxiety, and tension. If your insomnia is due to depression, see page 216, or anxiety, see page 158.

If psychological factors do not seem to be the cause, various foods, drinks, and medications may be responsible. There are numerous compounds in food and drink and well over 300 drugs that can interfere with normal sleep. If you are taking a medication, check with your doctor, pharmacist, or the *Physician's Desk Reference* to see if insomnia is a side effect.

If the insomnia is a side effect of a drug you are taking, your first step is to work with your physician to get off the medication.

Diet

A fundamental step for anyone experiencing insomnia is to eliminate dietary factors known to impair sleep processes. It is essential that the diet be free of natural stimulants such as caffeine and related compounds. Caffeine sources include coffee, black tea, green tea, soft drinks, chocolate, coffee-flavored ice cream, and hot cocoa. Alcohol must also be eliminated. It produces a number of effects that interfere with sleep.

Nocturnal Hypoglycemia

A special sleep-related problem is called *nocturnal hypoglycemia*. This afflicts people who don't have any trouble going to sleep, but wake up in the middle of the night with insomnia. This condition describes a low nighttime blood glucose level. A drop in the blood glucose level releases hormones like adrenaline, glucagon, cortisol, and growth hormone, which regulate glucose levels. These compounds stimulate the brain. They are a natural signal that it is time to eat. They can awaken individuals and keep them awake.

Good bedtime snacks to keep blood sugar levels steady throughout the night are complex carbohydrates such as oatmeal and other whole grain cereals, whole grain breads, and muffins. These foods will not only help regulate blood sugar levels, they actually can help promote sleep. Complex carbohydrates can increase the level of the natural sleep-promoting substance, serotonin, within the brain.

Valerian Root

Clearly, if a substance is to be used before sleep to help induce sleep, one that is effective without negative side effects would be optimal. A number of herbal sedatives are available. For insomnia sufferers, the extract of the valerian root is the best choice.

Studies have shown that taking valerian root compounds, rather than creating morning drowsiness, actually reduce it. Sleep quality improved.[1] The time required to get to sleep shortened. No hangover effect from the extracts was felt the next morning.[2]

Good clinical studies produced this evidence. A double-blind study on 128 patients reached the results noted above.[2] A study that followed up this work actually concluded that valerian extract reduced the time needed to fall asleep just as effectively as small doses of tranquilizers, without the side effects.[3]

The best valerian products are standardized to contain 8 percent valerenic acid. Most major health food store companies supply high-quality valerian extracts including Nature's Herbs, Nature's Way, Enzymatic Therapy, and Solaray. Take 150 to 300 milligrams, 30 to 45 minutes before retiring. If morning sleepiness occurs, reduce dosage. If dosage was not effective, make sure that you are eliminating other factors that disrupt sleep. Don't increase dosage until you implement the appropriate dietary and lifestyle changes.

Irritable Bowel Syndrome

Dr. Whitaker's Prescription for Irritable Bowel Syndrome:

1. Eliminate sugar from your diet.
2. Increase the amount of water-soluble fiber in the diet.
3. Eliminate food allergies.
4. Take one or two capsules of Peppermint-Plus, an enteric-coated peppermint oil product (Enzymatic Therapy), three times daily between meals.

Description

Irritable bowel syndrome (IBS) is a common condition in which the large intestine, or colon, fails to function properly. Estimates suggest that approximately 15 percent of the population have suffered from IBS.

IBS is known by a number of other names. Among them are nervous indigestion, spastic colitis, mucus colitis, and intestinal neurosis. IBS has characteristic symptoms which can include a combination of any of the following: abdominal pain and distension; more frequent bowel movements with pain; relief of pain with bowel movements; constipation; diarrhea; excessive production of mucus in the colon; symptoms of indigestion such as flatulence, nausea, or anorexia; and varying degrees of anxiety or depression.

Comments on Dr. Whitaker's Prescription for Irritable Bowel Syndrome

While deeply troubling to those afflicted with it, IBS is a health condition that is almost entirely food-related. The source of the river of good health may be discovered in a high-fiber diet that is low in refined carbohydrates and sugar.

Sugar usually has a detrimental effect on bowel function. White table sugar and sucrose are especially problematic for the individual with IBS. Those serious about healing IBS must avoid sugar.

Fiber intake is also especially important. The easiest prescription is to increase the amount of plant food consumed in the diet. All plants contain fibers. Fibers are the compounds of the plant that are not digested and assimilated. As such, these compounds are critically important for stool development.

For an individual with an "irritable" bowel, the optimal stool is both bulky and soft. This is a gentler stool to pass. The way to create such a stool is to increase the level of water-soluble fibers in the diet. These fibers are found in foods that, by and large, haven't received as much public acclaim for their value as fiber sources. The fiber in such high-visibility fiber foods as whole grains and wheat bran, for instance, is not water-soluble. Vegetables, beans, peas, and fruits are all excellent sources of water-soluble fiber. Oat bran is the high-profile exception in the water-soluble fiber category, and is very good for you.

The power of certain foods as basic fiber sources will surprise many. A single cup of cooked navy beans, for instance, has more fiber than ten slices of whole grain bread. A single pear has more fiber than four slices of whole grain bread. So does a serving of broccoli. In addition, a stool rich in water-soluble fiber will not only pass more gently, it will also help lower cholesterol levels.

Some individuals find that guaranteeing the level of fiber in their diets is easiest if they use a fiber supplement. If so, I recommend between 3 and 5 grams per day. Take the supplements an hour before going to bed. Make sure that the fiber formula you choose is rich in water-soluble fiber sources. Some sources of water-soluble fibers used in formulas are beets, carrots, pectin, psyllium seed husks, oat bran, and guar gum.

Food Allergies

For individuals with IBS, diet plays another important causal role in their health condition. Nearly 67 percent of individuals with IBS have at least one food allergy. Others have multiple food allergies.[1] In fact, IBS patients tend to have a symptom complex that parallels the classic food-allergy profile. These symptoms include fatigue and headaches. The elimination diet described in the section on food allergy (see page 245) is the best method of determining food allergies.

Peppermint Oil

If you have increased your intake of dietary fiber and eliminated food allergies and still have uncomfortable symptoms of IBS, you may want to take Peppermint-Plus, a special peppermint oil product in health food stores. This product, made by Enzymatic Therapy, provides peppermint oil in a special enteric-coated capsule. Enteric coating means that the capsule has been treated to ensure that it won't dissolve in your stomach. Without enteric coating, taking peppermint oil would cause a good case of heartburn. Peppermint-Plus is designed so the capsule dissolves and releases the peppermint oil only in the small intestines and colon.

Enteric-coated peppermint oil has been used in treating irritable bowel syndrome in Europe for many years. One double-blind crossover study concluded: "Peppermint oil in enteric-coated capsules appears to be an effective and safe preparation for symptomatic treatment of the irritable bowel syndrome."[2] The oil was found to relieve abdominal symptoms of the IBS. Peppermint oil works by relaxing the intestines and by helping the body eliminate gas. It may also work by destroying the yeast *Candida albicans.*

Many sufferers of the irritable bowel syndrome are told that it is a condition they just have to live with. Before giving up hope, I recommend enteric-coated peppermint oil. For best results, follow the recommendations on the bottle of Peppermint-Plus. Take one or two capsules between meals, three times daily. This product works extremely well for children over four years old who complain of colic.

Kidney Stones

Dr. Whitaker's Prescription for Kidney Stones:

Fluid intake
1. Drink two to three quarts of pure water daily.
2. Avoid coffee and alcohol.

Diet
1. Eat less animal protein and more fruits and vegetables.
2. Reduce fat and sugar consumption.
3. Avoid vitamin D-fortified dairy products.

Supplements
1. Take 1,000 milligrams of magnesium (preferably magnesium citrate) and 100 milligrams of vitamin B6 daily.
2. Use potassium citrate or Bicitra, when appropriate.

Description

Stones look good in your garden, make a secure path in your lawn, and small, thin ones skip well on a quiet lake (personal best, 14,

August 3, 1992). However, a stone in your urinary tract is very painful. Many equate the pain of passing a kidney stone to labor pains; since 75 to 80 percent of kidney stones are passed by men, some say that it's nature's way of evening the score.

Nearly 80 percent of kidney stones are made of calcium and oxalate, a normal acid breakdown product of many commonly eaten foods. Calcium and oxalate are both excreted in the urine and, if conditions favor it, they will condense into a stone. You can reduce the tendency for these two substances to coalesce into stones, and thus prevent the formation of these painful products of modern life.

Comments on Dr. Whitaker's Prescription for Kidney Stones

The National Institute of Diabetes and Digestive and Kidney Diseases and the Office of Medical Applications of Research from the National Institutes of Health convened the Consensus Development Conference on the Prevention and Treatment of Kidney Stones.[1] These experts recommended drinking plenty of water (my mother told me to do that), reducing calcium in the diet to less than 1,000 milligrams per day, and taking a thiazide diuretic. But if you follow these recommendations, you are going to make things worse.

At the time, it was thought that excess calcium in the diet would cause increased calcium in the urine, and therefore a tendency towards stones. Yet, according to most diet surveys, the overwhelming majority of Americans (including most kidney stone formers) don't consume nearly 1,000 milligrams of calcium a day. There has never been a scientifically controlled trial correlating reducing calcium with reduced formation of kidney stones. Recent studies published in the *New England Journal of Medicine* and the *Journal of the American Dietetic Association* have shown that an increase in dietary calcium is actually preventive against kidney stone formation, because calcium in the diet combines with oxalic acid in the gut and prevents oxalate absorption.[2] A diet low in calcium actually leads to greater stone formation.

Many kidney stone formers do have increased calcium in the urine, but it's not because of calcium in the diet, it is due to increased mobilization of calcium from the bone, which is causing osteoporosis. In short, if you followed the panel's recommendation and lowered your intake of dietary calcium, if you were an elderly woman, you would see two effects. First, you would not be reducing your chances of kidney stones. Second, you would be substantially increasing your chances of a hip fracture.

The panel also failed to mention the significant research demonstrating that reduced animal protein, a vegetarian diet, and supplementing the diet with magnesium, vitamin B6, and citrates are extremely effective in preventing kidney stones.

This panel also recommended the long-term use of one of the most dangerous diuretics available, the thiazides. Thiazide diuretics will reduce calcium excretion in the urine, and perhaps lead to reduced kidney stone formation, but they also dramatically lower potassium levels. They have been the cause of death from cardiac arrhythmia. They lower magnesium levels, probably the most important mineral for preventing kidney stones. These diuretics will elevate cholesterol levels and triglyceride levels. Increased risk for heart disease in addition to increased risk of osteoporosis are also possible outcomes of this recommendation.

Thiazide diuretics will cause diabetes in individuals who do not have it. In those who do, the drugs will dramatically worsen the effect of diabetes. The drugs will elevate uric acid levels, increasing the risk of gout.

Almost twenty years ago, a study called *MRFIT* (Multiple Risk Factor Intervention Trial) followed a large number of hypertensive patients allocated to the "aggressive" therapy arm of the study. Substantial increases of drugs were used to lower blood pressure. They were compared to an equal number of men in the less aggressive arm, but who were still receiving conventional treatment for high blood pressure. Those in the aggressive arm had a higher death rate (see High Blood Pressure, page 271). The culprit was thiazide diuretics. In 1988, a consensus panel goes on to recommend a drug that is more dangerous than the disease. This is the wrong advice.

Here are the recommendations the experts should have made. First, the amount and type of fluid intake is critical. Drink two to three quarts of pure water daily and avoid drinking coffee and alcohol. Dietary choices are critical. Eat less animal protein and more fruits and vegetables. Reduce fat and sugar consumption. Avoid vitamin D-fortified dairy products.

Now take some proactive steps. Take 1,000 milligrams of magnesium (preferably magnesium citrate) and 100 milligrams of vitamin B6 daily. Use potassium citrate or Bicitra when appropriate.

Taking magnesium and vitamin B6 (pyridoxine) daily will stop stones from developing, even in people who are extremely prone to kidney stones. The effectiveness of vitamin B6 and magnesium in this application is exceptionally well documented in the medical literature.[3] Magnesium makes calcium oxalate more soluble in the urine, and vitamin B6 reduces the production of oxalic acid in the body.

In 1974, Harvard physicians Edwin Prien and Stanley Gershoff gave 300 milligrams of magnesium oxide and 10 milligrams of vitamin B6 to 149 carefully selected patients with long-standing histories of recurrent kidney stone formation.[4] Prior to the administration of magnesium oxide and B6, this group produced an average of 1.3 stones per year. With magnesium and B6, stone production was reduced to only 0.1 stone per patient per year, a 92 percent reduction. Other studies have shown similar results.

If you look at the data on magnesium and vitamin B6, their effectiveness would so reduce the frequency of renal stones that all the lithotrypsy machines that many hospitals use to break up the stones would be useless; in fact, these vitamins and minerals could additionally break up their lithotrypsy profits.

The high rate of calcium-containing stones in affluent societies is directly associated with the following dietary patterns: low fiber, refined carbohydrates, high alcohol consumption, large amounts of animal protein, high fat, high calcium-containing food, high salt, and high vitamin D-enriched food.[5]

Eating more protein than the body requires is common among Americans. When protein ingestion is too high, it leads to increased calcium excretion in the urine. America's high protein intake is one of the main reasons we suffer from so many diet-related diseases, including those involving calcium metabolism like kidney stones and osteoporosis. Overconsumption of protein should be avoided; fresh fruit and vegetable intake should be increased.

Vegetarians have a reduced risk for developing kidney stones, and even among meat eaters, those who ate higher amounts of fresh fruits and vegetables had a lower incidence of kidney stones.[6] Also, a simple change, eating whole wheat bread instead of white, results in lower urinary calcium and reduced kidney stone formation in clinical studies.[7]

Excess body weight and faulty carbohydrate metabolism are high risk factors for stone formation; both lead to increased excretion of calcium in the urine. The common factor may be sugar (sucrose). Following sugar ingestion, there is a rise in urinary calcium. Refined carbohydrates should be restricted in the diet and replaced with complex carbohydrates like whole grains, legumes, and vegetables.[8]

If you are prone to kidney stone formation, avoid all dairy products fortified with vitamin D. Vitamin D causes increased absorption of calcium, but also increases the urinary calcium concentration. Increasing the amount of urinary calcium greatly increases the risk of stone formation. Compounding this negative effect is the fact that milk fortified with vitamin D results in lowered magnesium levels. Vitamin D-fortification of dairy products plays a definite role in kidney stone formation.[9]

Decreased urinary citrate is found in 20 to 60 percent of patients with kidney stones.[10] This is extremely important since citrate reduces urinary saturation of stone-forming calcium salts by forming complexes with calcium. If citrate levels are low, this inhibitory activity is not present and stone formation is more likely to occur. Citrate supplementation has been shown to be quite successful in preventing recurrent kidney stones. Take 450 milligrams of elemental potassium (as potassium citrate) daily. Or, have your doctor write you a prescription for Bicitra, a prescription form of sodium citrate, at a dose of one tablespoon (15 milliliters) per day.

Macular Degeneration

Dr. Whitaker's Prescription for Macular Degeneration:

1. Follow the Whitaker Wellness Program.
2. Take either *Ginkgo biloba* extract (40 milligrams, three times per day, of the 24 percent ginkgo flavonglycosides extract), or bilberry extract (80 to 160 milligrams, three times daily, of the 25 percent anthocyanidins extract).

Description

The macula is the portion of the eye responsible for fine vision. Degeneration of the macula is the leading cause of severe visual loss in the United States and Europe, in persons aged fifty-five years or older. The risk factors for macular degeneration include aging, atherosclerosis, and high blood pressure. There is no current medical treatment for the most common form of macular degeneration. Laser surgery is used for those individuals who develop a less common type of macular degeneration (exudative macular degeneration).

Comments on Dr. Whitaker's Prescription for Macular Degeneration

The origin of macular degeneration is ultimately related to damage caused by free radicals. As with most diseases related to free radical damage, prevention or treatment at an early stage is more effective than trying to reverse the disease process.

Numerous studies have shown that individuals consuming more fruits and vegetables are less likely to develop cataracts or macular degeneration, compared to individuals who do not regularly consume fruits and vegetables.[1] Fresh fruits and vegetables are rich in a broad range of antioxidant compounds, including vitamin C, carotenes, flavonoids, and glutathione. All of these antioxidants are critically involved in important mechanisms that prevent the development of macular degeneration.

In addition to eating a diet rich in antioxidants, it is essential to supplement the diet with additional antioxidant nutrients as directed in the Whitaker Wellness Program (see Chapter 2). Zinc supplementation has been shown to be of particular benefit in improving visual function in people with macular degeneration.

In a study conducted at the Department of Ophthalmology at the Utah School of Medicine, 151 patients with macular degeneration received either 100 milligrams of zinc or a placebo.[2] Those receiving the zinc had significantly less loss of vision.

Another key recommendation is to use either *Ginkgo biloba* extract (40 milligrams three times per day of the 24 percent ginkgo flavonglycoside extract) or bilberry extracts. Ginkgo has shown good results, but there is more support for bilberry (*Vaccinium myrtillus*).[3] This blue-black berry differs from an American blueberry in that its meat is also blue-black. The color is due to flavonoids known as *anthocyanosides*. These pigments are potent antioxidants and also work to improve blood flow to the eye.

Interest in bilberry was first aroused when British Royal Air Force pilots during World War II reported improved nighttime visual acuity on bombing raids after consuming bilberries. Subsequent studies showed that administration of bilberry extracts to healthy subjects resulted in improved nighttime visual acuity, quicker adjustment to darkness, and faster restoration of visual precision after exposure to glare.

In Europe, bilberry extracts are now part of the conventional medical treatment of many eye disorders, such as cataracts and macular degeneration, as well as retinitis pigmentosa, diabetic retinopathy, and night blindness. This use is supported by positive results in controlled clinical trials.[4]

The dosage for a bilberry extract is based on its content of anthocyanosides. The dose for an extract standardized to contain 25 percent anthocyanidins is 80 to 160 milligrams three times daily. Numerous manufacturers provide high quality bilberry products, including Bilberry extract (Enzymatic Therapy), Optimum Bilberry (Nature's Way), Bilberry with Ginkgo Biloba (Solgar), Bilberry (Natrol), and Bilberry-Power (Nature's Herbs).

Menopause

Dr. Whitaker's Prescription for Menopause:

1. Follow the Whitaker Wellness Program.
2. Develop a regular exercise program.

3. Use Barlean's High Lignan Flax Oil and increase the amount of phytoestrogens in the diet by consuming more soy foods, fennel, celery, parsley, nuts, and seeds.
4. Use a phytoestrogen-rich formula like Femtrol (Enzymatic Therapy), Change-O-Life (Nature's Way), or Femchange (Nature's Herbs).
5. If additional support is needed, take 300 milligrams of gamma-oryzanol each day.

Description

The skin of the head and neck of the fifty-year-old woman suddenly becomes warm and red. The feeling lasts for a couple of seconds. Sometimes it lasts longer, up to two minutes. The woman never knows when the feeling will come over her again. She doesn't know what is worse, suddenly being overcome with this sensation of heat, or the chills that sometimes follow.

For 65 to 75 percent of women in the United States, symptoms like these, known as *hot flashes,* will mark the advent of menopause. *Menopause* is the medical term that is given to denote the end of the child-bearing years and the cessation of menstruation.

Some women will feel other discomforts in association with hot flashes. These may include headache, increased heart rate, and insomnia. Hot flashes may also be accompanied by dizziness, weight gain, and fatigue. For most women, menopause arrives around the age of 50.

The signs and symptoms of the change are thought to be associated with altered functions in a part of the brain called the *hypothalamus.* The hypothalamus sits above the pituitary gland, in the center of the brain. There, it serves as the link between the nervous system and the hormonal or endocrine system. Compounds known as endorphins serve as chemical messengers between the brain and the endocrine system. They play a key role in the proper functioning of the hypothalamus. Release of pituitary hormones, rates of metabolism, body temperature, sleep patterns, libido, and mood alterations are all linked to the endorphin-hypothalamus relationship. They can all be affected during menopausal changes.

Menopause is a normal physiological process. The common medical view of menopause, however, is that it is a "condition" or "disease." With this perspective, the customary approach is to "attack the disease." Physicians often employ drug agents against the natural, shifting hormonal patterns in women. The chief weapon is hormone replacement therapy, which features varying combinations of estrogen and progesterone.

Hot flashes are usually most uncomfortable in the first one or two years after the hormonal changes of menopause commence. The body then begins to adapt to lower estrogen levels, and hot flashes typically subside.

Comments on Dr. Whitaker's Prescription for Menopause

Conventional American medicine in the past fifty years has tended to treat natural female processes as diseases. Giving birth, women were on their backs and frequently drugged, denied the benefits of gravity and their own active participation in labor. Forceps and Caesarean (C-section) delivery were common (and still are) compared to the rest of the Western world. "Man's way" was thought to be better than a woman's natural process; physicians were mostly men.

Mother's milk was also suspect. Infant formula advertisements had most physicians believing that manufacturers had one-upped Mother Nature. In general, women's natural processes became "women's problems." As the women's health movement provoked a review of the medical practices of the 1950s and 1960s, a rude discovery emerged. An unusually high number of surgeries were being performed on women's sex and birth-giving organs: hysterectomies, ovarectomies, mastectomies, episiotomies, and C-sections.

The women's health movement came to light with the 1971 publication of a book called *Our Bodies, Our Selves,* which played a seminal role in changing the way women looked at their own bodies. More women each year are entering medicine and becoming doctors. Men, however, remain in charge of the research establishment and the pharmaceutical companies.

Estrogen replacement therapy got its first big boost in 1966 in a book by Robert A. Wilson, M.D., called *Feminine Forever.* In it, he promoted the view that menopause is an estrogen-deficiency disease. The signs of this "disease," wrote Dr. Wilson, were that women became sexless "caricatures of their former selves." In short, a women would, if estrogen-deficient, become "the equivalent of a eunuch."[1] This sort of logic has emerged from a culture where aging is often viewed as a "youth-deficiency."

Wilson proposed what he thought was a simple cure: Women should have the normal supply of estrogen replaced. Instead of passing through their natural changes, the women would be "feminine forever."

Since Dr. Wilson's landmark book, the estrogen replacement research has moved in many directions. The issues include human vanity, the needs of pharmaceutical companies, major health risks, and possible promotion of cancer. The research is controversial and inconclusive.

Hormone Replacement Therapy

The healthy diet and lifestyle choices outlined in Chapter 2 are, in my opinion, the best ways to prevent the chronic problems often associated with menopause. These changes alone have been shown to provide some of the same beneficial effects of estrogen replacement therapy—without the risks. They are also the best way to maintain vitality during the aging process. Despite their value, these natural treatments are recommended less often than hormone replacement therapy.

American medicine should agree that promoting healthy diet and lifestyle choices should be at the heart of care for women during menopause. Instead, research debates are focused mostly on cost-benefit questions.

Hormone therapies of various kinds are recommended to women for a variety of reasons. The major source is birth control pills. Hormones are also prescribed for skin conditions, and they are increasingly prescribed for menopausal and post-menopausal women.

SIDE EFFECTS OF ESTROGEN THERAPY

Increased risk of cancer
Increased risk of gallstones
Increased risk for stroke or heart attack
Nausea
Symptoms similar to PMS
Breast tenderness
Depression
Liver disorders
Enlargement of uterine fibroids
Fluid retention
Blood sugar disturbances
Headache

Many chronic conditions are associated with long-term administration of estrogen. Women show an increased risk of developing certain cancers, principally, breast cancer. But a drug like estrogen, which must be administered from age 50 until death at 70, 80, or 90, is an extremely profitable product. A pharmaceutical firm wants science to say that the drug is valuable, because once a patient is on them, it is usually for life.

As in the research controversy over food additives (see page 274), we see a split between European research and research carried on in the United States. Most of the studies showing increased risk for breast cancer were performed in European countries. In the United States, most studies have shown negative.

Perhaps it is just that breast cancer risk in the United States is already so high that estrogen replacement therapy doesn't boost it further. Roughly one in nine American women are expected to develop breast cancer, the most common cancer in women in the United States. It's an awful rate. Yet the medical establishment here continues to enthusiastically recommend estrogen for various conditions and in hormone replacement therapy, and has for decades.

Experts have attempted to integrate the diverse results of the various studies on estrogen replacement therapy.[2] They have concluded that estrogen replacement therapy generally heightens the likelihood of cancer. The risk level for breast cancer rises between 1 and 30 percent.

The possible benefits of estrogen replacement therapy are diverse, such as relief of hot flashes and other uncomfortable menopausal symptoms. Another, less quantifiable benefit is that boasted by Dr. Wilson's book: "maintains femininity." Research has shown a significant reduction in osteoporosis. Furthermore, while early studies showed an increased risk for cardiovascular disease with estrogen use, more recent studies are indicating that estrogen may offer some protection against heart disease and strokes.[3]

We must evaluate this list from two perspectives: first, against the known risks; second, against the benefits of natural approaches. My own conclusion is that hormone replacement therapy may be of particular value to women who have a high risk of developing osteoporosis, or who already show signs of significant bone loss. (See Osteoporosis, page 314.) But the high rate of breast cancer in American women is argument enough that any risk should be avoided. Until a more conclusive study frees hormone replacement therapy from this killing shadow, long-term hormone therapy is not justified in most women.

Endorphins and Exercise

The endorphins which serve as messengers in the brain and endocrine system have become relatively well known in the past decade. Some exercise enthusiasts have a special relationship with these *endogenous opiates* or natural morphines. They are the body's own pain relieving and antidepressant compounds. We hear of people being "addicted to jogging." A runner will tell of moments when "the endorphins kick in."

The changing function of the hypothalamus during menopause provoked a group of Swedish researchers to look at the role of endorphins in hot flashes. They knew that exercise can increase endorphin levels. What would happen to hot flashes in women who began exercising? They set up a controlled study to test this.[4]

The researchers looked at 79 postmenopausal women who exercised on a regular basis. For the control group, they used 866 women, also postmenopausal, who did not regularly exercise. Women filled out elaborate questionnaires before and after the study. Extent of exercise was evaluated. Hot flashes were graded as mild, moderate, and severe.

The researchers found that just 3.5 hours per week of exercise led to no hot flashes whatsoever. With less exercise, hot flashes were still likely. The women who exercised were able to go through natural menopause without hormone replacement therapy. These results alone suggest that hot flashes are not best treated by estrogen replacement therapy in most cases. Physical activity presents an individual with a wide range of positive side effects. One is its positive effect on osteoporosis.

Soy Foods

In general, the dietary guidelines recommended in Chapter 2 are appropriate for menopause. I also recommend Barlean's High Lignan Flax Oil (see page 52) and increasing your intake of soy foods.

Soy is particularly rich in active estrogen-like substances known as *phytoestrogens.* Specifically, the isoflavones and phytosterols of soybeans produce a mild estrogenic effect. In a study of post-menopausal women, those women consuming the equivalent of 2/3 cup of cooked soybeans per day demonstrated signs of estrogenic activity when compared to a control group.[6] Specifically, the women consuming a variety of soy foods demonstrated an increase in the number of superficial cells that line the vagina. This increase offsets the vaginal drying and irritation common in postmenopausal women.

One cup of soybeans provides approximately 300 milligrams of isoflavone. This level is equivalent to about 0.45 milligrams of conjugated estrogens, or one tablet of Premarin. However, while estrogen replacement therapy may increase the risk for cancer, the consumption of soy foods is associated with a significant reduction in the risk of cancer.[5] The high intake of phytoestrogens is thought to explain why hot flashes and other menopausal symptoms rarely occur in cultures consuming a predominantly plant-based diet.

The ancient Chinese considered the soybean their most important crop and a necessity for life. Although the United States accounts for over 50 percent of the world's production, soy is used primarily for animal feed (protein meal) and for its oils. However, since the 1970s, there has been a marked increase in both the consumption of traditional soy foods such as tofu, tempeh, and miso, and in the development of "second-generation" soyfoods which simulate traditional meat and dairy products. Consumers can now find soy milk, soy hot dogs, soy sausage, soy cheese, and soy frozen desserts at their grocery stores.

Some other foods rich in phytoestrogens include fennel, celery, and parsley, and nuts and seeds. Fennel is particularly high in these compounds and possesses confirmed estrogenic action.[7] (If you have never had fennel, it is an absolutely delicious vegetable that can be lightly steamed or sautéed.)

Vitamin E and Vitamin C

High-dose vitamin E and C supplementation is of great benefit in relieving menopausal symptoms. There has been little research with these vitamins, but tremendous results have been noted in the few studies that have been done. For example, in the late 1940s, several clinical studies demonstrated that vitamin E is extremely effective in relieving hot flashes and menopausal vaginal complaints, when compared to a placebo.[8] Taking the amounts recommended in the Whitaker Wellness Program is sufficient.

Herbs

Many herbs historically used to tone and nourish the female glandular system during menopause are now known to contain phytoestrogens. While both synthetic and natural estrogens may pose significant health risks, including increasing the risk of cancer, gallbladder disease, and thrombo-embolic disease (stroke, heart attack), phytoestrogens have not been associated with these side effects. In fact, experimental studies in animals have demonstrated that phytoestrogens are extremely effective in inhibiting mammary tumors. The effect occurs not only because phytoestrogens occupy estrogen receptors, they also work through other unrelated anticancer mechanisms.[9]

The four most useful herbs in the treatment of hot flashes are angelica or dong quai (*Angelica sinensis*), licorice root (*Glycyrrhiza glabra*), chaste berry (*Vitex agnus-castus*), and black cohosh (*Cimicifuga racemosa*). These herbs have been used throughout history to lessen a variety of female complaints, including hot flashes.

These herbs are effective when taken individually, and combining them is thought to produce even greater benefit. Most major suppliers of herbal products feature formulas containing these herbs: Femtrol (Enzymatic Therapy), Change-O-Life (Nature's Way), and Femchange (Nature's Herbs). Take two capsules of any of these formulas three times daily.

Gamma-Oryzanol

If after one month additional support is needed, try gamma-oryzanol (ferulic acid), a growth-promoting substance found in grains and isolated from rice bran oil. In the treatment of hot flashes, its primary action is to enhance pituitary function and promote endorphin release by the hypothalamus. Gamma-oryzanol was first shown to be effective in menopausal symptoms, including hot flashes, in the early 1960s. Subsequent studies have further documented its effectiveness.

In one of the earlier studies, eight menopausal women and thirteen women who had their ovaries surgically removed were given 300 milligrams of gamma-oryzanol daily. At the end of the 38-day trial, over 67 percent of the women had a 50 percent or greater reduction in their menopausal symptoms.[10] In a more recent study, the benefits of a 300-milligrams-per-day dose of gamma-oryzanol was even more effective, 85 percent of the women reported improvement in their symptoms.[11]

Gamma-oryzanol is an extremely safe, natural substance. No significant side effects have ever been produced in experimental and clinical studies. In addition to being helpful in improving the symptoms of menopause, gamma-oryzanol has also been shown to be quite effective in lowering blood cholesterol and triglyceride levels.

Multiple Sclerosis

Dr. Whitaker's Prescription for Multiple Sclerosis:

1. Follow the Whitaker Wellness Program.
2. Take two tablespoons of flax oil daily.
3. Take *Ginkgo biloba* extract (24 percent ginkgo flavonglycoside content) at a dosage of 40 milligrams, three times daily.
4. Take a high-potency pancreatic enzyme supplement.

Description

Multiple sclerosis (MS) is a syndrome of progressive nervous system disturbances. The early symptoms of multiple sclerosis may include:

Muscular symptoms Feeling of heaviness, weakness, leg dragging, stiffness, tendency to drop things, clumsiness
Sensory symptoms tingling, "pins-and-needles" sensation, numbness, dead feeling, band-like tightness, electrical sensations
Visual symptoms blurring, fogginess, haziness, eyeball pain, blindness, double vision

Vestibular symptoms   light-headedness, feeling of spinning, sensation of drunkenness, nausea, vomiting
Genitourinary symptoms   incontinence, loss of bladder sensation,
loss of sexual function

Despite considerable research, there are still many questions
about MS. Consistent with mainstream medicine's belief in the germ
theory, research has focused on finding a viral cause for this disease.
Most current work, however, suggests immune or "host" disturbances.
(See Chapter 7 for a discussion of these two general approaches.)

In MS, the myelin sheath that surrounds nerves is destroyed. For
this reason, MS is classified as a *demyelinating disease.* Zones of de-
myelination (plaques) vary in size and location within the spinal cord.
Symptoms correspond in a general way to the distribution of the
plaques.

In about two-thirds of MS cases, onset is between ages 20 and 40.
The onset is rarely after 50. Women are affected slightly more often
than males (60 percent female to 40 percent male). The cause of MS remains to be definitively determined. Many causative factors have been
proposed, including viruses, autoimmune factors, and diet.

Comments on Dr. Whitaker's Prescription for Multiple Sclerosis

Dr. Roy Swank, Professor of Neurology, University of Oregon Medical School, has provided convincing evidence that a diet low in saturated fats, maintained over a long period of time (one study lasted
over thirty-four years), tends to halt the disease process with MS.[1]
Swank began successfully treating patients with his low-fat diet in
1948. Swank's diet recommends (1) a saturated fat intake of no more
than 10 grams per day; (2) a daily intake of 40 to 50 grams of polyunsaturated oils (margarine, shortening, and hydrogenated oils are not
allowed); (3) at least one teaspoon of cod liver oil daily; (4) a normal
allowance of protein; and (5) the consumption of fish three or more
times a week.

Swank's diet was originally thought to help patients with MS by
overcoming an essential fatty acid deficiency and by reducing the intake of saturated fats. Currently, it is thought that the beneficial effects
are probably a result of (1) decreasing platelet aggregation; (2) decreasing an autoimmune response; and (3) normalizing the decreased
essential fatty acid levels found in the serum, red blood cells, platelets,
and, perhaps most importantly, the cerebrospinal fluid in patients
with MS.

Linoleic acid, the essential fatty acid found in most vegetable oils, has been used as a treatment of MS. This has been investigated in three double-blind trials.[2] The results of the studies were mixed. Two showed an effect and one did not. A combined analysis of the three studies indicated that patients supplementing with linoleic acid had a smaller increase in disability. They also had reduced severity and duration of relapses than did controls. These studies used sunflower seed oil at a dosage of little more than one tablespoon per day. Other vegetable oils that primarily contain linoleic acid include safflower and soy.

Better results might have been attained in the double-blind studies with a few additional conditions. Dietary saturated fatty acids should have been restricted. Larger amounts of linoleic acid should have been used (at least two tablespoons per day). The studies would have showed even more positively if they had been of longer duration. In fact, one study found that normalization of fatty acid levels required at least two years of supplementation.

Even better results may be attained by using omega-3 oils as recommended in the Whitaker Wellness Program (see Chapter 2). Omega-3 oils are better because of their greater effect on platelets and the requirement for these oils in normal myelin integrity. Recommending omega-3 oils is consistent with Swank's protocol, which included the liberal consumption of fish and supplementation with cod liver oil, a rich source of omega-3 oils. Take two tablespoons of flax oil daily.

Antioxidants

Taking antioxidants at the levels recommended in the Whitaker Wellness Program is of great importance for the MS patient. MS is characterized by increased lipid peroxidation of nerve membranes. In addition, whenever the level of polyunsaturated fats is increased, so is the need for vitamin E, selenium, and other antioxidants.

I also recommend *Ginkgo biloba* extract (standardized to contain 24 percent ginkgo flavonglycosides) at a dosage of 40 milligrams, three times daily. Ginkgo is a potent antioxidant and also improves nerve function.

One final recommendation is to take Mega-Zyme (Enzymatic Therapy) or a similar high-potency pancreatic enzyme product. Studies in Germany have shown pancreatic enzyme preparations to produce good effects in reducing the severity and frequency of symptom flare-ups in MS.[3] Take two to four tablets of Mega-Zyme between meals.

Osteoarthritis

Dr. Whitaker's Prescription for Osteoarthritis:

1. Follow the Whitaker Wellness Program.
2. Take two tablets Armax (Enzymatic Therapy), three times daily.
3. Drink two 8-ounce glasses of water mixed with one tablespoon of powdered barley green juice. Use either Green Magma (Green Foods) or Kyo-Green (Wakunaga).
4. Apply capsaicin creams like Satogesic (Sato Pharmaceuticals), topically.

Description

To most physicians, the process of osteoarthritis is as inexorable as the movement of the evening sun. The job of the physician is to mute the pain of this disease.

The onset of osteoarthritis may be subtle. Just a little morning joint stiffness, most likely felt in the weight-bearing joints, the knees and the hips. Joints of the hands are also affected. This is an individual's signal that cartilage in the affected joints is slowly being destroyed.

The destroyed cartilage hardens. Bone spurs, small and large, can form. Deformity in the knuckles and joints becomes visible. For the individual, what was once stiffness is now better described as pain. Moving the limbs or fingers causes pain. Motion becomes restricted.

While there are exceptions, osteoarthritis is principally seen in the elderly. Degenerative changes from years of use are aggravated by the decreased ability in the elderly to repair. In the elderly, there is a slowing of the enzymes responsible for building up what age is tearing down. The availability of these enzymes, critically needed to provide this skilled biochemical labor, is also depleted.

The end result is not pleasant to anticipate. Roughly 80 percent of individuals over the age of fifty have osteoarthritis. Some 40 million Americans suffer from this condition. But this is not a necessary end-of-life experience.

Comments on the Whitaker Prescription for Osteoarthritis

Osteoarthritis can be halted. In many cases, this degenerative disease can be reversed through supportive natural healing. Unfortunately, the drugs that many physicians are prescribing to produce short-term benefits are actually accelerating the progress of joint destruction.

Nonsteroidal anti-inflammatory drugs (NSAIDs) such as aspirin, ibuprofen (Motrin), fenoprofen (Nalfon), indomethacin (Indocin), naproxen (Naprosyn), tolmetin (Tolectin), and sulindac (Clinoril), inhibit inflammation and pain. In the long run, however, they actually worsen the condition by inhibiting cartilage formation and accelerating cartilage destruction.[1]

In one study, physicians in Oslo, Norway, followed the course of 186 patients with X-rays of their hips.[2] Fifty-eight of the patients were taking Indocin, a powerful and very dangerous NSAID; 128 were not. Those taking the Indocin were found to have far more rapid destruction of the hip than the group that was not taking Indocin or any other NSAID. Similar results have been noted in other studies with aspirin and other NSAIDs.

When these drugs are used on a chronic basis, they can cause a number of additional negative effects. Included are gastrointestinal upset, headache, and dizziness. Close to 25,000 people a year have bleeding in the intestinal tract due to these drugs.

If current arthritis medications should be avoided, what is an arthritis sufferer to do? A naturally occurring substance found in high concentrations in joint structures appears to be nature's best remedy for osteoarthritis. This compound is glucosamine sulfate.

Glucosamine Sulfate

Glucosamine sulfate appears to be nature's best remedy for osteoarthritis. In the body, the main action of glucosamine on joints is to stimulate the manufacture of connective tissue. This is the fibrous network that holds everything together and is the primary substance of cartilage. Glucosamine is the first step to creating certain connective tissue components. Glucosamine is to connective tissue what wheat is to bread.

It appears that as some people age, they lose the ability to manufacture sufficient levels of glucosamine. The result is that cartilage loses its ability to hold water and act as a shock absorber. The inability to manufacture glucosamine has been suggested as the major factor leading to osteoarthritis. This link led researchers in Europe to ask an important question, "What would happen if individuals with osteoarthritis took glucosamine?" The results have been astonishing.

Numerous double-blind studies have shown that glucosamine sulfate is not only better than a placebo but also superior to commonly prescribed arthritis drugs.[3]

Glucosamine Sulfate versus Ibuprofen   In one study, Dr. Antonio Lopez Vaz from St. John Hospital in Oporto, Portugal, divided forty-eight patients, all with arthritis in only one knee, into two groups. One received 1.5 grams of glucosamine and the other received 1.2 grams of ibuprofen (the active component of Motrin, Advil, and Nuprin). They took these agents daily for eight weeks in a "head-to-head" trial.

The results say a lot about how two different type of substances can act. Those on ibuprofen had a rapid decrease in pain over the first two weeks. If the trial had ended then, ibuprofen would have appeared clearly as the winner. Hands down. The glucosamine sulfate users had less dramatic pain relief in the first two weeks. At the end of eight weeks, however, the arthritis pain of those on ibuprofen was on the rise again. In fact, after just four weeks, the glucosamine group had significantly less pain than the ibuprofen group.

A two-week head-to-head trial would not have proved the positive effect of glucosamine, which takes longer to be felt. At the end of two weeks, the negative effects of ibuprofen would not yet be noticed. This is how research results can be manipulated to serve a variety of special interests, not always the patient's.

Glucosamine Sulfate versus Arthritis Drugs   A group of Italian researchers compared glucosamine sulfate to Indocin in three groups of rats. The rats were induced with inflammation similar to rheumatic inflammation in humans.[4] Glucosamine was found to alter the inflammatory response in the three groups. But Indocin was much more potent. A dose of Indocin 50 to 300 times lower than of glucosamine was all that was needed.

The researchers then decided to factor toxicity into the picture. The toxicity of Indocin is 1,000 to 4,000 times greater than glucosamine. Glucosamine has no measured toxicity. The researchers concluded that treatment of inflammatory disorders with glucosamine is 10 to 30 times better than treatment with Indocin and stated: "Glucosamine sulfate can therefore be considered as a drug of choice for prolonged oral treatment of rheumatic disorders."[4]

Since osteoarthritis often requires long-term therapy, the effectiveness or potency of the therapy should be weighed against its potential toxicity. It makes little sense to dispense highly dangerous drugs when natural, nontoxic agents that increase the healing and repair of the joint surface are available. The drugs offer purely symptomatic relief. They may actually promote the disease process. Glucosamine sulfate addresses the cause of osteoarthritis. By getting at the root of the problem, glucosamine sulfate not only improves symptoms, including diminishing pain, it also helps the body repair damaged joints. This effect is outstanding, especially when glucosamine's safety and lack of side effects are considered.

Nutrient Supplementation

Glucosamine sulfate is extremely effective on its own, but it is just one part of a whole treatment plan. Most doctors seek the cure by prescribing a single agent, yet when the body sets out to heal itself, it needs and uses everything. The Whitaker Wellness Program must be used along with glucosamine sulfate for maximum benefit. Arthritis patients need a wide spectrum of nutrients, including high doses of antioxidants along with a low-fat, high-fiber diet.

Rather than a product containing glucosamine sulfate on its own, I recommend Armax (Enzymatic Therapy), a nutritional formula that also includes other important nutrients for healthy joints. Armax contains therapeutic levels of the trace mineral boron, which appears to be quite significant for osteoarthritis. Studies from a number of different countries have found that the lower the level of boron in the soil, the more often people develop osteoarthritis. Typically, the standard American diet is severely deficient in fruits and vegetables, the major food sources of boron. Hence, the intake of boron is insufficient in many Americans. Since the level of boron in foods is directly related to the level of boron in the soil, simply eating more fruits and vegetables may still not be enough to ensure adequate levels. Supplementing might be necessary.

Boron supplementation has been used in the treatment of osteoarthritis in Germany since the mid-1970s. This use was recently evaluated in a small, double-blind, clinical study. Of the patients given 6 milligrams of boron (as sodium tetraborate decahydrate), 71 percent improved, compared to only 10 percent in the placebo group.[5] The preliminary indication is that boron supplements are of value in treating osteoarthritis.

In addition to boron, Armax supplies other nutrients shown to be useful in arthritis, including PABA, niacinamide, pantothenic acid, zinc, manganese, and vitamin C.

Practical Guidelines

For my patients on nonsteroidal anti-inflammatory drugs, I eliminate these drugs over a one- to two-week period during which patients begin taking glucosamine sulfate. The effective dosage for glucosamine sulfate is 500 milligrams, three times daily. If I am prescribing Armax, the dosage is two tablets, three times daily. If I am recommending glucosamine sulfate on its own, I prescribe one 500-milligram capsule, three times daily.

Enzymatic Therapy was the first company to introduce glucosamine sulfate to the United States in its Armax and GS-500 formulas. Several other companies also supply glucosamine sulfate products to health food stores, or through nutritionally oriented physicians. Be sure to use glucosamine sulfate, and not glucosamine hydrochloride or n-acetylglucosamine. The scientific studies to date have been performed with the sulfate form. You may not see the same benefits from these other products.

Glucosamine sulfate is extremely safe and there are no contraindications or adverse interactions with other drugs. In rare instances, glucosamine sulfate may cause some gastrointestinal upset, such as nausea or heartburn. If this occurs, try taking it with meals.

The beneficial results of glucosamine supplementation are more obvious the longer it is used. Glucosamine sulfate is not an anti-inflammatory or pain-relieving drug; it doesn't directly "attack" the problem. It takes a while longer to produce results. But once it starts working, it will produce much better results compared to any drug that you may have taken previously.

Once you have achieved significant relief with glucosamine sulfate, try reducing the dosage by half. If you are still pain-free after one month at the lower dosage, you may be able to discontinue it altogether.

Two other recommendations are important:

1. Drink two 8-ounce glasses of water mixed with one tablespoon of powdered barley green juice. Use either Green Magma (Green Foods) or Kyo-Green (Wakunaga). These products are a rich source of plant enzymes, chlorophyll, and other beneficial substances.

2. Apply capsaicin creams like Satogesic (Sato Pharmaceuticals) topically. Capsaicin is a pain-relieving substance from red peppers. (It is discussed in greater detail under Rheumatoid Arthritis, page 342).

Osteoporosis

Dr. Whitaker's Prescription for Osteoporosis:

1. Follow the Whitaker Wellness Program.
2. Reduce intake of protein and sugar.
3. Take two tablets of OsteoPrime, twice daily.

Description

In 1994, the North American Menopause Society surveyed 833 women to identify the health issue that concerned them most. One-third (33 percent) said it was osteoporosis. The statistics on this condition are frightening. One in four postmenopausal women has osteoporosis. One third of all women will fracture their hips in their lifetime; one sixth of all men will. Between 12 and 20 percent of those who fracture hips will die as a result of this most traumatic of breaks in the human frame. Of those who survive, 50 percent will lose their ability to live independently. Long-term nursing home care will be the eventual outcome.

An examination of the list of known risk factors for osteoporosis begins to suggest why so many Americans are afflicted by this bone-loss condition.

MAJOR RISK FACTORS FOR OSTEOPOROSIS IN WOMEN

Postmenopausal
White or Asian
Premature menopause
Family history of osteoporosis
Short stature and small bones
Leanness
Low calcium intake
High protein diet
High refined sugar diet
Inactivity
Nulliparity (never pregnant)
Gastric or small-bowel resection
Long-term glucocorticosteroid therapy
Long-term use of anticonvulsants
Hyperparathyroidism
Hyperthyroidism
Smoking
Heavy alcohol use

More than 20 million people in the United States are affected by osteoporosis, which actually means *porous bones.* Bones become more brittle due to excessive bone loss. Age is a major factor. Bone loss in the American population accelerates after age forty. Women, particularly postmenopausal women, are at greater risk than men.

The bone loss is usually greatest in the hips, spine, and ribs, the key weight-bearing bones. Each year, 1.5 million osteoporosis-related fractures occur. Roughly 17 percent of these are hip fractures with their frequently catastrophic consequences.

Comments on Dr. Whitaker's Prescription for Osteoporosis

As a nation, we are literally losing our backbone. And our ribs and hips. Consider a statement about "care of the human frame" made by one of the leading scientists of this century, Thomas A. Edison:

The doctor of the future will give no medicine but will interest patients in care of the human frame, in diet, and in the cause and prevention of disease.

Edison died in 1931, and the future he imagined has still not arrived. My own work as a doctor is meant to support Edison's vision of a healthier future. The human suffering due to osteoporosis would be a lot less if more physicians followed Edison's advice.

Physical Activity

The most critical factor in the development of osteoporosis, the most important consideration in "care of the human frame," is exercise. A sedentary life in which the weight-bearing bones are not consciously used presents the highest risk for osteoporosis.

The effect of exercise has been shown to not only reverse bone loss but actually increase bone mass. One study looked at postmenopausal women who exercised moderately for just one hour, three times a week. These women spent 1.8 percent of the week in a moderate exercise program, 3 out of 168 hours in a week. With just this small level of commitment, the study showed, bone loss was prevented and bone mass increased.[1]

This finding does not stand alone in the research literature. Numerous studies have concluded that physical fitness is the major determining factor in the density of bones. Inactivity also increases the rates of secretion of both urinary and fecal calcium, the key mineral in bone formation. A significant negative calcium balance results.[2]

Two thoughts come to mind as I consider the health of our children and the future health of Americans. First, I am dismayed by reports of increasingly sedentary habits among young people. Perhaps a tax on the computer, video game, compact disk, and television industries can be levied to pool funds to pay for the hip replacements and long-term care of those who will be needing them in the year 2030. Call it not a "tax" but a "user fee."

On the other hand, the proliferation of sports activities for girls bodes well for developing the habit of physical activity in women. The 1970s' legal mandate for equal opportunity for girls in sports will prove to have a lasting healthcare benefit: More active women will mean less osteoporosis in women.

Diet

The health recommendations on osteoporosis that have reached the general public have focused on calcium. As noted in Chapter 2, the

FDA allows the calcium-osteoporosis claim. (The manufacturers of Tums have successfully created a belief that it is Tums, not calcium, that is actually one of the essential ingredients for bone formation.)

The focus on calcium reflects conventional medicine's single-agent approach, carried over into the realm of natural therapies. Instead of a drug, doctors want to prescribe a single vitamin, or a single mineral. This misses the point. The leading dietary player in the drama of osteoporosis is not calcium, it is the whole diet, as Edison indicated in his prescription for prevention of disease.

The high-meat diet of most Americans appears to be a major factor in osteoporosis. We know that during an individual's twenties, thirties, and forties, bone mass in meat-eaters and bone mass in vegetarians is roughly the same. Then the patterns for the two groups begin to differ. When a vegetarian reaches his or her fifties, bone loss is less than that of a meat-eater. As years go on, differences become more significant. In short, a vegetarian is less at risk for osteoporosis than a meat-eater.[3] The positive association between a vegetarian diet and lower risk of osteoporosis exists whether or not the vegetarian also consumes dairy products. The healthy association exists for both vegans (who eat no meat, no dairy, no eggs) and lacto-ovo vegetarians.[6]

The high-protein character of a meat diet seems to be the most significant source of the difference in bone loss. High protein and high phosphates are associated with an increase in urinary calcium. One study looked at the effects of raising the protein content of a diet 300 percent, from 47 grams to 142 grams. (A protein level of about 150 grams is common for an American diet.) The result of this high protein: The excretion of calcium in the urine doubles.[2]

Refined sugar is another "bouncer" for calcium.[5] As with proteins, phosphates, and a sedentary lifestyle, sugar promotes excretion of dietary calcium. The American diet matches, gram for gram, its protein and sugar intake.

The havoc on bones is increased by the stimulant coffee and its ·depressant cousin, alcohol. Both types of drinks promote a negative calcium balance. Smoking, friend of the coffee drinker and the barfly, also harms the body's calcium balance.[4]

An individual sits down with a burger. Bone loss implicated. Drink a sugary, carbonated soda high in phosphates. Bone loss double-whammy. Finish off the meal with a sweet dessert. Bone loss implicated. Feeling a little full? Head home and "veg out" in front of the TV. Bone loss implicated. Crank up a little coffee to stay awake for a late show. Bone loss implicated. Oops! A little heartburn. Take a Tums.

Calcium is not the central issue. Calcium deficiency and bone loss are symptoms of larger dietary problems.

Supplemental Nutrients

Bone is dynamic, living tissue. It is constantly being broken down and rebuilt, even in adults. The focus should not be on calcium alone. Calcium is among over two dozen nutrients that are necessary for optimal bone health.

A good foundation for an osteoporosis supplement program is to follow the guidelines in Chapter 2. The next step I recommend was developed by two of the leading nutrition-oriented physicians in the world, Dr. Alan Gaby and Dr. Jonathan Wright. For years, these doctors have taught intensive seminars designed to give conventional medical doctors the opportunity to begin to make up for the lack of nutrition education in their medical training.

These two leading physicians turned their attention to osteoporosis in the late 1980s and developed a product, called OsteoPrime, which I use in my clinic. In addition to the supplements in the Whitaker Wellness Program, I recommend that patients with osteoporosis, or at risk for it, take two tablets of OsteoPrime (Enzymatic Therapy), twice daily.

Dr. Gaby has written a book *Preventing and Reversing Osteoporosis* (Prima Publishing, Rocklin, CA, 1994), which I strongly recommend for anyone who wants to learn more about this condition. My brief discussion of important supplemental nutrients is based on his work.

Calcium   Many experts are recommending a daily calcium intake of 1,500 milligrams. This typically means that supplementation in the range of 1,000 to 1,200 milligrams is required. Supplementation of calcium has been shown to be effective in reducing bone loss in postmenopausal women.[7]

Magnesium   In osteoporosis, magnesium supplementation is as important as calcium supplementation. Women with osteoporosis have lower bone magnesium content than people without osteoporosis. They also have other indicators of magnesium deficiency.[8] In human magnesium deficiency, there is a decrease in serum concentration of vitamin D (1,25-(OH)2D3). This form of the vitamin is its most active form in supporting proper utilization of calcium. In fact, magnesium (or boron) deficiencies may result in the low levels of active vitamin D3 found in people with osteoporosis.[9]

The relationship between vitamin D and magnesium has a surprising twist when we look at vitamin D in the form most of us are used to, the "fortified with vitamin D" form in milk and other dairy products. While intake of magnesium is associated positively with active vitamin D levels, consumption of artificially fortified dairy foods actually results in decreased absorption of magnesium.[10]

Using dairy as a source of calcium has an additional problem. Between 27 and 47 percent of women with osteoporosis cannot tolerate milk. A look at the incidence of osteoporosis in cultures with diverse dietary habits reveals that the rate of osteoporosis is highest among milk-drinking cultures. It is lowest in those cultures that do not drink milk. My conclusion is that milk may not be an appropriate food to prevent osteoporosis.[11]

Vitamin B6, Folic Acid, and Vitamin B12   A good way to understand the role of specific nutrients in preventing osteoporosis is to look at a compelling theory about the origins of this condition. We know that osteoporosis is marked by losses of the mineral or inorganic phases of bone. The focus on calcium exemplifies this. We also know that in osteoporosis there is a loss of the organic or nonmineral phase. The *homocysteine theory* takes both of these losses into account.

If the amino acid methionine is not properly converted into cysteine, homocysteine levels will increase in the body. Homocysteine is shown to be problematic in a number of conditions, including osteoporosis. Concentrations of homocysteine are high in postmenopausal women. High levels are associated with the organic development of a defective bone matrix.

The likelihood of high levels of homocysteine can be reduced if methionine can be properly converted into cysteine. Vitamin B6, folic acid, and vitamin B12 are all important in this conversion. They are necessary for metabolism of homocysteine. Supplementation of folic acid has been shown to decrease homocysteine levels. Deficiencies of these necessary vitamins, common in the elderly and postmenopausal women, may lead to osteoporosis.[12] Interestingly, when folic acid is supplemented homocysteine metabolism is supported, even in women who do not show a folic acid deficiency using standard laboratory criteria.

Silicon   Silicon is responsible for cross-linking collagen strands. It contributes greatly to the strength and integrity of the connective tissue matrix of bone. We know that silicon concentrations are increased at calcification sites, the "construction sites" in growing bone. For this reason, adequate levels of silicon may be necessary before bone remodeling can take place. It is not known whether the typical American diet provides adequate amounts of silicon. It is fair to say that in patients with osteoporosis, or where accelerated bone regeneration is desired, silicon requirements may be increased. Supplementation may be indicated.

Boron   In treating osteoporosis, the trace mineral boron should be considered. While the spotlight has fallen on calcium, boron's role is only now being appreciated.[13] Just 3 milligrams of supplemental boron per day has been shown to reduce calcium excretion by almost half (44 percent).

Boron's positive benefits do not end here. It appears to be required to activate certain hormones, as well as vitamin D. Boron, like magnesium, may be required in the conversion of vitamin D within the kidney to its most active form (1,25-(OH)2D3). In addition, supplemental boron (in the study noted above) dramatically increased levels of the most biologically active estrogen, 17 beta-estradiol. In some postmenopausal women, supplementation of boron has been shown to mimic the effects of estrogen therapy.[15]

The importance of taking supplemental boron is evident from studies of American consumption patterns of boron-containing foods. Fruits and vegetables are the main dietary sources of boron. In the Second U.S. National Health and Nutrition Examination, researchers concluded that only one in ten Americans eats the recommended amounts of these foods. The recommendation is for two fruit and three vegetable servings each day. In fact, the study concluded that only 51 percent ate a single serving of vegetables a day.[14]

To be assured of an adequate dose, supplementing 3 to 5 milligrams of boron per day should be sufficient.

Estrogen

One of the most publicized effects of estrogen is its role in maintaining bone health and preventing osteoporosis. (The pros and cons of estrogen replacement therapy is covered at length under Menopause, page 303.) As noted there, I do not usually recommend estrogen replacement therapy. Natural approaches are much better—without the side effects.

There is one exception. I believe the benefits of hormonal therapy significantly outweigh its risks in women who are susceptible to osteoporosis and in women who have already experienced significant bone loss. To get a sense of your risk, take the following self-test.

Self-Test: Determining Your Risk of Osteoporosis

Choose the item in each category that best describes you, and fill in the point value for that item in the space to the right. You may choose more than one item in categories marked with an asterisk.

	Points	*Score*
Frame Size		
Small-boned or petite	10	_____
Medium frame, very lean	5	_____
Medium frame, average or heavy build	0	_____
Large frame, very lean	5	_____
Large frame, heavy build	0	_____
Ethnic Background		
Caucasian	10	_____
Asian	10	_____
Other	0	_____

Activity Level
How often do you walk briskly, jog, engage in aerobics/sports, or perform hard physical labor, of a duration of at least 30 continuous minutes?

Seldom	30	_____
1–2 times per week	20	_____
3–4 times per week	5	_____
5 or more times per week	0	_____
Smoking		
Smoke 10 or more cigarettes a day	20	_____
Smoke fewer than 10 cigarettes a day	10	_____
Quit smoking	5	_____
Never smoked	0	_____
Personal Health Factors*		
Family history of osteoporosis	20	_____
Long-term corticosteroid use	20	_____
Long-term anticonvulsant use	20	_____
Drink more than 3 glasses of alcohol each week	20	_____
Drink more than 1 cup of coffee per day	10	_____
Seldom get outside in the sunlight	10	_____
For women only:		
Had ovaries removed	10	_____
Premature menopause	10	_____
Had no children	10	_____
Dietary Factors*		
Consume more than 4 oz. of meat on a daily basis	20	_____
Drink soft drinks regularly	20	_____
Consume the equivalent of 3–5 servings of vegetables each day	–10	_____
Consume at least 1 cup of green leafy vegetables each day	–10	_____
Take a calcium supplement	–10	_____
Consume a vegetarian diet	–10	_____
Total score		_____

*If applicable, choose more than one item in this category.

Premenstrual Syndrome

Dr. Whitaker's Prescription for Premenstrual Syndrome (PMS):

1. Follow the Whitaker Wellness Program.
2. Follow the guidelines for enhancing detoxification in Chapter 4.
3. If no significant improvement is noted after two months, add 15 milligrams of pyridoxal-5-phosphate daily.

Description

The natural shift in hormones as women move through their menstrual cycle often includes an elevated estrogen-to-progesterone ratio. This shifting ratio appears to be the major hormonal factor in the frequently ill-defined symptoms of a condition known as *PMS*.

This condition, called *premenstrual syndrome* or *premenstrual tension*, can make its presence felt in many ways. As the more descriptive term premenstrual tension implies, PMS can mean irritability, backache, headache, and generalized tension. In other women, PMS appears as depression or decreased energy. Sex drive can be altered. Abdominal bloating and swelling of the fingers and toes are other symptoms.

For women between thirty and forty years of age, roughly one in three will be affected by PMS. Of those affected, about 10 percent will be debilitated by it.

Comments on the Whitaker Prescription for Premenstrual Syndrome

PMS is one of the health conditions most effectively dealt with by following the diet and supplement guidelines in the Whitaker Wellness Program (see Chapter 2). Nutrition-oriented physicians will recommend a battery of dietary changes for individuals with PMS. The aim is to help normalize hormonal levels.

REDUCE OR ELIMINATE

> Refined carbohydrates (sugars, honey, white flour)
> Other concentrated carbohydrates (maple sugar, dried fruit, fruit juices)
> Salt
> Fats, especially naturally and synthetically saturated fats
> Milk and dairy products

Caffeine-containing foods and beverages (coffee, tea, chocolate, sodas)

Alcohol

INCREASE AND FEATURE

Proteins, especially from vegetables and legumes

Essential fatty acids

Vegetables

A common occurrence in PMS is decreased liver function. For this reason, the detoxification protocols recommended in Chapter 4 may provide additional support.

Some of the nutrients recommended in the Whitaker Wellness Program have been shown to have special value in improving the symptoms of PMS in a number of studies. The most important appear to be vitamin B6, magnesium, and vitamin E.

Vitamin B6

The first use of vitamin B6 in the management of cyclical conditions in women was in the successful treatment of depression caused by birth control pills, as noted in several studies in the early 1970s. These results led researchers to determine the effectiveness of vitamin B6 in relieving PMS symptoms. Since 1975, there have been at least a dozen double-blind clinical trials. The majority of these studies demonstrated a positive effect. For example, in one double-blind, cross-over trial, 84 percent of the subjects had a lower symptoms score during the B6 treatment period.[1] Although PMS has multiple causes, B6 supplementation alone appears to benefit most patients.[2] In another study, premenstrual acne flare-up was reduced in 72 percent of 106 affected young women taking 50 milligrams pyridoxine daily for one week prior and during the menstrual period.[3]

However, not all double-blind studies of vitamin B6 have been positive.[4] These negative results may have been caused by many factors, such as the inability of some women to convert B6 to its active form due to a deficiency in another nutrient (such as vitamin B2). These results suggest that supplementing pyridoxine by itself may not result in adequate clinical results for all women suffering this disorder.

Too much vitamin B6 (in excess of 250 milligrams per day for several months) can cause neurological problems in some people. Therefore, I recommend no more than 150 milligrams per day. If you do not gain benefit from taking this amount daily after two months, you may be having difficulty converting vitamin B6 into its active form, pyridoxal-5-phosphate. To overcome this conversion difficulty, take 15 milligrams of this form of vitamin B6 daily.

Magnesium

Magnesium deficiency is strongly implicated as a causative factor in premenstrual syndrome. Red-blood-cell magnesium levels in PMS patients have been shown to be significantly lower than in normal subjects.[5] The deficiency is characterized by excessive nervous sensitivity with generalized aches and pains, and a lower premenstrual pain threshold. One clinical trial of magnesium in PMS showed a reduction of nervousness in 89 percent of the subjects, breast tenderness was reduced in 96 percent, and there was less weight gain (fluid retention) in 95 percent.[6] In another study, magnesium supplementation successfully relieved premenstrual mood changes.[7]

Vitamin E

Most of the research on vitamin E and PMS has focused primarily on breast tenderness. However, vitamin E has been shown to produce a significant reduction of other PMS symptoms in double-blind studies. In one study, nervous tension, headache, fatigue, depression, and insomnia were all significantly reduced.[8]

Prostate Enlargement (BPH)

Dr. Whitaker's Prescription for Prostate Enlargement:

1. Follow the Whitaker Wellness Program.
2. Eat 1/4 to 1/2 cup of raw pumpkin seeds daily.
3. Take 160 milligrams, twice daily, of the saw palmetto berry extract standardized to contain 85 to 95 percent fatty acids and sterols.

Description

Over half of all men over forty years of age in the United States will develop an enlarged prostate or benign prostatic hyperplasia (BPH). Often, the first sign of BPH is the need to get up in the middle of the night to urinate. Force and caliber of urination diminish. In BPH, the proper function of the bladder is obstructed by the swollen prostate. If left untreated, the prostate can pinch off the flow of urine. This condition, called *uremia,* is potentially life-threatening.

BPH is distinguished from prostatitis (see page 328), which is marked by pain during urination and sometimes a discharge from the penis. In prostatitis, the prostrate becomes inflamed or infected.

BPH must also be distinguished from prostate cancer. About 10 percent of men will develop prostate cancer at some time in their life. Of these, roughly one-fourth, or 2.5 percent of all men, will die of prostate cancer.

Diagnosing BPH

The usual methods for diagnosing BPH, and for distinguishing between BPH and prostate cancer, are inexact. The most common test is a digital exam in which a physician inserts a gloved finger into the rectum, where the lower part of the prostate can be felt. The classic sign of BPH is an enlarged or "boggy" prostate. The gland may be two to three times its normal size. With prostate cancer, the prostate is generally harder than normal, and the physician will usually have difficulty in distinguishing the gland's border.

Another trait in physical diagnosis of prostate conditions is the sensitivity of the gland. With BPH, the boggy prostate is nonsensitive, whereas the gland infected with prostatitis will usually feel tender upon exam.

Physical examination is not ultimately reliable for a couple of reasons. With BPH, the gland may not yet be swollen enough for this relatively crude diagnostic procedure. And if indeed a diagnosis as serious as cancer is suggested, further tests will be needed.

Another test is an ultrasound, which can give a definitive reading on whether or not you have BPH. Also, a type of protein that is produced by the prostate provides a useful method of distinguishing between BPH and prostate cancer. The protein is called prostate-specific antigen (PSA). In normal men, the level of this "marker" is roughly 4 nanograms per milliliter. For men with prostate cancer, the blood level of this protein will be over 250 percent higher. A simple blood test is all that is needed. The PSA test is not foolproof. Cancer is not always indicated by an elevated PSA level. BPH can move PSA levels higher. Some 90 percent of the time, however, PSA levels of 10 nanograms per milliliter or higher prove to be a good indicator of cancer. I recommend this test annually, plus a physical exam, for any men over the age of fifty who have a known risk, such as a relative who has had prostate cancer. The PSA test, while it is not perfect, has gained the endorsement of the American Cancer Society, the American Urological Association, and other physicians' groups.

Conventional Treatment

There are two conventional treatments of BPH. One is mechanical and surgical; the other is pharmaceutical.

The idea behind the surgical procedure is simple. If there is not a big enough hole for the urine to get through, create a bigger hole. The procedure is called trans-urethral resection of the prostate (TURP). The procedure is fraught with complications. First, the action does not address the more fundamental question: Why is the prostate getting bigger? Second, this procedure often makes matters worse. It should only be utilized if absolutely necessary.

In recent years, this relatively primitive bit of anatomical carpentry has taken second fiddle to a drug (mentioned in Chapter 1) called Proscar. This is the first agent that the FDA has so far approved for treatment of BPH. It has many problems associated with it. First, it is not very effective. Second, it is so toxic that the FDA recommends that pregnant women not be exposed to the semen of men who are on Proscar, due to the risk of birth defects. Third, the saw palmetto extract has demonstrated much better results.

Comments on Dr. Whitaker's Prescription for Prostate Enlargement (BPH)

The Whitaker Wellness Program will reduce the risk of BPH by addressing underlying risk factors such as elevated dietary cholesterol levels, low zinc and vitamin B6 status, essential fatty acid deficiency, and lack of physical activity.

In addition, an old folk remedy for BPH is to eat 1/4 to 1/2 cup of raw pumpkin seeds each day. This recommendation appears to be scientifically sound. We know that there is a high zinc and essential fatty acid content in pumpkin seeds. Both zinc and essential fatty acid supplementation have been shown to improve prostate function.[1]

In many cases, simply following the Whitaker Wellness Program and eating pumpkin seeds will bring about clinical improvement in BPH. If additional support is necessary, the fat-soluble extract of saw palmetto berries appears to be the best treatment.

Saw Palmetto Berry Extract (Serenoa repens)

The saw palmetto berry extract, derived from a scrubby palm tree from the West Indies, has been proven clinically to be more effective than Proscar, without the side effects.[2] That's the long and short of it.

The therapeutic value of this berry, like that of pumpkin seeds, has a long folk history. Native Americans and herbalists of the lower eastern seaboard of the United States from South Carolina to Florida, and in the West Indies where the palm is native, have long hailed the berry's reputation an as an aphrodisiac and sexual rejuvenator. Therein lies the suggestion of a possible link between BPH and impotence. This connection has not, to my knowledge, been explored in clinical trials, as it was apparently commonly explored in the homes and fields of the people of these regions.

However, like the pumpkin seed, saw palmetto has been used for centuries in treating problems of the prostate. Here, a great deal of modern scientific inquiry, together with modern methods for extraction and standardization, have supported the ancient use. A purified, fat-soluble extract was developed which contains 85 to 95 percent fatty acids and sterols. Over a dozen double-blind clinical studies have proved its effectiveness in improving the signs and symptoms of an enlarged prostate.

Studies show the saw palmetto extract to be effective in nearly 90 percent of patients. The effects will usually be felt in four to six weeks. The standard dosage of the fat-soluble saw palmetto extract (standardized to contain 85 to 95 percent fatty acids and sterols) is 160 milligrams, twice daily. If you want the best results, make sure you are using the right extract at the right dosage. Several manufacturers provide the saw palmetto extract, including Enzymatic Therapy, Solaray, Pro-Sanoa, Klabin Marketing, and Nature's Herbs.

The saw palmetto extract is completely safe. No significant side effects have ever been reported in clinical trials of the extract or with direct ingestion of saw palmetto berries. Detailed toxicology studies on the extract have been carried out on mice, rats, and dogs, which also indicate that the extract has no toxic effects.

The UroFlow Test

The urinary flow (or UroFlow) test is a measurement that we routinely perform at the Whitaker Wellness Institute in men over the age of fifty. It is a relatively inexpensive and quick measurement of prostate function. The subject simply urinates into a funnel, which drains into a beaker attached to a computerized weighing scale. The readout of the urinary flow gives the peak flow rate per second, followed by the average flow rate, as well as the total volume expelled. In addition, it will show one of the characteristic signs of prostate enlargement— dribbling.

A healthy peak urinary flow is anywhere from 35 to 50 milliliters per second. As the prostate enlarges and begins to obstruct the bladder, the high, peaked wave spreads out as both the peak flow and the average flow rate decline. We recommend that men over age fifty get a baseline Uroflow test, and repeat the test every one or two years.

In my patients with prostate enlargement, we also use the Uroflow test to measure improvement. Following are three Uroflow tests on the same gentleman. The tremendous improvement came about simply by using the saw palmetto extract.

The UroFlow Test

ENDOTEK UROFLOW   Date: 12-1-92

Summary:
Chart Speed:	6.6 cm/ml
Flow Time:	0:10 min:sec
Uro Vol:	76 ml
Peak Flow:	14 ml/sec
Peak Time:	0:03 min:sec
Avg Flow:	07 ml/sec
Total Time:	0:18 min/sec

ENDOTEK UROFLOW   Date: 1-20-93

Summary:
Chart Speed:	6.6 cm/ml
Flow Time:	0:12 min:sec
Uro Vol:	145 ml
Peak Flow:	18 ml/sec
Peak Time:	0:03 min:sec
Avg Flow:	12 ml/sec
Total Time:	0:20 min/sec

ENDOTEK UROFLOW   Date: 4-13-93

Summary:
Chart Speed:	6.6 cm/ml
Flow Time:	0:13 min:sec
Uro Vol:	236 ml
Peak Flow:	31 ml/sec
Peak Time:	0:04 min:sec
Avg Flow:	17 ml/sec
Total Time:	0:14 min/sec

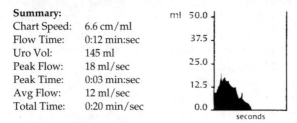

Prostatitis

Dr. Whitaker's Prescription for Prostatitis:

Acute prostatitis
1. Antibiotics are essential.
2. Take bromelain (1,800 to 2,000 m.c.u.) at a dosage of 400 to 500 milligrams, three times daily, on an empty stomach to enhance the effectiveness of the antibiotic.

Chronic prostatitis
1. Take 150 milligrams of zinc daily for one month, and 45 milligrams per day thereafter.

2. Take two capsules of Hydrastine (Enzymatic Therapy), three times daily between meals, with a large glass of water.
3. Take two tablets of Cernilton, three times daily.

Description

The condition known as *prostatitis* most often starts like this. An unusual, microscopic critter that is part bacteria, part virus is sexually transmitted. An infection grows. This infection becomes known to the carrier as pain during urinary discharge. The individual may run a fever. Perhaps there will be a discharge from the penis.

These are signs of the inflammation or infection of the prostate gland, otherwise known as prostatitis. A sample of urine or prostatic fluid will show the signs of this infection.

A wide variety of bacterial, viral, and other organisms can cause prostatitis. But this unusual viral-bacterial "critter," called *Chlamydia trachomatis,* is the most serious offender.[1] This organism is a parasite and lives within human cells. This characteristic shows its virus-like nature. But its physical structure is more like that of bacteria. It is of growing concern in sexually transmitted disease centers. Untreated, it can cause infertility. In women, chlamydia can lead to scarring of the fallopian tubes and pelvic inflammatory disease. Previous chlamydia infection is associated with a large percent of female infertility. In men, the seminal vessels (epididymus and vas deferens) become infected.

Comments on Dr. Whitaker's Prescription for Prostatitis

In the case of acute prostatitis or confirmed chlamydial infection, antibiotics are necessary. Serious scarring and blockage can occur without effective treatment. Chlamydia is sensitive to tetracyclines and erythromycin, but because it lives within human cells it is often quite difficult to totally eradicate the organism with antibiotics alone. Bromelain may help improve the effectiveness of antibiotics when they are necessary.

Bromelain refers to a mixture of enzymes from pineapple. Bromelain has been shown in clinical studies to increase serum levels of a variety of antibiotics (amoxycillin, tetracycline, and penicillin) in many different tissues and body fluids.[2] If you are taking an antibiotic for a male genitourinary infection (or for any reason), it is a good idea to take bromelain with your medication. The standard dosage of bromelain is based on its m.c.u. (milk clotting unit) activity. The most beneficial range of activity appears to be 1,800 to 2,000 m.c.u. The dosage for this range would be 400 to 500 milligrams, three times daily on an empty stomach.

Goldenseal

In chronic prostatitis due to chlamydia, I recommend goldenseal as a possible alternative to standard antibiotics. Berberine, the active compound in goldenseal, has shown antimicrobial activity against bacteria, protozoa, and fungi.[3]

Its action against some of these organisms is actually stronger than that of most antibiotics commonly used. In addition, researchers have shown berberine to prevent the adherence of bacteria to human cells.[4] By blocking adherence, infection is thwarted. Berberine has also been shown to activate the immune system, particularly macrophages.[5] These cells are responsible for engulfing and destroying bacteria, viruses, tumor cells, and other particulate matter.

Some suggestions on the possible value of berberine come from research on this natural agent with another infection caused by *Chlamydia trachomatis*. Researchers have examined the use of berberine in patients with an eye disease called *trachoma*.[6] In one study, they compared the effects of berberine (0.2 percent) to a commonly used drug, sulphacetamide (20 percent).

The results showed a pattern of effects that may exemplify head-to-head comparisons between drugs and natural agents. I call this pattern of effects the hare and the tortoise pattern. The drug (the hare in this scenario) jumps off to a fast lead. In this case, the sulphacetamide showed the best initial improvements of the trachoma, but it was administered at 100 times the concentration of berberine. The sulphacetamide was developed to directly attack the chlamydia.

Meantime, the patients on berberine saw positive effects, but more slowly. In fact, mild eye symptoms persisted in patients with berberine even after they had disappeared in many of the individuals on the drug.

If the trial were stopped at this point, sulphacetamide would be declared the winner. In short, the desire for fast relief in our speeded-up world may be the reason so many doctors prescribe the drug.

Over the long run the tortoise wins, in this case the berberine. The patients on sulphacetamide had a high rate of recurrence. Even in tests shortly after the drug was first administered, tests showed positive for chlamydia, even though the patients were not experiencing the symptoms of the infection. The drug had fooled the patients into believing that the infection was gone.

In contrast, the patients given berberine did not suffer a relapse, even a full year after treatment. After administration, the cultures from these subjects were shown to be negative for chlamydia. The activity of berberine, unlike that of sulphacetamide, does not directly attack chlamydia. It appears instead to stimulate some host defense mechanism. The berberine's long-term effect, which appears to be more curative than the drug, comes from stimulating the body's ability to heal itself. This clinical outcome, together with some of berberine's other characteristics, suggest that it may be useful in treating chlamydia-related prostatitis.

For best results, goldenseal extracts standardized for berberine content are preferred. I also recommend that goldenseal be used in conjunction with bromelain. Enzymatic Therapy is the only company I know that has put goldenseal and bromelain together in one capsule. Their product, Hydrastine, provides 200 milligrams of an 8 percent alkaloid extract of goldenseal along with 100 milligrams of bromelain and 100 milligrams of vitamin C. Take two to four capsules, three times daily between meals, with a large glass of water.

Zinc

Many men with prostate disorders are deficient in zinc. Zinc is critical to male sex hormone synthesis and action, sperm formation and motility, and overall prostate function. The prostate concentrates then secrete zinc so that the mineral can function in sperm motility, as well as the prevention of infection. In fact, the prostate has the highest concentration of zinc of any body tissue. In addition to promoting sperm motility, prostatic fluid also contains a powerful zinc-containing, anti-infective substance. Frequent prostate infections are often a sign of lack of zinc within the prostate.

The recommendation to eat 1/4 to 1/2 cup of pumpkin seeds each day applies to prostatitis as well as BPH (see page 324). In addition, in chronic prostatitis, I recommend a daily intake of 150 milligrams of zinc for one month and 45 milligrams thereafter.

Flower Pollen

Cernilton, a flower pollen extract, has been used to treat prostatitis and BPH for more than twenty-five years in Europe.[7] It has been shown to be quite effective in several double-blind clinical studies in the treatment of prostatitis due to inflammation or infection.[8] In one study published in the *British Journal of Urology*, thirteen of fifteen patients with chronic prostatitis that was unresponsive to antibiotics had either complete and lasting relief of symptoms or a tremendous improvement.

The extract has been shown to exert some anti-inflammatory action and produce a contractile effect on the bladder while simultaneously relaxing the urethra. Cernilton is available in health food stores. (If you cannot find it, call Cernitin American at 1-800-831-9505.) The standard dosage for Cernilton is two tablets, three times daily.

Psoriasis

Dr. Whitaker's Prescription for Psoriasis:

1. Follow the Whitaker Wellness Program.
2. Follow the recommendations on enhancing digestion in Chapter 3.
3. Follow the recommendations on enhancing detoxification in Chapter 4.
4. Take one teaspoon of desiccated shark cartilage (Cartilade), three times daily.
5. Apply CamoCare (Abkit), Simicort (Enzymatic Therapy), or Psoractin (Strata Dermatologics) to affected areas twice daily.

Description

Psoriasis is a skin condition which is likely to have the following origins. The body's digestion of proteins may be incomplete or the gut's ability to handle proteins may be impaired. If so, the bacteria in the gut create toxic compounds which are implicated in the development of the condition. Some of these compounds are toxic amino acids called *polyamines*. These are seen in elevated levels in individuals with psoraisis.[1] Two have particularly descriptive names: *putrescine* and *cadaverine*. A third polyamine also found in higher levels is *spermidine*.

In addition, the liver's detoxification mechanisms may be impaired. The level of polyamines and other toxins may be too high for the liver to successfully filter them out of the blood. Alternatively, a liver overburdened with other challenges may not be as effective in filtering these compounds.

These toxins get into the bloodstream. Individuals begin to know something is wrong when a rash reddens on their skin. Plaques of overlapping silvery scales may build up. The topical problem is that the skin cells are dividing at a rate roughly 1,000 times greater than normal. The rate is too fast for the skin's sloughing action. The cells accumulate, forming the plaque. The problem can be exacerbated by elevated levels in the blood of saturated fats and arachidonic acid, which are known to increase the production of the inflammatory compounds linked to this wild overgrowth of skin cells.

Psoriasis generally forms on the scalp or on the backside of the wrists, elbows, knees, and ankles. This inflamed condition may also appear in places of repeated trauma. The affected areas are sharply bordered.

Comments on Dr. Whitaker's Prescription for Psoriasis

One sign that we will have come a long way toward true health reform in this country would be if doctors, encountering psoriasis, asked themselves what is going on with the person's health to cause that? The itching of psoriasis is actually a person's body screaming to them that there's something amiss inside the body.

An old-time saying among naturopathic physicians says that "all health begins in the gut." A good case can be made that proper diet, digestion, and elimination will go a long way toward taking care of many health problems. Psoriasis is certainly one of them.

Diet

Animal foods are a triple-whammy to the body in the creation of psoriasis. First, a high-meat diet is linked to constipation. Constipation gives the bacteria in the gut a long time to create havoc-wreaking compounds. Second, meat is the main contributor to the excessive and damaging protein consumption that typifies the average American diet. The overabundance of proteins creates the elevated levels of trouble-making polyamines in the blood. Second, a high consumption of meats means elevated levels of saturated fats and arachidonic compounds. These stimulate skin cell division.

The best therapeutic diet is described in the Whitaker Wellness Program (see Chapter 2). Eliminating meats altogether, except fish, is recommended for optimal results. The value of fish is in its polyunsaturated oils, such as the omega-3 oils. The ingestion of these oils should be increased. Flax oil is also an excellent source, either in a dietary or supplemental form. Other supplemental oils may also prove beneficial. In fact, several double-blind studies have shown that supplementing the diet with 10 to 12 grams of EPA oils results in significant improvement of psoriasis.[2]

Another critical element is increasing dietary fiber. One study in a Swedish hospital looked at the effects of vegetarian diets and fasting (detoxification) on various inflammatory conditions.[3] Remarkable improvements were noted in individuals with psoriasis.

The positive benefits of the high-fiber diet are as numerous as are the negative effects of the high-meat diet. Gut-derived toxins, such as the polyamines and bacterial byproducts, are known to be associated with low-fiber diets.[4] Elimination is enhanced with increased dietary consumption of fiber.

The gut bacteria are put on a diet that promotes elimination, so they don't have as much time to convert into polyamines. Fiber strengthens the body's defense against the production of toxic compounds; in fact, fiber components bind the bowel toxins. Plant foods such as whole grains, legumes, and vegetables enhance this process. Such a diet also cuts back protein consumption.

Alcohol and the Liver

A basic task of the big sponge organ, the liver, is to take in and filter the blood. If the liver is overburdened, it can do a bad job.

The last thing an overworked liver want to see coming its way is alcohol. The liver would be much better off if it never made alcohol's acquaintance at all. Studies have shown conclusively that alcohol consumption can considerably worsen psoriasis.[5] Alcohol is also implicated in increasing the absorption into the bloodstream of toxins from the gut. Elimination of alcohol is critical to treatment of psoriasis.

Taking a load off the liver is one way to enhance its effectiveness in detoxification. Another is to help stimulate its healthy function. The extract of the milk thistle weed (*Silybum marianum*) is a great tool (see Chapter 4). This herb has a number of characteristics that suggest a positive role in psoriasis. It is known to improve liver function, inhibit inflammation, and reduce excessive cellular proliferation. Silymarin has been shown to be effective against psoriasis.[6] The standard dose is 70 to 210 milligrams, three times a day.

Shark Cartilage

Jane was 65 and had as bad a case of psoriasis as I have seen. Her legs were solid with the fiery red patches, which were also on her chest, back, and arms. She had seen a university-based dermatologist without success; her visit to me was a last resort. I started her on a shark cartilage supplement, and her improvement was immediate and miraculous. Her arms and trunk cleared completely, and the legs cleared to just a few bald patches.

The shark's skeleton is made out of cartilage, which, though very much alive, has no blood vessels. Cartilage draws in oxygen and nutrients from its surface and contains proteins that block the development of new blood vessels. This unique characteristic of cartilage is one of the reasons why shark cartilage supplements will fade psoriasis patches and seem to inhibit growth of cancer tumors. Both of these conditions require the proliferation of new blood vessels.

The National Cancer Institute initially planned to do research on shark cartilage in January and February of 1992 with studies on Karposi's sarcoma tumor in rats. This cancer occurs frequently in AIDS patients. However, NCI officials told Dr. William Lane, the developer of the product, that they did not want to appear to be "endorsing" the product by studying it. (Of course, they have no problem studying a drug.)

A survey of users of shark cartilage yielded interesting results. Although not scientific, these results are encouraging: 106 cancer patients (78.3 percent) reported fair, good, or excellent results; 140 of 158 arthritis patients (88.6 percent) reported fair, good, or excellent results; and 25 of 30 psoriasis patients (83.3 percent) reported fair, good, or excellent results.

You can get shark cartilage at health food stores (look for the tradename Cartilade) or directly from Ocean Health Products, Inc., P.O. Box 860, Putney, VT 06346, 1-800-477-5108.

Desiccated shark cartilage is nontoxic, and doesn't even taste bad. It has a slightly fishy odor and can be mixed with fruit juice, water, or applesauce. Take one teaspoon of Cartilade, three times a day.

Topical Creams

A number of excellent all-natural creams can be used in place of cortisone creams in the topical relief of psoriasis (just as they can be used with eczema). Preparations containing extracts of licorice and German chamomile are the most active. CamoCare (Abkit) is worth a try and so is Simicort (Enzymatic Therapy). Both contain ingredients (chamomile extract in CamoCare; and chamomile, licorice, and allantoin in Simicort) that have demonstrated an effect equal to or superior to cortisone when applied topically. Unlike cortisone creams, these topical agents are without side effects.

Another good topical formula to try contains fumaric and lauric acid esters. The product name is Psoractin (Strata Dermatologics). Topically applied fumaric acid esters are a popular treatment for psoriasis in Europe.

Rheumatoid Arthritis

Dr. Whitaker's Prescription for Rheumatoid Arthritis:

1. The first step is therapeutic fasting or an elimination diet followed by careful reintroduction of foods. Note any symptom-producing foods.
2. Eliminate all animal products from the diet, with the exception of cold-water fish.
3. Follow the Whitaker Wellness Program.
4. Take one to two servings of Green Magma (Green Foods) or Kyo-Green (Wakunaga), powdered drink mixes of the dried juice of young barley leaves, one tablespoon, once or twice daily.
5. Follow the recommendations for enhancing digestion in Chapter 3.

6. Take a 10X USP pancreatic enzyme product at a dosage of 500 to 1,000 milligrams, three times a day, 10 to 20 minutes before meals.
7. Take Curazyme (Enzymatic Therapy), or similar curcumin and bromelain combination, to provide a dosage of 400 to 600 milligrams of each, three times daily between meals.
8. Take desiccated shark cartilage like Cartilade (Cartilage U.S.A.), as directed.
9. Apply capsaicin-containing creams topically.

Description

Rheumatoid arthritis is a chronic condition that continues to befuddle researchers. A simple causal factor has not been found. Most of the conventional therapies are of short-term value at best. Many make the condition worse.

The first signs of this condition tend to appear gradually. An individual, usually between twenty and forty years of age, will begin to feel joint stiffness or vague pain in the joints.[1] Other individuals may feel a low-grade fever, fatigue, or weakness. But the reason for these signs and symptoms will not yet be clear to the individual.

Then, several weeks later, some of the individual's joints will become warm, tender, and swollen. In about a third of those afflicted, the signs will be confined to just one or two joints.[1] More often, the swelling will appear in a symmetrical fashion. Both wrists may be involved, or both hands, or both ankles. The skin around the affected joints turns a purplish color. For a minority of individuals, the onset can appear quite rapidly. If the disease progresses, the swelling will become a visible deformity. The hands and feet are most often affected.

Rheumatoid arthritis is an example of a condition where the body is actually at war with itself. This is called an *autoimmune condition*. In such conditions, for a single reason or a pattern of reasons, the immune system begins attacking the body's own tissues. In rheumatoid arthritis, antibodies develop to target the joint tissues. The result is the chronic inflammatory character of this arthritis. The condition develops in women three times as often as in men. Between 1 and 3 percent of the population will suffer from this potentially debilitating internal conflict.

Researchers have looked high and low to discover what triggers this autoimmune reaction. Some of the leading candidates are genetic factors and obscure microorganisms. A cluster of possibilities are food-related: allergies, diet and lifestyle factors, and abnormal bowel permeability. Low levels of antioxidants are a risk factor. The picture that has emerged thus far is of a multifactorial disease. Common sense suggests that a multifactorial response would be recommended.

NSAIDs, Corticosteroids, and Disease-Modifying Drugs

Standard medical treatment has focused on suppressing symptoms, with three tiers of successively more risky drug therapies. For rheumatoid arthritis, treatment usually involves aspirin and other NSAIDs (nonsteroidal anti-inflammatory drugs). The effect of this treatment is a net-negative. The symptoms may be suppressed so the individual feels less pain for a time. But in the long run, these drugs actually make the condition worse.[2]

NSAIDs can cause ulcers, the ultimate form of permeability: perforation, holes in the GI tract. Many harmful agents can pass into the system, and do, where they cause harm. Each year, 20,000 individuals with rheumatoid arthritis who are on NSAIDs end up in the hospital due to these side effects. Each year, 2,600 people with this disease will die because of the NSAID therapies.[3]

For many people with rheumatoid arthritis, NSAIDs do not prove at all effective in controlling symptoms. The next line of attack is usually long-term administration of corticosteroids. Most experts and medical textbooks, aware of the harmful side effects in such long-term administration, clearly state that such a therapeutic course is "ill-advised." Yet the practice continues.

Like NSAIDs, corticosteroids ("steroid" anti-inflammatory drugs) are used to suppress symptoms and control inflammation. These agents are so powerful that, even at lower doses, a handful of side effects are not just possible, they are expected. On less than 10 milligrams per day, an individual will feel increased appetite. Salt and water will be retained. The individual will gain weight. And the person will get sick more often. Research shows an increased susceptibility to infections in rheumatoid arthritis patients on corticosteroids.

The extent and type of side effects from corticosteroids is a function of both the dose and the length of administration. Too much of a corticosteroid in a short period of time is not the causal factor. The side effects noted above reflect chronic use.

If the dose is stepped up, a whole cascade of problems can emerge. There are cosmetic problems, such as acne and increasing facial hair on women. Individuals may begin to feel muscle cramps and weakness. The individual's skin may thin and weaken. Peptic ulcers may develop. Blood pressure may rise, with its attendant risks. Diabetes can develop. So can osteoporosis. Susceptibility to blood clot formation increases. Meantime, over one half (57 percent) of individuals on corticosteroids feel depression, or other mental or emotional disturbances. This is not surprising, considering the onslaught of side effects overlaid on their original disease.

A third tier of drug therapy is used if both of these toxic approaches fail. These are disease-modifying drugs. Methotrexate, cyclophosphamide, penicillamine, hydroxychloroquine, azathioprine, and gold therapy are examples. These measures are more toxic. And they don't replace NSAIDs or corticosteroids. They are administered simultaneously.

A long-term study is necessary to get a good sense of the risks and benefits of this aggressive drug treatment. A recent study in the prominent British journal *The Lancet* looked at 112 patients who were on drug therapy after a twenty-year interval.[4] Over one third (35 percent) had died. Another fifth (19 percent) were severely disabled. Most of the mortality and morbidity was directly related to rheumatoid arthritis and its treatment. Just 18 percent were able to carry on normal lives.

There may be some short-term benefits from these drugs. But clearly, in the long run, these therapies are not curing rheumatoid arthritis. When side effects are taken into consideration, a cost-benefit analysis results in a clear net-negative outcome.

Comments on Dr. Whitaker's Prescription for Rheumatoid Arthritis

The known outcomes of conventional treatment are the best argument for employing the natural approach. What I recommend may not be as "easy" as taking aspirin or popping pills. A serious, habit changing intervention for individuals with rheumatoid arthritis is the best course, starting today.

The first step in my prescription is a therapeutic fast, followed by careful reintroduction of foods to rule out food allergies. (Chapter 4 describes a fast. See Food Allergies for a description of the elimination diet, page 245.) These steps should be followed by a vegetarian diet. I recommend this step, this commitment, as a simple yet extremely effective measure to get off the drugs.

A study conducted in Norway at the Oslo Rheumatism Hospital took two groups of patients suffering from rheumatoid arthritis.[5] One group followed a therapeutic diet (the treatment group); the other group (the control group) was allowed to eat as they wished. Both groups started the study by visiting a "health farm," or what we in America call a "spa," for four weeks.

The treatment group began their therapeutic diet by fasting for seven to ten days. Dietary intake during the fast consisted of herbal teas, garlic, vegetable broth, a decoction of potatoes and parsley and the juice from carrots, beets, and celery. No fruit juices were allowed.

Patients with rheumatoid arthritis have historically benefited from fasting. However, strict water fasting should only be done under direct medical supervision.[6] Fasting decreases the absorption of allergic food components. It also reduces the levels of inflammatory mediators. A juice fast or a fast similar to the one used in this study is safer than a water fast and may actually yield better results. Short-term fasts of three to five days duration are recommended during acute worsening of rheumatoid arthritis.

After the fast, the patients reintroduced specific food items every second day. If they noticed an increase in pain, stiffness, or joint swelling within two to forty-eight hours, this food was omitted from the diet for at least seven days before being reintroduced a second time. If the food caused worsening of symptoms after the second time, it was permanently omitted from the diet.

The results of the thirteen-month study indicated that short-term fasting followed by a vegetarian diet resulted in "a substantial reduction in disease activity" in many patients. The researchers concluded that the improvements were due primarily to elimination of food allergies and changes in dietary fatty acids.

Additional studies have also shown the value of eliminating food allergies for some individuals with rheumatoid arthritis.[7] Certain foods pop up regularly as problematic. The nightshade family is on this list. These foods include tomatoes, potatoes, eggplants, peppers, and tobacco. Food additives can be a problem. And many "staple" foods in the customary American diet are also on this list: wheat, corn, meat, and dairy products.

Don't be overwhelmed by the thought of giving up all these foods. First, a return to good health rarely comes in drug form; it certainly doesn't for those with rheumatoid arthritis. Second, there is a huge world of food choices out there, once a person breaks out of the fence of his or her habits and begins to explore. Finally, helping your arthritis will also strengthen your immune system in general. You won't be as likely to be sick as often.

Some European countries actually cover "spa therapy" in their national health plans. Taking the time to retreat and focus on engaging dietary and lifestyle habit changes is helpful. Although I have not seen statistics on this, I would bet that this investment of money proves cost-effective for these governments in the long run.

Food Digestion

Many autoimmune diseases have a common denominator in elevated levels of circulating "immune complexes" which then are deposited in body tissues. Diseases where this is found include rheumatoid arthritis, lupus erythematosus, periarteritis nodosa, scleroderma, ulcerative colitis, Crohn's disease, and multiple sclerosis. The trick is to keep these complexes out of the bloodstream. That means working on digestion so they are better metabolized and eliminated.

Help comes from some natural agents (described in Chapter 3), which assist the pancreas in its digestive tasks. The agents are pancreatic enzymes. Individuals with rheumatoid arthritis tend to be deficient in pancreatic enzymes.[8] Experimental and clinical studies have shown that preparations of protease enzymes lower levels of circulating immune complexes. Clinical improvements have followed this decrease. Supplementing the diet with pancreatic enzymes helps people feel better. I recommend 500 to 1,000 milligrams of a 10X pancreatin product (see page 71), three times each day, 20 minutes before meals.

An individual with rheumatoid arthritis may be deficient in another key digestive agent, hydrochloric acid.[9] I recommend the self-test for possible hydrochloric acid need (described in Chapter 3).

Dietary Fats

Research is increasingly coming clear on why rheumatoid arthritis should be added to the list of serious health conditions affected by intake of problematic fatty acids. Some of these acids are servants of the inflammatory process. They form inflammatory compounds, known as *thromboxanes* and *leukotrienes*. Animals fats, especially arachidonic acid and saturated fats, appear to be the most devout of these servants of the inflammatory process.

The good news is that by choosing what you eat, you can keep the animal fats away, and send in instead plant oils and omega-3 oils from fish that not only don't increase inflammation but actually inhibit it. EPA and GLA supplements have been shown to produce benefit when used in high doses.[10] My recommendation with rheumatoid arthritis is, in addition to using flax oil as detailed in the Whitaker Wellness Program, take enough fish oil capsules to provide 1.8 grams of EPA each day. Once significant benefit has been achieved, the dosage of fish oils can be cut in half.

Antioxidants

Rheumatoid arthritis is characterized by a tremendous amount of oxidative damage. Because antioxidants are known to prevent oxidative damage, researchers have long postulated that low levels of antioxidants may be a significant risk factor for developing rheumatoid arthritis.

Results from a recent study seem to support this hypothesis. The study followed 1,419 adult Finnish men and women over a twenty-year period.[1] Blood levels of vitamin E, beta-carotene, and selenium were determined. Those individuals who developed rheumatoid arthritis had lower levels of these antioxidant nutrients, compared to individuals who did not develop rheumatoid arthritis. The sum of these antioxidants were totaled into what the researchers termed the *antioxidant index*. The researchers found a highly significant link between a low antioxidant index and the likelihood of developing rheumatoid arthritis.

This research suggests that individuals with rheumatoid arthritis should make sure that their diet is rich in foods high in antioxidants and that they take additional supplements as recommended in Chapter 2. To further boost antioxidant levels in rheumatoid arthritis, I recommend using either Green Magma (Green Foods) or Kyo-Green (Wakunaga). These products are powdered drink mixes made of the dried juice of young barley leaves. Take one to two servings each day.

The Whitaker Wellness Program

My wellness program will go a long way in providing the nutritional support required by a person with rheumatoid arthritis. Its focus is on plant foods, the inclusion of omega-3 fatty acids, provides exceptional levels of dietary antioxidants.

Curazyme

Curazyme (Enzymatic Therapy) is a combination of curcumin, the yellow pigment of *Curcuma longa* (turmeric), and bromelain, the anti-inflammatory enzyme from pineapple. Both of these compounds have been shown to be of benefit in the treatment of rheumatoid arthritis and other inflammatory conditions. In one double-blind clinical trial in patients with rheumatoid arthritis, curcumin (1,200 milligrams per day) was compared to phenylbutazone (300 milligrams per day).[11] The improvements in the duration of morning stiffness, walking time, and joint swelling were comparable in both groups. However, it must be pointed out that while phenylbutazone is associated with significant adverse effects, curcumin has not been shown to produce any side effects at the recommended dosage level.

The recommended dosage for curcumin and/or bromelain (1,200 to 1,800 m.c.u.) in inflammation is 400 to 600 milligrams of each, three times a day on an empty stomach, twenty minutes before meals.

Shark Cartilage

Rheumatoid arthritis depends upon the generation of new blood vessels. This need implies that factors like shark cartilage, which inhibits the generation of new blood vessels (angiogenesis), may offer some therapeutic benefit. (The value of this agent is described under Psoriasis, page 334.) A survey of users of shark cartilage demonstrated that 140 of 158 (88.6 percent) arthritis patients reported fair, good, or excellent results.

You can get shark cartilage at health food stores (look for the trade name Cartilade) or at a discount from Ocean Health Products, Inc., P.O. Box 860, Putney, VT 06346, 1-800-477-5108).

For best results, here is what I recommend for using shark cartilage in cases of rheumatoid arthritis:

1. *As a retention enema:* Add 2 1/2 rounded teaspoons of Cartilade to 2/3 cup of body-temperature water. Pour mixture into an enema bag. Insert mixture into the body as a retention. Hold fluid for at least 30 minutes, longer if possible.

2. *For oral absorption:* Mix one teaspoon of Cartilade in juice, water, or applesauce and consume this twice a day.

Red Pepper

Cayenne pepper (*Capsicum frutescens*) contains a pungent principle known as *capsaicin.* When applied to the skin, capsaicin is known to stimulate and then block the transmission of the pain impulse. It does this by depleting the nerves of a messenger substance called *substance P* (the P stands for pain). In addition to playing a key role in the pain impulse, substance P has also been shown to activate inflammatory mediators into joint tissues in both osteoarthritis and rheumatoid arthritis.

In one study of seventy patients with osteoarthritis and thirty-one with rheumatoid arthritis, the subjects were instructed to apply 0.025 percent capsaicin cream or its vehicle (placebo group) to painful knees four times daily.[12] Pain relief was assessed using visual analog scales for pain and relief, a categorical pain scale, and physicians' global evaluations. Most of the patients continued to receive their arthritis medications. Significantly more relief of pain was reported by the capsaicin-treated patients than the placebo patients, throughout the study. After four weeks of capsaicin treatment, patients with either rheumatoid arthritis or osteoarthritis demonstrated mean reductions in pain of 57 percent and 33 percent, respectively. Overall evaluations indicated that 80 percent of the capsaicin-treated patients experienced a reduction in pain. A slight, transient, burning sensation was felt at the sites of application by twenty-three of the fifty-two capsaicin-treated patients, but only two patients withdrew from treatment because of this side effect.

The product used in this study was a nonprescription topical capsaicin product known as Zostrix. A stronger product, Zostrix HP, contains 0.075 percent capsaicin, three times the amount found in Zostrix. Both products are expensive. A 2-ounce tube of Zostrix HP costs about $45. However, several companies now offer capsaicin-containing products at a more reasonable price. For example, Sato

Pharmaceuticals makes a 2-ounce arthritis formula content, Satogesic, with 0.04 percent capsaicin that retails for about $5. (Call the company at 310-793-0509 for information on distributors in your area.)

Sinus Infection

Dr. Whitaker's Prescription for Sinus Infection:

1. Eliminate food allergies.
2 Take 1,000 milligrams of vitamin C, or as much as your bowel will tolerate (see page 41) every waking hour.
3. Use goldenseal and bromelain in combination at recommended levels.
4. Take measures to promote mucus drainage.

Description

The mucous membranes of the sinus swell up. Drainage of the sinus is blocked. A key pathway for the body to get rid of problematic fluids is closed. Behind this barrier, bacteria normally present in the sinuses overgrow. An infection takes hold in the sinus cavities around the eyes and nose. The individual hit with this pattern of infectious activity feels pain or pressure in the head. A yellow-green mucous discharge from the nose results. The diagnosis: sinusitis.

The cause of sinusitis can vary. In the person for whom this process is a rare occurrence, acute sinus infection is generally preceded by a common cold. Other individuals have repeated and chronic experience of these symptoms. For them the likely cause is allergies or other forces that induce swelling and fluid retention in the mucous membranes.

In either the acute or chronic condition, the body's normal method of protecting against infection through discharge from the nose is obstructed. Your body wants to discharge problematic substances from the nose. But the exit is blocked.

A conventional approach to the problem is to shrink the swelling with antihistamine nasal sprays. This can provide short-term relief. But while "fast, fast, fast" relief may be its selling point, "long-lasting" relief is not. Something caused the swelling. What is it? The antihistamines don't address this question. In fact, a rebound effect often results from these sprays. The shrinkage under the influence of the spray confuses the body for a moment and the swelling returns, creating even greater congestion.

With chronic sinusitis conditions, antibiotics are commonly prescribed. However, the bacteria didn't cause the problem; they took advantage of a situation conducive to their overgrowth. Those who take antibiotics for chronic sinusitis often have to take repeat courses.

The results of some studies question whether antibiotics are, in fact, any better than doing nothing at all. One such study was recently published in the *Journal of Allergy and Clinical Immunology*.[1] Some subjects were given an antibiotic, either amoxicillin, amoxiciloin clavlanate potassium, or trimethoprim-sulfamethoxazole. Others were given no therapy. The percentage of responders and nonresponders was similar in each group.

Comments on Dr. Whitaker's Prescription for Sinus Infection

My prescription is twofold. First, assist the body in draining mucus. Second, keep conditions from developing which will swell up the sinus and provide the mucous reservoir in which bacteria can multiply. Focus on keeping the condition from recurring.

First, if you are already feeling some sinus pain, I suggest three simple, common sense, inexpensive, natural measures for acute conditions. The technological implements for these medical procedures are less sophisticated than those used to create antihistamines and antibiotics. The medicine chest includes hot or warm water, towels, gravity, a bulb syringe, and some exotic medical agents called salt and baking soda.

Strategy number one features gravity. On page 175, I describe the postural drainage technique. With sinusitis, use a warm towel or a hot water bottle in the place of a poultice. A poultice should not be used on the face.

Strategy number two involves warming a concoction of two cups of water, a teaspoon of salt, and a pinch of baking soda. Pinch one nostril and breathe in the mix through the other. This "washes" the nostril. The sensation can be a little unpleasant at first but it gets easier. Or, alternatively, use a bulb syringe to squirt the water in the nostril. Then gently blow your nose. This can help rinse out the offending agents.

Another technique involves heated water and a towel. Heat the water until it is steaming, then place the towel over your head to create a tent and hold your tented head over the steaming water. Breathe in the steam for at least 10 minutes; this will help open up the nasal passages. I recommend doing this twice a day. Some find it helpful to put a little Vick's VapoRub or White Flower Balm in the water.

Even for those with a rare, acute condition, these simple techniques should be all your body needs to work the infection out of your system.

Chronic Sinusitis

Chronic sinus problems require a solution that focuses on finding the "chronic" cause. Most long-term problems are associated with allergies. Some are from foods. Some are airborne. A good place to start, in an acute phase of a chronic problem, is to immediately discontinue eating the group of foods most associated with development of sinusitis. These are milk, wheat, eggs, citrus, corn, and peanut butter. This prescription, however, does not determine the allergens that are most prominent for a given individual with sinusitis. For these individuals, I recommend reading and following the recommendations in the section on food allergies (see page 342). The problematic substances must be isolated and eliminated.

I also recommend use of immune-enhancing herbs, including goldenseal and bromelain. (I discussed these herbs under Bronchitis and Pneumonia, page 174.) Follow the same recommendations to help strengthen your immune system against sinus infection.

Stroke

Dr. Whitaker's Prescription for Stroke:

1. Follow the recommendations for Cerebral Vascular Insufficiency (see page 189).
2. For individuals with a history of high blood pressure (page 269) or atherosclerosis (page 88), follow the recommendations in those sections.
3. For high-risk individuals, follow standard medical treatment, using a coumadin preparation and aspirin in a dose of at least 900 milligrams per day.

Description

A stroke is basically the end-stage of one or more chronic health problems. Specifically, a portion of the cerebral vascular system moves beyond "insufficiency" to "dangerous." Suddenly blood, and the oxygen it carries, cannot make it to the brain. Alternatively, blood escapes the vascular system and leaks outside the walls of the blood vessels in the brain. A part of the brain is damaged.

Strokes hit individuals and families of victims as a sudden shock. But the process that leads to them has been underway and probably giving warnings for a long while before it happens. Epidemiological statistics report "stroke" as the third leading cause of death for Americans, behind heart disease and cancer. But an understanding of stroke suggests that most often they result from a long history of atheroscle-rosis or high blood pressure. The cause of death, the finger that pulls the trigger known as stroke, is more likely the slower process of in-creasing cerebral vascular insufficiency.

A third of the people who suffer a stroke die from it. Another third suffer permanent handicaps. The final third have no lasting effects.

Comments on Dr. Whitaker's Prescription for Stroke

Standard medical treatment of stroke focuses on preventing the end-stage of this long process in which the brain's supply of blood, and therefore oxygen and nutrients, is impaired. The treatment focuses on preventing the formation of blood clots. The main agents are coumadin preparations like Warfarin. Aspirin at 900 milligrams per day is generally recommended, along with these drug agents, because of aspirin's blood-thinning effect.[1]

If patients are at high risk of a stroke, I think the standard recom-mendation is sound. However, while focusing on the proximate cause (the blood clot), this therapy neglects more basic causal factors, like atherosclerosis or conditions leading to high blood pressure. I strongly recommend that individuals follow my recommendations for cerebral vascular insufficiency. Those with atherosclerosis or high blood pres-sure should also follow the recommendations in those sections.

An agent of particular value in my program for those who have a chance to recover from a stroke is the long-term use of *Ginkgo biloba* ex-tract. This remarkable herb is described at length in the section on cere-bral vascular insufficiency. Researchers have reported its positive value in individuals who have had strokes. Ginkgo was shown to improve blood flow and blood viscosity in these patients.[2] Note that ginkgo can be taken side-by-side with prescription medicines. I recommend 40 milligrams, three times per day, of the 24 percent ginkgo flavonglycoside extract.

If you are prescribed aspirin as part of a medical plan for recov-ering from a stroke, going too easy on the aspirin dose will lose its ef-fect. Some doctors prescribe low-dose aspirin for those with a past experience of transient ischemic attacks. We know, however, that less than 900 milligrams per day is not effective.[1]

Ulcer

Dr. Whitaker's Prescription for Ulcer:

1. Take two to four 380-milligrams chewable tablets of DGL (degly-cyrrhizinated licorice) twenty minutes before meals three times daily.

2. Follow the Whitaker Wellness Program.
3. Avoid milk products and eliminate all food allergies.

Description

It is a remarkable fact of the body's activity that the acid secreted by the stomach does not eat right through the stomach lining. After all, stomach acids are strong enough to break down meat or animal flesh. Why don't these powerful acids also then break down the human flesh that contains these foods during this part of the digestive process? The reason is that the tissues of these digestive organs have some protective characteristics that are just as remarkable as our digestive acids are potent.

Mucoprotective substances provide a protective lining for these cavities and passages. In addition, when harsh stomach juices come in contact with the stomach walls and intestinal linings, special secretions are emitted to neutralize the acids. Intestinal cells are constantly renewed. When all of these protective factors are functioning properly, these sensitive surfaces are protected from ulceration by stomach acids.

For people with ulcers, a loss of the protective lining allows the acids to burn a hole, or *ulcer*. If the acids burn the lining of the stomach, the result is called a *gastric ulcer*. If the burn is on the initial section of the small intestine, it is called a *duodenal ulcer*. These are both forms of *peptic ulcers*.

Not surprisingly, the first signs a person may have of an ulcer is a burning sensation. Some call it "heartburn." Others feel an ache or gnawing pain. The onset usually comes between forty-five minutes and an hour after mealtime.

Conventional Treatment

Current medical treatment focuses on one part of the equation: the level of stomach acids. One step is to counter the levels of gastric acid by taking antacids. These over-the-counter medications can often bring great relief to the ulcer sufferer.

A more severe step is to take drugs which block the secretion of stomach acids in the first place. This drug strategy targets the histamines that give stomach walls a message to secrete acids. If these agents could be blocked from "landing" on their receptor sites in the stomach, acid output could be greatly released.

A group of anti-ulcer drugs called H2-receptor antagonists were developed. Common examples of these drugs are Tagamet (cimetidine), Zantac (ranitidine), Pepcid (famotidine) and Axid (nizatidine).

In most cases, the successful interference in the activity of the histamines brings immediate relief.

However, the success of these drugs depends on their disruption of the body's natural digestive process. Stomach acids are necessary for proper digestion. Without proper digestion, even the best of diets can go down the tube without being assimilated, or, alternatively, have trouble going down the tube. In fact, diarrhea and constipation are among the common side effects of the H2-receptor antagonists. Impaired digestion can lead to nutrient deficiencies. Nausea is also common.

The list of possible side effects of the H2-receptor antagonists does not end here. Physiological effects of this drug include breast enlargement in men, headache, dizziness, insomnia, depression, osteoporosis, liver damage, and impotence. These drugs are also associated with an additional range of adverse reactions when combined with other drugs.

Manufacturers of this class of prescription-only drugs are pushing to have them approved for over-the-counter purchase. This does not seem wise. These drugs may have a reputation of being relatively safe, but they interfere with a vital bodily function, and they can create some dangerous side effects.

Peptic ulcers can be extremely dangerous. The ulcerated lining of the skin can perforate. Fluids can move into the body, where they don't belong. Hemorrhage and obstruction are two other potential complications. All these require immediate hospitalization. An individual with a peptic ulcer should be under the care of a physician, even if he or she is following my prescription.

Comments on Dr. Whitaker's Prescription for Ulcer

Therapies for ulcer have to focus on more than one part of the whole picture that leads to ulcers. They need to address why the stomach acids are overpowering the protective forces in the stomach and intestine. What is causing these forces to be out of balance? Is there some way to assist the protective factors to do their job more efficiently and effectively?

First, we know that the imbalance between the acids and protective factors is associated with a number of diet and lifestyle causes. Alcohol and cigarette smoking are linked to development of peptic ulcers. A low-fiber diet, nutrient deficiency and stress are also implicated. The Whitaker Wellness Program in Chapter 2 addresses all of these causes. It goes a long way toward preventing and treating peptic ulcers.

Another strategy for removing the cause of an ulcer is removal of food allergies. A great deal of evidence points to food allergy as a prime causative factor in ulcers.[1] Research also gives evidence that treating peptic ulcers and preventing new ulcers by removing food allergies is also very effective.[2] This therapeutic approach will likely produce many positive side effects.

Many people soothe peptic ulcers by drinking milk. This is an example of a "home remedy" that might actually be doing a person harm. Allergies are known to be a major causal factor in development of ulcers, and milk is a highly allergic food. Milk is known to greatly increase stomach acid production and aggravate ulcer symptoms.[3] Population studies show that the rate of peptic ulcer is higher when the consumption of milk is high in the population. In short, milk for treating ulcers is a natural remedy that should be discarded.

DGL

The preventive recommendations above are the best steps toward creating a long-term, ulcer-free environment in your stomach and duodenum. But what of treating the burning ulcer that has already happened?

One approach is to stimulate the protective abilities of the stomach and duodenum. Such an approach, if successful, is without the harmful side effect of interfering with the production of digestive acids. A remarkable natural agent, altered to remove a problematic compound, has been shown to successfully target this protective mechanism. Studies have shown it to be both safer and superior to Tagamet and Zantac, the most popular of the H2-receptor antagonists. This safer agent is a form of the licorice root called *deglycyrrhizinated licorice*, or DGL.

First, the licorice root is altered. Licorice normally contains a compound called *glycyrrhizin*. This agent produces some of the same effects in the human as the endogenous hormone known as *aldosterone.* It can elevate blood pressure and lower potassium levels. Researchers in Europe developed a way to remove glycyrrhizin from the licorice root and make the licorice into a chewable tablet. In this form, DGL has been used throughout Europe for years to treat stomach ulcers. No side effects are associated with it.

How does DGL work? Rather than decreasing stomach acid secretion, it enhances the normal defense mechanisms of the stomach and intestinal cells. DGL is known to increase the number of the cells with the protective responsibility of forming the mucosal lining. DGL appears to increase the life span of the intestinal tract cells. It also enhances blood flow to the lining of the intestinal tract. By way of comparison, Tagamet and Zantac each mildly debilitate the activities of these important protective cells.

Does this licorice substance really stop the pain? Is it any better than the drugs? Here is the report from one large study. Researchers found 874 patients with chronic duodenal ulcers. Some were given DGL, some Tagamet, and some antacids. In six weeks, 77 percent of the ulcers of the subjects on DGL had healed. This compared to 63 percent of those on Tagamet. But on the incidence of recurrence, the DGL patients, whose protective forces had been stimulated, showed a reduced incidence of relapse.[4]

This study does not stand alone. Several other well-designed studies reached the same conclusion: A preparation from a root of a plant known to most of us as a penny candy will have more success in healing an ulcer than H2-receptor antagonists, antacids, and other anti-ulcer drugs.[5] The major advantage is in the lowered rate of relapse.

The chewable form is not only recommended, it may be necessary. Michael T. Murray, N.D., a naturopathic physician who helped bring the research on DGL to the attention of the American public, suggests that the anti-ulcer benefits of DGL may be linked to its effects on the salivary glands. In short, DGL may promote release of salivary compounds which in turn stimulate the growth and regeneration of the cells lining the stomach and intestine. Therefore, in order for DGL to be effective it needs to mix with saliva. That is why it is important to take DGL in the form of a chewable tablet.

In my practice, I have my patients stop taking their anti-ulcer drugs immediately. You should definitely discuss such a change with your physician. I recommend between two and four 380-milligrams chewable tablets, 20 to 40 minutes before meals. The length of administration, to give an ulcer a chance to heal, should be eight to sixteen weeks, depending on the response. The product is available at health food stores from Enzymatic Therapy (DGL) and Nature's Herbs (DGL-Power). Alternatively, your physician can order the DGL product (Rhizinate) from Phyto-Pharmica (1-800-533-2370).

Anti-Arthritis Drugs

An additional factor often associated with the breakdown of the defenses protecting the stomach lining are a number of the drugs used in treating arthritis. If you are on anti-arthritis drugs and have ulcers, I suggest you read the relevant chapter of this book, depending on the type of arthritis you have. Work with your physician to make the changes needed to limit or end your arthritis drugs. Use DGL to help protect or restore the stomach lining.

Vaginitis

Dr. Whitaker's Prescription for Vaginitis:

1. See a physician for proper diagnosis.
2. Follow the Whitaker Wellness Program.
3. Follow the recommendations on enhancing the immune system in Chapter 7.
4. If due to yeast (*Candida albicans*), follow recommendations under Candidiasis, page 176.
5. Insert *Lactobacillus acidophilus* into vagina as directed.
6. Douche, or insert a vaginal implant of betadine, boric acid, or tea tree oil.

Description

The vaginal environment is an extremely sensitive part of the female's host terrain. The infections of the vagina known as *vaginitis* actually involve many microorganisms that are normal inhabitants of the vagina and cervix of a healthy woman. The problem comes when the ecology of the vagina gets out of balance.

Many factors can influence the ecological balance of the vagina. Sugar intake is one. The presence of blood, antibodies, and other compounds in vaginal secretions can throw off the balance. The acid-base ratio, or pH, can become distorted. The presence or absence of various organisms, particularly lactobacilli, can be a key factor. The impact of these factors can be mediated or worsened depending on a women's general immune status.

Vaginitis will likely make itself known to a woman as itching, which can be quite painful. Urination may be painful. A woman may notice an unusual discharge. A vaginal odor may be an early sign that something is out of balance.

I strongly recommend that women with vaginitis see a physician. My reason is that the complications of untreated vaginitis can be severe. The itching may be a sign of a sexually transmitted disease, involving an organism like *Neisseria gonorrhea, Herpes simplex,* or *Chlamydia.* Untreated infections by the more common organisms, which account for 90 percent of vaginitis, can ascend up the genital tract. These can lead to tubal scarring, infertility, and ectopic pregnancies. The more common organisms are *Candida albicans, Trichomonas vaginalis* and *Gardenerella vaginalis.*

An estimated 7 percent of all visits to gynecologists is for vaginitis. The treatment most physicians recommend is antibiotics.

Remember that a number of microorganisms that overgrow in vaginitis are actually, in more limited presence, a part of the ecology of a healthy vagina. The antibiotics do not discriminate. What biota they can kill, they will. Not surprisingly, antibiotics can significantly alter the microecology of the vagina.

One outcome associated with the vastly expanding use of antibiotics in the past twenty years has been the growing incidence of *candidal vaginitis*. The candida microorganism is opportunistic and takes over terrain where other microorganisms have been killed off by antibiotic administration. Steroids and oral contraceptives have also contributed to the growing problem. The increasing incidence of diabetes mellitus is associated with candidal growth in recent years.

Diagnosis of a candidal infection can only be made accurately through microscopic examination of vaginal secretions, or, alternatively, culturing out the secretions. Signs, besides itching, may include a "cottage-cheese"-like discharge. Such a discharge is a strong suggestion that a candidal infection exists. However, it should be pointed out that a woman can have a candidal infection without such a discharge.

Comments on Dr. Whitaker's Prescription for Vaginitis

The health of the host terrain and the general immune status of the woman in balancing the vaginal environment provides one therapeutic lead. Therefore, following the Whitaker Wellness Program (see Chapter 2) will go a long way toward preventing most cases of vaginal infection. I also recommend reading the chapter on enhancing immune function, for those with noncandidal infections. The specific effect achieved by conscious attention to general health issues is in balancing the proteins, electrolytes, water, nutrients, and other components that constitute vaginal secretions.

A key dietary culprit is excessive sugar intake. Yeast infections such as *Candida albicans* thrive off the increased levels of sugar in vaginal excretions of women whose diets include high levels of sugars. I recommend that individuals with candidal vaginitis follow the suggestions in the section on candidiasis, page 176.

Natural Agents for Acute Symptoms

Attention to general wellness is the critical factor in preventing vaginitis and creating a long-term resolution of this health condition. The natural medicine chest also includes some excellent agents for addressing acute concerns. Regardless of the type of vaginitis, I recommend that a woman introduce the health-promoting bacteria

Lactobacillus acidophilus into the vagina. Either place a capsule or two of *L. acidophilus* product into the vagina, or douche with one-half teaspoon of *L. acidophilus* in a cup of warm water.

Betadine   Most of us came to learn of the antibiotic value of iodine when it was used topically on us as children to clean out a cut. We learned that iodine could sting. This may, indirectly, have lead many of us to learn for the first time that the body can heal on its own. After the first iodine experience, many a child learned to keep a wound quiet in order to not experience iodine's stinging!

One iodine preparation, *povidone iodine* (Betadine), has been developed to maintain an antibiotic effect without stinging or staining side effects. This substance is used in hospitals for wound cleaning or as preparation for surgery. A study over a quarter century ago produced a remarkable outcome. A full 100 percent of candidal vaginitis, 80 percent of trichomonas vaginitis and 93 percent of combinations were successfully treated with betadine douches.[1] The recommended mix is one part Betadine to 100 parts water. Douching with betadine twice daily for two weeks has proven effective against most organisms.[2]

Boric Acid   A shorter treatment which has fared well in head-to-head trials with nystatin, a common prescription drug, utilizes boric acid.[3] Place a 500- to 600-milligram capsule of boric acid in the vagina twice daily. Note that this therapy should not be continued more than a week, since boric acid can cause irritation to the vaginal lining.

Tea tree Oil   This powerful antibiotic agent has also been shown to be a medicinal douche. I recommend the 20 percent teatree oil from Desert Essence. Mix one teaspoon with a pint of warm water. Daily douches may be all that is necessary.

This natural oil is harvested from a tree that is native to Australia. Teatree oil has been shown to be effective against a number of common pathogens involved with vaginitis, including *Candida albicans* and *Trichomonas*.[4] One controlled study involved a weekly in-office treatment.[5] The treatment regime began with a thorough washing of the perinuem, labia, and vagina. The study used a commercial preparation called pHisoHex. Once dried, the area was then washed with a 1 percent teatree oil solution. Finally, a tampon was inserted which was saturated with teatree oil in a 40 percent solution. The women took the tampon out after twenty-four hours. Treatment usually took four to six weeks. The program was found to be highly effective.[5]

Varicose Veins

Dr. Whitaker's Prescription for Varicose Veins:

1. Follow the Whitaker Wellness Program. In particular, consume a diet high in fiber and exercise regularly.
2. Avoid standing in one place for long periods of time (use elastic support stockings if standing is necessary).
3. Take 150 to 300 milligrams of pycnogenols (procyanidolic oligomers) daily, or two capsules of Cellu-Var (Enzymatic Therapy), twice daily.
4. Eat foods that enhance fibrinolytic activity and take 500 milligrams of bromelain, three times daily between meals.

Description

The condition called varicose veins is a particular curse on a culture caught up in "looking good." Generally, these dilated, superficial veins in the legs pose little threat of physical harm. An individual may feel a heaviness in the legs, some coldness, a tingling sensation, or some aching discomfort. But from the perspective of vanity, varicose veins rank right up there with male pattern baldness.

For individuals in England and the United States, varicose veins are viewed simply as a sign of aging. Over 50 percent of middle-aged American adults will have varicose veins. The incidence is particularly high in women, where the risk is four times as great. For obese people, the likelihood of having varicose veins is also much higher.[1]

Speculation on cause is wide-ranging. One commonly held theory, certainly a major contributing factor, notes the strain on the venous system in the legs which comes from long periods of standing. Pressure can increase up to ten times in a person who stands for a long period of time. Regular heavy lifting is also implicated. Individuals with jobs requiring these behaviors are most at risk. We also know that a pregnant woman's pushing during labor can increase venous pressure on legs. This may also be a contributing factor.

Another line of thinking on the origins of varicose veins suggests that genetically weak veins or valves are a major predisposing factor. Risk increases with the loss of tissue tone, loss of muscle mass, and weakening of the walls of veins, all of which are enhanced during the aging process. Others researchers point to the straining in defecation that is a result of low-fiber diets. Some evidence suggests that varicose veins may be more likely to appear following damage to veins that resulted from inflammation. Any and all of these factors may be involved in a given individual's development of this condition.

What is known for certain is that veins are fairly frail structures. If a defect in the venous wall appears, the vein "balloons" out under the pressure of the blood. This can damage the valves in the vein, which are not made for the newly widened circumference in dilated veins. Blood becomes more static. Veins bulge.

While the problem most associated with varicose veins is that they are unappealing cosmetically, a more serious version of the condition exists. Instead of affecting a surface vein, a deeper vein dilates. This type of a varicose vein can lead to stroke, heart attack, pulmonary embolism, and thrombophlebitis.

These very serious conditions are sometimes associated with the diminished ability of an individual with varicose veins to break down fibrin. Fibrin then deposits in tissue near varicose veins. The skin becomes hard and lumpy due to the presence of fibrin and fat.

In the case of severe varicose veins, one of two procedures are often recommended by conventional doctors and may be necessary. One, called sclerotherapy, involves hardening the vein by injection of sodium chloride or another agent. The other is stripping of the vein. I recommend the former over the latter, if it is possible. Consult an expert in the field, usually a vascular surgeon, for an evaluation and always seek a second opinion.

Comments on Dr. Whitaker's Prescription for Varicose Veins

A damaged venous valve does not heal, regardless of therapies. However, new varicose veins can be prevented and there is evidence that some natural agents can improve the look of small varicose or "spider" veins. My suggested approach is multifaceted. Included are dietary and exercise measures, the use of agents that can strengthen blood flow and the integrity of the venous walls, a topical cream, and some compounds to help increase the breakdown of fibrin.

Diet and Exercise

One of the most important insights into the origins of varicose veins did not flow from elaborate biochemical or physiological analysis. It came instead from studies of the incidence of this condition in various populations. As noted above, these visible renditions of venous maps favor the legs of middle-aged and older denizens of the United States and England.[1] Varicose veins are rarely seen elsewhere in the world.

What distinguishes these two populations? The most obvious is their low-fiber diets that are high in refined foods, and relatively sedentary lifestyles. The high statistics on the high incidence of varicose veins are relative to these dietary and lifestyle choices. They do not express the likelihood of varicose veins for all human beings.

One way that such a diet may be a causal factor in varicose veins is that such foods may not provide enough of the nutrients required to optimize the integrity of the venous walls. However, this is not the major way that this diet is implicated. Individuals eating a low-fiber, high-refined-carbohydrate diet have to strain more during bowel movements. Their stools are smaller and harder. The straining blocks the flow of blood back up through the veins in the legs. Over time, this pressure may weaken vein walls. Varicose veins and hemorrhoids may result. In addition, straining during defecation is associated with weakening of the walls of the large intestine, producing diverticuli (outpouches) in the colon.[2]

What difference does a high fiber diet make? Fiber components attract water. This keeps the stool soft, gelatinous, and bulky. Diets rich in legumes, fruits, vegetables, and grains promote the colon muscle activity (peristalsis) that assists with defecation. Less straining is needed. The risk of varicose veins and related disorders diminishes. As with so many conditions, a high-fiber diet is the most important over-the-counter (of the grocery store) prescription for restoring health.

A second general measure is to be physically active. Exercise like walking, bike riding, and jogging promotes the contraction of leg muscles to get the pooled blood back into circulation. If standing for long periods of time can be avoided, do so. For those who are required to stand for hours on end, elastic compression stockings may be helpful.

Bioflavonoids and Botanicals

One approach to limiting the damage of varicose veins is to supply veins with all the nutrients that will allow them to be as strong as possible. A long list of natural agents have been shown to provide important support in at least one of two ways. They may promote blood flow. This limits wear and tear in veins. Or they may serve to improve venous support structures.

Pycnogenols Several clinical studies have looked at the value of supplementing a standardized extract of either grapeseed skin (*Vitis vinifera*) or the bark of Landes' pine as a therapy for varicose veins. Favorable results have been observed in both blood flow and in venous appearance.[3]

The active agents in these very different members of the vegetable kingdom are *pycnogenols*. These are also known as *procyanidolic oligomers* (PCOs) or *leukocyanidins*. They are complexes of flavonoids (polyphenols). In general, pycnogenols are known to have a number of beneficial activities. They increase intracellular levels of vitamin C. Capillary permeability and fragility is decreased. They help bind collagen structures and inhibit destruction of collagen. Pycnogenols also act as free radical scavengers.

A number of companies offer products containing pycnogenols, including Solgar, Solaray, Country Life, and KAL. These can be found in health food stores. The standard dosage of the grapeseed or pinebark extract should be 150 to 300 milligrams per day. This assumes that the extract has a procyanidin content of 85 to 95 percent.

Cellu-Var   The list of bioflavonoids and botanicals besides pycnogenols which have been shown to exert positive effect on varicose veins is long. Some of the top items are citrus bioflavonoids, hesperidin, and rutin. The extracts of bilberry, hawthorn, horse chestnut, gotu kola, butcher's broom, and *Ginkgo biloba* are also useful.

Because of the wealth of options from nature, I prefer to use a product that offers the combined activity of a number of these agents: gotu kola (*Centella asiatica*), butcher's broom (*Ruscus aculeatus*) and horse chestnut (*Aesculus hippocastanum*). All of these botanicals are standardized for potency, at levels at which they have been independently shown in clinical trials to exert a positive effect on varicose veins.[4]

Cellu-Var (Enzymatic Therapy) improves blood flow and venous tone to help get rid of the symptoms of tingling, heaviness, pain, and coldness of the legs. Small varicose veins sometimes disappear altogether. It is particularly effective when combined with Cellu-Var Cream before bed. I recommend two capsules of Cellu-Var twice each day.

Foods and Nutritional Agents

Studies have shown that individuals with varicose veins have a reduced ability to break down fibrin.[5] Potentially dangerous lumpy deposits develop in the skin near the veins. To assist the body in dealing with fibrin, I recommend that individuals with varicose veins increase their consumption of foods known to increase the breakdown of fibrin, or fibrinolytic activity, in the blood. Among these are garlic, onions, cayenne pepper, and ginger.[6] In short, get accustomed to spicier foods! These agents also help other cardiovascular conditions.

One agent in particular, the protein-digesting compound from pineapple called *bromelain*, deserves special mention. I recommend a dosage of 500 milligrams three times per day, between meals, for its fibrinolytic activity.[7] In addition, bromelain has been shown to be of particular value when a vein becomes inflamed (thrombophlebitis) or in recovery from surgery for varicose veins.[8] One study looked at 180 individuals on whom operations for varicose veins were performed.[9] Every other patient was given supplemental bromelain. In just two weeks, over two-thirds of those who received bromelain (65 of 90) had no severe bruises. Only one-third (32 of 90) of those who received no bromelain were without severe bruises.

Appendix

About the Whitaker Wellness Institute

Julian M. Whitaker, M.D., is the founder and director of the Whitaker Wellness Institute in Newport Beach, California. Dr. Whitaker graduated from Dartmouth College in Hanover, New Hampshire, in 1966, received his medical training at Emory University Medical School in Atlanta, Georgia, and completed a surgical medical internship at Grady Memorial Hospital in Atlanta in 1971. He continued his postgraduate medical training in surgery at the University of California at San Francisco. In 1973, he entered private practice and changed the course of his professional direction.

Switching from surgery as the focus of his approach, Dr. Whitaker began to practice preventive medicine using dietary and lifestyle changes, and exercise as his primary treatment tools for patients with heart disease, diabetes, high blood pressure, obesity, and other chronic degenerative diseases.

In 1979, he opened the Whitaker Wellness Institute. Since that time, approximately 15,000 patients have successfully been treated. The cornerstone of the Whitaker Wellness Institute is a five-day residential program designed to provide in-office treatment and education. Approximately 80 to 100 patients attend this program each month.

This five-day program is recommended as a second opinion for those who are candidates for invasive techniques for heart disease such as angiogram, angioplasty, or bypass surgery. It is also recommended for the diabetic and high blood pressure patient who desires to reduce or eliminate medication.

The program focuses on learning how to incorporate the Whitaker Wellness Program into your life. If appropriate, EDTA chelation therapy is also incorporated into the program (at an additional charge).

Patients are housed across the street from our office at the Sheraton Hotel in Newport Beach, California. Many of the activities take place in the hotel. Meals are specially prepared by a chef who has worked with Dr. Whitaker for many years. The Sheraton kindly extends to our patients a significant discount for a class A resort hotel. Hotel accommodations are paid directly to the Sheraton.

TYPICAL DAY AT THE WHITAKER WELLNESS INSTITUTE

7:30 A.M.	Vital signs taken by nurse
8:30 A.M.	Breakfast
9:30 A.M.	Educational seminar with Dr. Whitaker
11:00 A.M.	Supervised exercise
12:00 NOON	Lunch
1:00 P.M.	Nutrition/Food preparation session
2:00 P.M.	Private consultations with the doctor
5:00 P.M.	Stress management and relaxation session
6:00 P.M.	Dinner

Evenings are free

MEDICAL ASSESSMENT

- Complete history and physical exam with emphasis on the cardiovascular system
- Two complete laboratory panels include chemistry panel, complete blood cell count, thyroid profile, and cardiovascular risk assessment
- Resting electrocardiogram with interpretation
- Exercise tolerance test to determine appropriate exercise level
- Oxygen therapy

BREAKDOWN OF FEES

Medical assessments	$1,348.00
Laboratory (approximate)	300.00
Hotel accommodations (6 nights)	429.00
Daily meals	250.00
Total	$2,327.00

ADDITIONAL CHARGES AND INFORMATION

- All laboratory charges are billed directly to you or your insurance company by the laboratory.
- Diabetics have an additional laboratory charge of $150.
- Magnesium injections are routinely given at $15 per injection; typically two to four injections per patient.

- Nutritional supplements are recommended for each patient. Most purchase the supplements before leaving the Institute.
- Companions are encouraged to join the patient in the program. The only fee for companions is for meals ($250). If medical attention is required, the companion is billed accordingly.
- If additional testing is necessary, we will bill your insurance.

INSURANCE INFORMATION

The majority of the medical charges are covered by most private medical insurance plans. Although you will be responsible for payment, our office, as a courtesy, will submit your claim to your insurance carrier.

DEPOSIT AND CANCELLATION INFORMATION

- A deposit of $750 is to be submitted with your application 30 days prior to the start date of the session to guarantee admission in the session of your choice.
- If cancellations are made less than five working days prior to the start date of a session, a $250 penalty is drawn.

For more information on the Whitaker Wellness Institute, call or write:

Whitaker Wellness Institute
4321 Birch Street, Suite 100
Newport Beach, CA 92660
1-800-283-4584

References

Chapter 1

1. Wortis J and Stone A: The addiction to drug companies. Biol Psychiatry 32:847–9, 1992.
2. Ensor PA: Projecting future drug expenditures—1992. Am J Hosp Pharm 49:140–5, 1992.
3. Dickson M: The pricing of pharmaceuticals: An international comparison. Clin Ther 14:604–10, 1992.
4. Consumers Union: Pushing drugs to doctors. Consumer Reports 57:87–94, 1992.
5. American College of Physicians: Position Paper. Physicians and the pharmaceutical industry. Annals Int Med 112:624–6, 1990.
6. Waud DR: Pharmaceutical promotions—A free lunch? New Engl J Med 327:351–3, 1992.
7. Wilkes MS, Doblin BH, and Shapiro MF: Pharmaceutical advertisements in leading medical journals: Expert's assessments. Annals Int Med 116:912–9, 1992.
8. Safavi KT and Hayward RA: Choosing between apples and apples: Physicians' choices of prescription drugs that have similar side effects and efficacies. J Gen Intern Med 7:32–7, 1992.
9. Hemila H: Vitamin C and the common cold. Br J Nutr 67:3–16, 1992.
10. Stampfer MJ, et al.: Vitamin E consumption and the risk of coronary disease in women. New Engl J Med 328:1444–8, 1993.
11. Rimm EB: Vitamin E consumption and the risk of coronary heart disease in men. New Engl J Med 328:1450–5, 1993.
12. Roufs JB: Safety of amino acids in human subjects: A summary prepared for Honorable Henry Waxman, Chairman, House Subcommittee on Health and Environment. Townsend Letter 124:1068–73, 1993.
13. Collin J: FDA handed defeat by federal judge on GLA supplement seizure. Townsend Letter 95:397, 406–8, 1991.
14. Keller K. Legal Requirements for the use of phytopharmaceutical drugs in the Federal Republic of Germany. J Ethnopharamacol 32:225–9, 1991.
15. Kleijnen J and Knipschild P. Drug profiles—*Ginkgo biloba*. Lancet 340:1136–9, 1993.
16. McCaleb RS: Food ingredient safety evaluation. Food Drug Law J 47:657–65, 1992.
17. Boccafoschi and Annoscia S: Comparison of *Serenoa repens* extract with placebo by controlled clinical trial in patients with prostatic adenomatosis. Urologia 50:1257–68, 1983.

    Cirillo-Marucco E, et al.: Extract of *Serenoa repens* (Permixon) in the early treatment of prostatic hypertrophy. Urologia 5:1269–77, 1983.

    Tripodi V, et al.: Treatment of prostatic hypertrophy with *Serenoa repens* extract. Med Praxis 4:41–6, 1983.

    Emili E, Lo Cigno M, and Petrone U: Clinical trial of a new drug for treating hypertrophy of the prostate (Permixon). Urologia 50:1042–8, 1983.

    Greca P and Volpi R: Experience with a new drug in the medical treatment of prostatic adenoma. Urologia 52:532–5, 1985.

Tasca A, et al.: Treatment of obstructive symptomatology caused by prostatic adenoma with an extract of *Serenoa repens:* Double-blind clinical study versus placebo. Minerva Urol Nefrol 37:87–91, 1985.

Crimi A and Russo A: Extract of *Serenoa repens* for the treatment of the functional disturbances of prostate hypertrophy. Med Praxis 4:47–51, 1983.

Champault G, Patel JC, and Bonnard AM: A double-blind trial of an extract of the plant *Serenoa repens* in benign prostatic hyperplasia. Br J Clin Pharmacol 18:461–2, 1984.

Champault G, et al.: Medical treatment of prostatic adenoma. Controlled trial: PA 109 versus placebo in 110 patients. Ann Urol 18:407–10, 1984.

Mattei FM, Capone M, and Acconcia A.: *Serenoa repens* extract in the medical treatment of benign prostatic hypertrophy. Urologia 55:547–52, 1988.

Chapter 2

1. Ferraro KF and Albrecht-Jensen CM: Does religion influence health? J Scientific Study Religion 30:193–203, 1991.
2. National Research Council: Diet and Health. Implications for Reducing Chronic Disease Risk. National Academy Press, Washington, D.C., 1989.
3. National Research Council: Recommended Dietary Allowances, 10th edition. National Academy Press, Washington, D.C., 1989.
4. Enstrom JE, et al.: Vitamin C intake and mortality among a sample of the United States population. Epidemiol 3(3):194–202, 1992.
5. Hennekens CH and Gaziano JM: Antioxidants and heart disease: Epidemiology and clinical evidence. Clin Cardiol 16 (supplement 1):10–15, 1993.

     Stahelin HB, et al.: Plasma antioxidant vitamins and subsequent cancer mortality in the 12-year followup of the prospective Basel Study. Am J Epidemiol 133:766–75, 1991.

     Diplock AT: Antioxidant nutrients and disease prevention: An overview. Am J Clini Nutr 53:189S–93S, 1991.
6. Shils ME and Young VR: Modern Nutrition in Health and Disease, 7th edition. Lea and Febiger, Philadelphia, 1988.

     Cheraskin E: Vitamin C—Who Needs It? Arlington Press, Birmingham, AL, 1993.
7. Ginter E: Optimum intake of vitamin C for the human organism. Nutr Health 1:66–77, 1982.
8. Pauling L: Vitamin C and the Common Cold. Freeman, San Francisco, 1970.

     Cathcart RF: The third face of vitamin C. J Orthomol Med 7:197–200, 1992.
9. Werbach MR: Nutritional Influences on Illness, 2nd edition. Third Line Press, Tarzana, CA, 1993.
10. Gey KF, et al.: Inverse correlation between plasma vitamin E and mortality from ischemic heart disease in cross-cultural epidemiology. Am J Clin Nutr 53:326S–34S, 1991.
11. Purvis JR and Movahed A: Magnesium disorders and cardiovascular disease. Clin Cardiol 15:556–68, 1992.
12. Gullestad L, et al.: Oral versus intravenous magnesium supplementation in patients with magnesium deficiency. Magnes Trace Elem 10:11–6, 1991.

     Lindberg JS, et al.: Magnesium bioavailability from magnesium citrate and magnesium oxide. J Am Coll Nutr 9:48–55, 1990.
13. Iimura O, Kijima T, Kikuchi K, et al.: Studies on the hypotensive effect of high potassium intake in patients with essential hypertension. Clin Sci 61 (supplement 7):77s–80s, 1981.

     Khaw KT and Barrett-Connor: Dietary potassium and blood pressure in a population. Am J Clin Nutr. 39:963–8. 1984.

     Skrabal F, Aubock J, and Hortnagl H: Low sodium/high potassium diet for prevention of hypertension: Probable mechanisms of action. Lancet ii:895–900, 1981.

     Meneely G and Battarbee H: High sodium-low potassium environment and hypertension. Am J Card 38:768–81, 1976.

14. Schauss A: Dietary Fish Oil Consumption and Fish Oil Supplementation. In: A Textbook of Natural Medicine. Pizzorno JE and Murray MT (eds). Bastyr College Publications, Seattle, 1991. ppV:Fish Oils:1–7.

    Simopoulos AP: Summary of the NATO Advanced Research Workshop on Dietary w3 and w6 Fatty Acids: Biological effects and nutritional esssentiality. J Nutr 119:521–8, 1989.

    Von Schacky C: Prophylaxis of atherosclerosis with marine omega-3 fatty acids: A comprehensive strategy. Annals Int Med 107:890–9, 1987.

    Bjerve KS, et al.: Clinical studies with alpha-linolenic acid and long-chain n-3 fatty acids. Nutrition 8:130–2, 1992.

    Bierenbaum ML, et al.: Reducing atherogenic risk in hyperlipemic humans with flaxseed supplementation: A prelimary report. J Am Coll Nutr 12:501–4, 1993.
15. Horrobin DF: Fatty acid metabolism in health and disease: The role of delta-6-desaturase. Am J Clin Nutr 57:732S–6S, 1993.
16. Leaf A: Health claims: Omega-3 fatty acids and cardiovascular disease. Nutr Rev 50:150–4, 1992.

    Simopoulus AP: Omega-3 fatty acids in health and disease and in growth and development. Am J Clin Nutr 54:438–63, 1991.

    Leaf A and Weber PC: Cardiovascular effects of n-3 fatty acids. New Eng J Med 318:549–57, 1988.
17. Adlercreutz H, et al.: Determination of urinary lignans and phytoestrogen metabolites, potential antiestrogens and anticarcinogens, in urine of women in various habitual diets. J Steroid Biochem 25:791–7, 1986.

    Serraino M and Thompson LU: The effect of flaxseed supplementation on early risk markers for mammary carcinogenesis. Cancer Letters 60:135–42, 1991.
18. Kremer J, et al.: Effects of manipulation of dietary fatty acids on clinical manifestation of rheumatoid arthritis. Lancet i:184–7, 1985.

    Magaro M, et al.: Influence of diet with different lipid composition on neutrophil composition, on neutrophil chemiluminescence, and disease activity in patients with rheumatoid arthritis. Annals Rheum Dis 47:793–6, 1988.

    Darlington LG: Do diets rich in polyunsaturated fatty acids affect disease activity in rheumatoid arthrits? Annals Rheum Dis 47:169–72, 1988.

    Levanthal LJ, et al.: Treatment of rheumatoid arthritis with gammalinoleic acid. Annals Int Med 119:867–73, 1993.
19. Trowell H, Burkitt D, and Heaton K: Dietary Fibre, Fibre-depleted Foods and Disease. Academic Press, New York, 1985.

    U.S. Dept of Health and Human Services: The Surgeon General's Report on Nutrition and Health. Prima, Rocklin, CA, 1988.

    National Research Council: Diet and Health: Implications for Reducing Chronic Disease Risk. National Academy Press, Washington, D.C., 1989.
20. Ryde D: What should humans eat? Practitioner 232:415–8, 1985.

    Eaton SB and Konner M: Paleolithic nutrition: A consideration of its nature and current implications. New Engl J Med 312:283–9, 1985.

Chapter 3

1. Rafsky HA and Weingarten M: A study of the gastric secretory response in the aged. Gastroent May:348–52, 1946.

   Davies D and James TG: An investigation into the gastric secretion of a hundred normal persons over the age of sixty. Brit J Med i:1–14, 1930.
2. Mojaverian P, et al.: Estimation of gastric residence time of the Heidelberg capsule in humans. Gastroenterol 89:392–7, 1985.

   Wright JV: A proposal for standardized challenge testing of gastric acid secretory capacity using the Heidelberg capsule radiotelemetry system. J John Bastyr Col Nat Med 1:2:3–11, 1979.
3. Wright JV: Dr. Wright's Guide to Healing with Nutrition. Keats Publishing, New Canaan, CT, 1990, pp. 30–50.

4. Barrie SA: Heidelberg pH capsule gastric analysis. In: Pizzorno JE and Murray MT: A Textbook of Natural Medicine. JBC Publications, Seattle, 1985.

   Bray GW: The hypochlorhydria of asthma in childhood. Br Med J i:181–97, 1930.

   Rabinowitch IM: Achlorhydria and its clinical significance in diabetes mellitus. Am J Dig Dis 18:322–33, 1949.

   Carper WM, et al.: Gallstones, gastric secretion and flatulent dyspepsia. Lancet i:413–5, 1967.

   Rawls WB and Ancona VC: Chronic urticaria associated with hypochlorhydria or achlorhydria. Rev Gastroent Oct:267–71, 1950.

   Gianella RA, Broitman SA, and Zamcheck N: Influence of gastric acidity on bacterial and parasitic enteric infections. Ann Int Med 78:271–6, 1973.

   De Witte TJ, Geerdink PJ, and Lamers CB: Hypochlorhydria and hypergastrinaemia in rheumatoid arthritis. Ann Rheum Dis 38:14–17, 1979.

   Ryle JA and Barber HW. Gastric analysis in acne rosacea. Lancet ii:1195–6, 1920.

   Ayres S: Gastric secretion in psoriasis, eczema, and dermatitis herpetiformis. Arch Derm Jul:854–9, 1929.

   Dotevall G and Walan A: Gastric secretion of acid and intrinsic factor in patients with hyper and hypothyroidism. Acta Med Scand 186:529–33, 1969.

   Howitz J and Schwartz M: Vitiligo, achlorhydria, and pernicious anemia. Lancet i:1331–4, 1971.

5. Graham DY, Smith JL, and Patterson DJ: Why do apparently healthy people use antacid tablets? Am J Gastroenterol 78:257–60, 1983.

6. Taylor GA, et al.: Gastrointestinal absorption of aluminum in Alzheimer's disease: Response to aluminum citrate. Age Aging 21:81–90, 1992.

   Bolla KI, et al.: Neurocognitive effects of aluminum. Arch Neurol 49:1021–6, 1992.

   Flaten TP: Geographical associations between aluminum and drinking water and death rates with dementia (including Alzheimer's disease), Parkinson's disease and amyotrophic sclerosis in Norway. Environ Geochem Health 12:152–7, 1990.

   Perl DP, et al.: Intraneuronal aluminum accumulation in amyotrophic lateral sclerosis and Parkinsonism-dementia of Guam. Science 217:1053–5, 1982.

7. Weberg R and Berstad A: Gastrointestinal absorption of aluminum from single doses of aluminum-containing antacids in man. Eur J Clin Invest 16:428–32, 1986.

   Weberg R, Berstad A, Aaseth J, and Falch JA: Mineral-metabolic side effects of low-dose antacids. Scand J Gastroenterol 20:741–6, 1985.

8. Nicar MJ and Pak CYC: Calcium bioavailability from calcium carbonate and calcium citrate. J Clin Endocrinol Metabol 61:391–3, 1985.

9. Editorial: Citrate for calcium nephrolithiasis. Lancet i:955, 1986.

10. Cushner HM, Copley JB, and Foulks CJ: Calcium citrate, a new phosphate-binding and alkalinizing agent for patients with renal failure. Curr Ther Res 40:998–1004, 1986.

11. Rubinstein E, et al.: Antibacterial activity of the pancreatic fluid. Gastroenterol 88:927–32, 1985.

12. Innerfield I: Enzymes in Clinical Medicine. McGraw Hill, New York, 1960.

    Ransberger K: Enzyme treatment of immune complex diseases. Arthr Rheum 8:16–9, 1986.

13. Taussig S, et al.: Bromelain, a proteolytic enzyme and its clinical application: A review. Hiroshima J Med Sci 24:185–93, 1975.

14. Oelgoetz AW, et al.: The treatment of food allergy and indigestion of pancreatic origin with pancreatic enzymes. Am J Dig Dis Nutr 2:422–6, 1935.

Chapter 4

1. Passwater RA and Cranton EM: Trace Elements, Hair Analysis and Nutrition. Keats, New Canaan, CT, 1983.

   Rutter M and Russell-Jones R (eds): Lead versus Health: Sources and Effects of Low-Level Lead Exposure. John Wiley, New York, 1983.

   Yost KJ: Cadmium, the environment and human health: An overview. Experentia 40:157–64, 1984.

Gerstner BG and Huff JE: Clinical toxicology of mercury. J Toxicol Environ Health 2:471–526, 1977.

Nation JR, et al.: Dietary administration of nickel: Effects on behaviour and metallothionien levels. Physiol Behavior 34:349–53, 1985.

Editorial: Toxicologic consequences of oral aluminum. Nutr Rev 45:72–4, 1987.

2. Schwartz BS, et al.: Decrements in neurobehavioral performance associated with mixed exposure to organic and inorganic lead. Am J Epidemiol 137:1006–21, 1993.

Marlowe M, et al.: Hair mineral content as a predictor of learning disabilities. J Learn Disabil 17:418–421, 1977.

Pihl R and Parkes M: Hair element content in learning disabled children. Science 198:204–6, 1977.

David O, Clark J, and Voeller K: Lead and hyperactivity. Lancet ii:900–3, 1972.

David O, Hoffman S, and Sverd J: Lead and hyperactivity: Behavioral response to chelation: A pilot study. Am J Psychiatry 133:1155–1188, 1976.

Benignus V, et al.: Effects of age and body lead burden on CNS function in young children: EEG spectra. EEG and Clin Neurophys 52:240–8, 1981.

Rimland B and Larson G: Hair mineral analysis and behavior: An analysis of 51 studies. J Learn Disabil 16:279–285, 1983.

3. Ruff HA, et al.: Declining blood lead levels and cognitive changes in moderately lead-poisoned children. JAMA 269:1641–6, 1993.

4. Hunter B: Some food additives as neuroexcitors and neurotoxins. Clin Ecol 2:83–9, 1984.

Seaton A, Jeelinek EH, and Kennedy P: Major neurological disease and occupational exposure to organic solvents. Quart J Med 305:707–12, 1992.

Cullen MR (ed): Workers with Multiple Chemical Sensitivities. Hanley & Belfus, Philadelphia, 1987.

Stayner LT, Elliott L, Blade L, et al.: A retrospective cohort mortality study of workers exposed to formaldehyde in the garment industry. Am J Ind Med 13:667–81, 1988.

Kilburn KH, Warshaw R, Boylen CT, et al.: Pulmonary and neurobehavioral effects of formaldehyde exposure. Arch Environ Health 40:254–60, 1985.

Sterling TD and Arundel AV: Health effects of phenoxy herbicides. Scand J Work Environ Health 12:161–73, 1986.

Lindstrom K, Riihimaki H, and Hannininen K: Occupational solvent exposure and neuropsychiatric disorders. Scan J Work Environ Health 10:321–3, 1984.

5. Flora SJS, et al.: Protective role of trace metals in lead intoxication. Toxicol Lett 13:51–6, 1982.

Hsu HS, Krook L, Pond WG, and Duncan JR: Interaction of dietary calcium with toxic levels of lead and zinc in pigs. J Nutrit 105:112–68, 1975.

Petering HG: Some observations on the interaction of zinc, copper, and iron metabolism in lead and cadmium toxicity. Environ Health Perspect 25:141–5, 1978.

Papaioannou R, Sohler A, and Pfeiffer CC: Reduction of blood lead levels in battery workers by zinc and vitamin C. J Orthomol Psychiatry 7:94–106, 1978.

Flora SJS, Singh S, and Tandon SK: Role of selenium in protection against lead intoxication. Acta Pharmacol et Toxicol 53:28–32, 1983.

Tandon SK, et al.: Vitamin B complex in treatment of cadmium intoxication. Annals Clin Lab Sci 14:487–92, 1984.

Bratton GR, et al.: Thiamin (vitamin B1) effects on lead intoxication and deposition of lead in tissue: Therapeutic potential. Toxicol Appl Pharmacol 59:164–72, 1981.

Flora SJS, Singh S, and Tandon SK: Prevention of lead intoxication by vitamin B complex. Z Ges Hyg 30:409–11, 1984.

Shakman RA: Nutritional influences on the toxicity of environmental pollutants: A review. Arch Environ Health 28:105–33, 1974.

6. Imamura M and Tung T: A trial of fasting cure for PCB-poisoned patients in Taiwan. Am J Ind Med 5:147–53, 1984.

7. Bloom WL: Fasting as an introduction to the treatment of obesity. Metabolism 8:214–20, 1959.

Duncan GG, et al.: Intermittent fasts in the correction and control of intractable obesity. Am J Med Sci 245:515–20, 1963.

Duncan GG, et al.: Contraindications and therapeutic results of fasting in obese patients. Ann NY Acad Sci 131:632–6, 1965.

Suzuki J, et al.: Fasting therapy for psychosomatic disease with special reference to its indications and therapeutic mechanism. Tohoku J Exp Med, 118 (supplement):245–59, 1976.

Lithell H, et al.: A fasting and vegetarian diet treatment trial on chronic inflammatory disorders. Acta Derm Venereol 63:397–403, 1983.

Sundquist T, et al.: Influence of fasting on intestinal permeability and disease activity in patients with rheumatoid arthritis shows normalization during fasting. Scand J Rheumatol 11:33–8, 1982.

Kroker GF, Stroud RM, Marshall R, et al.: Fasting and rheumatoid arthritis: A multicentre study. Clin Ecol 2:3:137–44, 1984.

Boehme DL: Preplanned fasting in the treatment of mental disease: Survey of the current Soviet literature. Schizophr Bull 3:2:288–96, 1977.

8. Padova C, et al.: S-adenosyl-L-methionine antagonizes oral contraceptive-induced bile cholesterol supersaturation in healthy women: Preliminary report of a controlled randomized trial. Am J Gastroenterol 79:941–4, 1984.

Frezza M, et al.: Reversal of intrahepatic cholestasis of pregnancy in women after high-dose S-adenosyl-L-methionine (SAM) administration. Hepatol 4:274–8, 1984.

Bombardieri G, et al.: Effects of S-adenosyl-methionine (SAM) in the treatment of Gilbert's syndrome. Curr Ther Res 37:580–5, 1985.

Mazzanti R, et al.: On the antisteatosic effects of S-adenosyl-L-methionine in various chronic liver diseases: A multicenter study. Curr Ther Res 25:25–32, 1979.

9. Barak AJ, et al.: Dietary betaine promotes generation of hepatic S-adenosylmethionine and protects the liver from ethanol-induced fatty infiltration. Alcohol Clin Exp Res 17:552–5, 1993.

Zeisel SH, et al.: Choline, an essential nutrient for humans. FASEB J 5:2093–8, 1991.

10. Wisniewska-Knypl J, et al.: Protective effect of methionine against vinyl chloride-mediated depression of non-protein sulfhydryls and cytochrome P-450. Toxicol Lett 8:147–52, 1981.

Ruffmann R and Wendel A: GSH rescue by N-acetylcysteine. Klin Wochenschr 69:857–62, 1991.

11. Ballatori N and Clarkson TW: Dependence of biliary excretion of inorganic mercury on the biliary transport of glutathione. Biochem Pharmacol 33:1093–8, 1984.

Murakami M and Webb MA: A morphological and biochemical study of the effects of L-cysteine on the renal uptake and nephrotoxicity of cadmium. Br J Exp Pathol 62:115–30, 1981.

Baker DH and Czarnecki-Maulden GL: Pharmacolic role of cysteine in ameliorating or exacerbating mineral toxicities. J Nutr 117:1003–10, 1987.

12. Hikino H, et al.: Antihepatotoxic actions of flavonolignans from *Silybum marianum* fruits. Planta Medica 50:248–50, 1984.

Vogel G, Trost W, Braatz R, et al.: Studies on pharmacodynamics, site and mechanism of action of silymarin, the antihepatotoxic principle from *Silybum marianum* (L.) Gaert. Arzneim.-Forsch 25:179–85, 1975.

Wagner H: Antihepatotoxic flavonoids. In: Plant Flavonoids in Biology and Medicine: Biochemical, Pharmacological, and Structure-Activity Relationships. Cody V, Middleton E and Harbourne JB (ed). Alan R. Liss, Inc, New York, NY, 1986, pp. 545–558.

13. Sarre H: Experience in the treatment of chronic hepatopathies with silymarin. Arzneim-Forsch 21:1209–12, 1971.

Canini F, et al.: Use of silymarin in the treatment of alcoholic hepatic steatosis. Clin Ter 114:307–14, 1985.

Salmi HA and Sarna S: Effect of silymarin on chemical, functional, and morphological alteration of the liver: A double-blind controlled study. Scand J Gastroenterol 17:417–21, 1982.

Boari C, et al.: Occupational toxic liver diseases: Therapeutic effects of silymarin. Min Med 72:2679–88, 1985.

Ferenci P, et al.: Randomized controlled trial of silymarin treatment in patients with cirrhosis of the liver. J Hepatol 9:105–13, 1989.

14. Valenzuela A, et al.: Selectivity of silymarin on the increase of the glutathione content in different tissues of the rat. Planta Med 55:420–2, 1989.

Chapter 5

1. Tucker DM, et al.: Nutrition status and brain function in aging. Am J Clin Nutr 52:93–102, 1990.
2. Werbach M: Nutritional Influences on Mental Illness: A Sourcebook of Clinical Research. Third Line Press, Tarzana, CA, 1991.
3. Benton D and Roberts G: Effect of vitamin and mineral supplementation on intelligence of a sample of schoolchildren. Lancet i:140–3, 1988.
4. Constantinidis J: The hypothesis of zinc deficiency in the pathogenesis of neurofibrillary tangles. Med Hypoth 35:319–23, 1991.
5. Constantinidis J: Treatment of Alzheimer's disease by zinc compounds. Drug Devel Res 27:1–14, 1992.
6. Boosalis MG, Evans GW, and McClain CJ: Impaired handling of orally administered zinc in pancreatic insufficiency. Am J Clin Nutr 37:268–71, 1983.
7. Fairbanks VF and Beutler E: Iron. In: Modern Nutrition in Health and Disease, 7th edition. Shils ME and Young VR (eds). Lea and Febiger, Philadelphia, 1988, pp. 193–226.
8. Craig GM, Elliot C, and Hughes KR: Masked vitamin B12 and folate deficiency in the elderly. Br J Nutr 54:613–9, 1985.
9. Levitt AJ and Karlinsky H: Folate, vitamin B12 and cognitive impairment in patients with Alzheimer's disease. Acta Psychiatry Scand 86:301–5, 1992.
   Abalan F and Delile JM: B12 deficiency in presenile dementia. Biol Psychiatry 20:1247–51, 1985.
   Cole MG and Prchal JF: Low serum vitamin B12 in Alzheimer-type dementia. Age Aging 13:101–5, 1984.
10. Bolla KI, et al.: Neurocognitive effects of aluminum. Arch Neurol 49:1021–6, 1992.
    Grammas P and Caspers ML: The effect of aluminum on muscarinic receptors in isolated cerebral microvessels. Res Commun Chem Pathol Pharmacol 72:69–79, 1991.
    Flaten TP: Geographical associations between aluminum and drinking water and death rates with dementia (including Alzheimer's disease), Parkinson's disease, and amyotrophic sclerosis in Norway. Environ Geochem Health 12:152–7, 1990.
11. Perl DP and Brody AR: Alzheimer's disease: X-ray spectometric evidence of aluminum accumulation in neurofibrillary tangle-bearing neurons. Science 208:297–99, 1980.
    Caster WO and Wang M: Dietary aluminum and Alzheimer's disease—A review. Sci Total Environ 17:31–6, 1981.
12. Kleijnen J and Knipschild P: Drug Profiles—*Ginkgo biloba*. Lancet 340:1136–9, 1993.
13. Kleijnen J and Knipschild P: *Ginkgo biloba* for cerebral insufficiency. Br J Clin Pharmacol 34:352–8, 1992.
14. Vorberg G: *Ginkgo biloba* extract (GBE): A long-term study of chronic cerebral insufficiency in geriatric patients. Clin Trials J 22:149–157, 1985.
    Gessner B, Voelp A, and Klasser M: Study of the long-term action of a *Ginkgo biloba* extract on vigilance and mental performance as determined by means of quantitative pharmaco-EEG and psychometric measurements. Arzneim-Forsch 35:1459–65, 1985.
    Hofferberth B: Effect of *Ginkgo biloba* extract on neurophysiological and psychometric measurement in patients with cerebroorganic syndrome—A double-blind study versus placebo. Arzneim-Forsch 39:918–22, 1989.
    Hindmarch I and Subhan Z: The psychopharmacological effects of *Ginkgo biloba* extract in normal healthy volunteers. Int J Clin Pharmacol Res 4:89–93, 1984.
15. Warburton DM: Clinical psychopharmacology of *Ginkgo biloba* extract. In: Rokan (*Ginkgo Biloba:* Recent Results in Pharmacology and Clinic). Funfgeld EW (ed). Springer-Verlag, New York, 1988, pp. 327–45.

16. Zeisel SH and Canty DJ: Choline phospholipids: Molecular mechanisms for human diseases: A meeting report. J Nutr Biochem 4:258–63, 1993.
17. Little A, et al.: A double-blind, placebo-controlled trial of high-dose lecithin in Alzheimer's disease. J Neurol Neurosurg Psychiatry 48:736–42, 1985.

    Rosenberg G and Davis KL: The use of cholinergic precursors in neuropsychiatric diseases. Am J Clin Nutr 36:709–20, 1982.

    Sitaram N, et al.: Choline: Selective enhancement of serial learning and encoding of low imagery words in man. Life Sci 22:1555–60, 1978.
18. Kalimi M and Regelson W: The Biological Role of Dehydroepiandrosterone. de Gruyter, New York, 1990.
19. Flood JF and Roberts E: Dehydroepiandrosterone sulfate improves memory in aging mice. Brain Res 448:178–81, 1988.

    Flood JF, Smith GE, and Roberts E: Dehydroepiandrosterone and its sulfate enhance memory retention in mice. Brain Res 447:269–78, 1988.

Chapter 6

1. Seyle H: Stress in Health and Disease. Buttersworth, London, UK, 1976.
2. Benson H: The Relaxation Response. William Morrow, New York, 1975.
3. Brown ML: Present Knowledge in Nutrition, 6th edition. Washington, D.C., 1990.
4. Britton SW and Silvette H: Further experiments on cortico-adrenal extract: Its efficacy by mouth. Science 74:440–1, 1931.
5. Hikino H: Traditional remedies and modern assessment: The case of ginseng. In: The Medicinal Plant Industry. Wijeskera ROB (ed). CRC Press, Boca Raton, FL, 1991, Chapter 11, pp. 149–66.

    Farnsworth NR, et al.: Siberian ginseng (Eleutherococcus senticosus): Current status as an adaptogen. Econ Med Plant Res 1:156–215, 1985.
6. Saito H, Yoshida Y and Takagi K: Effect of Panax ginseng root on exhaustive exercise in mice. Jap J Pharmacol 24:119–27, 1974.
7. Brekhman II and Dardymov IV: New substances of plant origin which increase nonspecific resistance. Ann Rev Pharmacol 9:419–30, 1969.

    Brekhman II and Dardymov IV: Pharmacological investigation of glycosides from ginseng and Eleutherococcus. Lloydia 32:46–51, 1969.

Chapter 7

1. Cousins N: Anatomy of an Illness. Bantam Books, New York, 1979.
2. Dillon KM and Minchoff B: Positive emotional states and enhancement of the immune system. Intern J Psychiatry Med 15:13–7, 1986.

    Martin RA and Dobbin JP: Sense of humor, hassles, and immunoglobulin A: Evidence for a stress-moderating effect of humor. Int J Psychiatry Med 18:93–105, 1988.
3. Vollhardt LT: Psychoneuroimmunology: A literature review. Am J Orthopsychiatry 61:35–47, 1991.

    Kiecolt-Glaser JK and Glaser R: Psychoneuroimmunology: Can psychological interventions modulate immunity? J Consult Clin Psychol 60:569–75, 1992.
4. Irwin M, et al.: Reduction of immune function in life stress and depression. Biol Psych 27:22–30, 1990.

    O'Leary A: Stress, emotion, and human immune function. Psychol Bull 108:363–82, 1990.
5. Kusaka Y, Kondou H, and Morimoto K: Healthy lifestyles are associated with higher natural killer cell activity. Prev Med 21:602–15, 1992.

    Nekachi K and Imai K: Environmental and physiological influences on human natural killer cell activity in relation to good health practices. Jap J Cancer Res 83:789–805, 1992.

6. Sanchez A, et al.: Role of sugars in human neutrophilic phagocytosis. Am J Clin Nutr 26:1180–4, 1973.

Ringsdorf W, Cheraskin E, and Ramsay R: Sucrose, neutrophil phagocytosis and resistance to disease. Dent Surv 52:46–8, 1976.

7. Palmblad J, Hallberg D, and Rossner S: Obesity, plasma lipids and polymorphonuclear (PMN) granulocyte functions. Scand J Heamatol 19:293–303, 1977.

8. Chandra RK: Effect of vitamin and trace-element supplementation on immune responses and infection in elderly subjects. Lancet 340:1124–7, 1992.

9. National Research Council: Diet and Health. Implications for Reducing Chronic Disease Risk. National Academy Press, Washington, D.C., 1989.

10. Brown MB (ed): Present Knowledge in Nutrition, 6th Edition. Nutrition Foundation, Washington, DC, 1990.

Beisel WR: Single nutrients and immunity. Am J Clin Nutr 35:S417–68, 1982.

Alexander M, Newmark H and Miller R: Oral beta-carotene can increase the number of OKT4+ cells in human blood. Immunol Lett 9:221–4, 1985.

Vojdani A and Ghoneum M: In vivo effect of ascorbic acid on enhancement of human natural killer cell activity. Nutr Res 13:753–64, 1993.

11. Dardenne M, et al.: Contribution of zinc and other metals to the biological activity of the serum thymic factor. Proc Natl Acad Sci 79:5370–3, 1982.

Bogden JD, et al.: Zinc and immunocompetence in the elderly: Baseline data on zinc nutriture and immunity in unsupplemented subjects. Am J Clin Nutr 46:101–9, 1987.

12. Boukaiba N, et al.: A physiological amount of zinc supplementation: Effects on nutritional, lipid, and thymic status in an elderly population. Am J Clin Nutr 57:566–72, 1993.

13. Cazzola P, Mazzanti P, and Bossi G: In vivo modulating effect of a calf thymus acid lysate on human T-lymphocyte subsets and CD4+/CD8+ ratio in the course of different diseases. Curr Ther Res 42:1011–7, 1987.

Kouttab NM, Prada M, and Cazzola P: Thymomodulin: Biological properties and clinical appliactions. Medical Oncol and Tumor Pharmacother 6:5–9, 1989.

14. Fiocchi A, et al.: A double-blind clinical trial for the evaluation of the therapeutic effectiveness of a calf thymus derivative (Thymomodulin) in children with recurrent respiratory infections. Thymus 8:831–9, 1986.

15. Bauer R and Wagner H: *Echinacea* species as potential immunostimulatory drugs. Econ Med Plant Res 5:253–321, 1991.

Foster S: *Echinacea:* Nature's Immune Enhancer. Healing Arts Press, Rochester, VT, 1991.

16. Schoneberger D: The influence of immune-stimulating effects of pressed juice from *Echinacea purpurea* on the course and severity of colds: Results of a double-blind study. Forum Immunol 8:2–12, 1992.

Chapter 8

1. Laville M, et al.: Decreased glucose-induced thermogenesis at the onset of obesity. Am J Clin Nutr 57:851–6, 1993.

Rampone AJ and Reynolds PJ: Obesity: Thermodynamic principles in perspective. Life Sci 43:93–110, 1988.

2. National Research Council: Diet and Health. Implications for Reducing Chronic Disease Risk. National Academy Press, Washington, D.C., 1989.

Kawate R, et al.: Diabetes mellitus and its vascular complications in Japanese migrants on the island of Hawaii. Diabetes Care 2:161–70, 1979.

3. Spiller GA (ed): Dietary Fiber in Human Nutrition. CRC Press, Boca Raton, FL, 1992.

Anderson JW and Bryant CA: Dietary fiber: Diabetes and obesity. Am J Gastroenterol 81:898–906, 1986.

Trowell H, Burkitt D, and Heaton K: Dietary Fibre, Fibre-depleted Foods and Disease. Academic Press, New York, 1985.

4. Hylander B and Rossner S: Effects of dietary fiber intake before meals on weight loss and hunger in a weight-reducing club. Acta Med Scand 213:217–20, 1983.

   Rossner S, et al.: Weight reduction with dietary fibre supplements: Results of two double-blind studies. Acta Med Scand 222:83–8, 1987.

   El-Shebini SM, et al.: The role of pectin as a slimming agent. J Clin Biochem Nutr 4:255–62, 1988.

   Krotkiewski M: Effect of guar gum on body-weight, hunger ratings and metabolism in obese subjects. Br J Nutr 52:97–105, 1984.

5. Halama WH and Maudlin JL: Distal esophageal obstruction due to a guar gum preparation. South Med J 85:642–6, 1992.

6. Dietz WH and Gortmaker SL: Do we fatten our children at the television set? Pediatrics 75:807–12, 1985.

7. Thompson JK, et al.: Exercise and obesity: Etiology, physiology, and intervention. Psychol Bull 91:55–79, 1982.

8. van Gaal L, et al.: Exploratory study of coenzyme Q10 in obesity. In: Biomedical and Clinical Aspects of Coenzyme Q10, vol 4. Folkers K and Yamamura Y (eds). Elsevier Science Publishers, Amsterdam, 1984, pp. 369–73.

9. Baba N, Bracco EF, and Hashim SA: Enhanced thermogenesis and diminished deposition of fat in response to overfeeding with diet containing medium-chain triglyceride. Am J Clin Nutr 35:678–82, 1982.

10. Hill JO, et al.: Thermogenesis in humans during overfeeding with medium-chain triglycerides in man. Amer J Clin Nutr 44:630–4, 1986.

    Hill JO, et al.: Thermogenesis in man during overfeeding with medium-chain triglycerides. Metabol 38:641–8, 1989.

11. Seaton TB, et al.: Thermic effect of medium-chain and long-chain triglycerides in man. Am J Clin Nutr 44:630–4, 1986.

12. Acheson K, Jequier E, and Wahren J: Influence of B-beta-adrenergic blockade on glucose-induced thermogenesis in man. J Clin Invest 72:981–6, 1983.

13. Pasquali R and Casimirri F: Clinical aspects of ephedrine in the treatment of obesity. Int J Obes 17 (supplement 1):S65–8, 1993.

    Arch JRS, Ainsworth AT, and Cawthorne MA: Thermogenic and anorectic effects of ephedrine and congeners in mice and rats. Life Sci 30:1817–26, 1982.

    Massoudi M and Miller DS: Ephedrine: a thermogenic and potential slimming drug. Proc Nutr Soc 36:135A, 1977.

14. Dulloo AG and Miller DS: The thermogenic properties of ephedrine/methylxanthine mixtures: Animal studies. Am J Clin Nutr 43:388–94, 1986.

15. Astrup A, et al.: Pharmacology of thermogenic drugs. Am J Clin Nutr 55 (supplement 1):246S–48S, 1992.

    Dulloo AG, Seydoux J, and Girardier L: Potentiation of the thermogenic antiobesity effects of ephedrine by dietary methylxanthines: Adenosine antagonism or phosphodiesterase inhibition? Metabol 41(11):1233–41, 1992.

    Dulloo AG and Miller DS: The thermogenic properties of ephedrine/methylxanthine mixtures: Human studies. Int J Obesity 10:467–81, 1986.

16. Astrup A, et al.: The effect and safety of an ephedrine/caffeine compound compared to ephedrine, caffeine and placebo in obese subjects on an energy restricted diet: A double blind trial. Int J Obes 16:269–77, 1992.

    Daly PA, et al.: Ephedrine, caffeine and aspirin: Safety and efficacy for the treatment of human obesity. Int J Obes 17 (supplement 1):S73–S78, 1993.

17. Kalow W: Variability of caffeine metabolism in humans. Arzneim-Forsch 35:319–24, 1985.

18. Chee H, Romsos DR, and Leveille GA: Influence of (-)-hydroxycitrate on lipigenesis in chickens and rats. J Nutr 107:112–9, 1977.

    Sullivan AC, et al.: Effect of (-)-hydroxycitrate upon the accumulation of lipid in the rat. I. Lipogenesis. Lipids 9:121–8, 1974.

19. Rao RN and Sakariah KK: Lipid-lowering and antiobesity effect of (-)-hydroxycitric acid. Nutr Res 8:209–12, 1988.

20. Drenick EJ: Exogenous thyroid hormones to accelerate weight loss. Obes Bariatric Med 4:244–50, 1975.

    Abraham GK, et al.: The effects of triiodothyronine on energy expenditure, nitrogen balance, and rates of weight and fat loss in obese patients during prolonged caloric restriction. Int J Obes 9:433–42, 1985.

Rozen R, Abraham G, Falcou R, and Apfelbaum M: Effects of a "physiological" dose of triiodothyronine on obese subjects during a protein-sparing diet. Int J Obes 10:303–12, 1986.

Acne

1. Michaelsson G, Vahlquist A, and Juhlin L: Serum zinc and retinol-binding protein in acne. Br J Dermatol 96:283–6, 1977.
2. Michaelsson G, Juhlin L, and Ljunghall K: A double-blind study of the effect of zinc and oxytetracycline in acne vulgaris. Br J Dermatol 97:561–5, 1977.

   Cunliffe WJ, et al.: A double-blind trial of a zinc sulphate/citrate complex and tetracycline in the treatment of acne. Br J Dermatol 101:321–5, 1979.

   Dreno B, et al.: Low doses of zinc gluconate for inflammatory acne. Acta Derm Venereol 69:541–3, 1989.
3. Kugman A, et al.: Oral vitamin A in acne vulgaris. Int J Dermatol 20:278–85, 1981.
4. Michaelsson G and Edqvist L: Erythrocyte glutathione peroxidase activity in acne vulgaris and the effect of selenium and vitamin E treatment. Acta Derm Venerol (StockH) 64:9–14, 1984.

   Snider B and Dieteman D: Pyridoxine therapy for premenstrual acne flare. Arch Dermatol 110:103–1, 1974.

Age Spots

1. Eskelinen A and Santalahti J: Natural cartilage polysaccharides for the treatment of sun-damaged skin in females: A double-blind comparison of Vivida and Imedeen. J Int Med 20:227–33, 1992.

   Lassus J, et al.: Imedeen for the treatment of degenerated skin in females. J Int Med 19:147–52, 1991.

Anemia

1. Mahan LK and Arlin M: Krause's Food, Nutrition, and Diet Therapy, 8th edition. Saunders, Philadelphia, 1992.

   Shils ME and Young VR: Modern Nutrition in Health and Disease, 7th edition. Lea and Febiger, Philadelphia, 1988.

Angina

1. Graboys TD, et al.: Results of a second opinion program for coronary artery bypass surgery. JAMA 268:2537–40, 1992.

   Graboys TD, et al.: Results of a second opinion program for coronary artery bypass surgery. JAMA 258:1611–4, 1987.
2. Alderman EL, et al.: Ten-year follow-up of survival and myocardial infarction in the randomized coronary artery surgery study (CASS). Circ 82:1629–46, 1990.

   CASS Principle Investigators and Their Associates: Myocardial infarction and mortality in the coronary artery surgery study (CASS) randomized trial. New Engl J Med 310:750–8, 1984.

CASS Principle Investigators and Their Associates: Coronary artery surgery (CASS)—A randomized trial of coronary artery bypass surgery. Circ 68:939–50, 1983.

3. White CW, et al.: Does visual interpretation of the coronary angiogram predict the physiologic importance of a coronary stenosis? New Eng J Med 310:819–24, 1984.

4. Winslow CM, et al.: The appropriateness of performing coronary artery bypass surgery. JAMA 260:505, 1988.

5. Hueb W: Two- to eight-year survival rates in patients who refused coronary artery bypass grafting. Am J Cardiol 63:155–9, 1989.

6. Clarke NE, et al.: Treatment of angina pectoris with disodium ethylene diamine tetraacetic acid. Am J Med Sci 232:654–66, 1956.

   Clarke NE: Atherosclerosis, occlusive vascular disease and EDTA. Am J Cardiol 6:233–6, 1960.

   Clarke NE, et al.: Treatment of occlusive vascular disease with disodium ethylene diamine tetraacetic acid (EDTA). Am J Med Sci 239:732–44, 1960.

7. Steinberg D, et al.: Beyond cholesterol: Modifications of low-density lipoprotein that increase its atherogenicity. N Engl J Med 320:915–24, 1989.

8. Cranton EM and Frackelton JP: Current status of EDTA chelation therapy in occlusive arterial disease. J Adv Med 2:107–19, 1989.

   Olszwer E and Carter JP: EDTA chelation therapy: A retrospective study of 2,870 patients. J Adv Med 2:197–211, 1989.

   Olszewer E, Sabbag FC, and Carter JP: A pilot double-blind study of sodium-magnesium EDTA in peripheral vascular disease. J Nat Med Assoc 82:173–7, 1988.

   Olszewer E and Carter JP: EDTA chelation therapy in chronic degenerative disease. Med Hypoth 27:41–9, 1988.

   Casdorph HR: EDTA chelation therapy: Efficacy in arteriosclerotic heart disease. J Hol Med 3:53–9, 1981.

9. Sloth-Neilsen J, et al.: Arteriographic findings in EDTA chelation therapy on peripheral atherosclerosis. Am J Surg 162:122–5, 1991.

   Guldager B, et al.: EDTA treatment of intermittent claudication: A double-blind, placebo-controlled study. J Int Med 231:261–7, 1992.

10. Ritchie JL, et al.: Coronary angioplasty: Statewide experience in California. Circ 88:2735–43, 1993.

11. Ornish D, et al.: Can lifestyle changes reverse coronary heart disease? Lancet 336:129–33, 1990.

12. Cherchi A, et al.: Effects of L-carnitine on exercise tolerance in chronic stable angina: A multicenter, double-blind, randomized, placebo-controlled, crossover study. Int J Clin Pharm Ther Toxicol 23:569–72, 1985.

    Orlando G and Rusconi C: Oral L-carnitine in the treatment of chronic cardiac ischaemia in elderly patients. Clin Trials J 23:338–44, 1986.

    Kamikawa T, et al.: Effects of L-carnitine on exercise tolerance in patients with stable angina pectoris. Jap Heart J 25:587–97, 1984.

    Pola P, et al.: Use of physiological substance, acetylcarnitine, in the treatment of angiospastic syndromes. Drugs Exptl Clin Res X:213–7, 1984.

    Folkers K and Yamamura Y (eds): Biomedical and Clinical Aspects of Coenzyme Q10, vols 1–4, Elsevier Science Publishers, Amsterdam, vol. 1:1977, vol. 2:1980, vol. 3:1982, vol. 4:1984.

    Littarru GP, Ho L, and Folkers K: Deficiency of coenzyme Q10 in human heart disease: Part II. Int J Vit Nutr Res 42:413, 1972.

    Kamikawa T, Kobayashi A, Yamashita T, et al.: Effects of coenzyme Q10 on exercise tolerance in chronic stable angina pectoris. Am J Cardiol 56:247, 1985.

13. Turlapaty PDMV and Altura BM: Magnesium deficiency produces spasms of coronary arteries: Relationship to etiology of sudden death ischemic heart disease. Sci 208:199–200, 1980.

    Altura BM: Ischemic heart disease and magnesium. Magnesium 7:57–67, 1988.

    Iseri L: Role of magnesium in cardiac tachyarrhythmias. Am J Cardiol 65:47k–50k, 1990.

    Teo KK and Yusuf S: Role of magnesium in reducing mortality in acute myocardia. Drugs 46:347–1993.

14. Ammon HPT and Handel M: Crataegus, toxicology and pharmacology. Planta Medica 43:101–120,318–22, 1981.
    O'Conolly VM, et al.: Treatment of cardiac performance (NYHA stages I to II) in advanced age with standardized crataegus extract. Fortschr Med 104:805–8, 1986.
    Leuchtgens H: Crataegus Special Extract WS 1442 in NYHA II heart failure: A placebo-controlled, randomized, double-blind study. Fortschr Med 111(20–21): 352–4, 1993.
15. Osher HL, Katz KH, and Wagner DJ: Khellin in the treatment of angina pectoris. New Eng J Med 244:315–21, 1951.
    Anrep GV, Kenawy MR, and Barsoum GS: Coronary vasocilator action of khellin. Am Heart J 37:531–42, 1949.
16. Conn JJ, Kisane RW, Koons RA, and Clark TE: Treatment of angina pectoris with khellin. Ann Int Med 36:1173–8, 1952.

Anxiety

1. Werbach MR: Nutritional Influences on Mental Illness. Third Line Press, Tarzana, CA, 1991.
2. Heulluy B: Random trial of L.72 with diazepam in cases of nervous depression. Center for Therapeutic Research and Documentation, Paris, France, January 1985.

Asthma

1. Kaliner M and Lemanske R: Rhinitis and asthma. JAMA 268:2807–29, 1992.
2. Sly RM: Asthma mortality, East and West. Annals Allergy 69:81–4, 1992.
3. Brostoff J and Challacombe SJ (eds): Food Allergy and Intolerance. Saunders, Philadelphia, 1987.
4. Lindahl O, Lindwall L, Spangberg A, et al.: Vegan diet regimen with reduced medication in the treatment of bronchial asthma. J Asthma 22:45–55, 1985.
5. Olusi SO, et al.: Plasma and white blood cell ascorbic acid concentrations in patients with bronchial asthma. Clin Chimica Acta 92:161–6, 1979.
6. Anderson R, et al.: Ascorbic acid in bronchial asthma. SA Med J 63:649–52, 1983.
    Spannhake EW and Menkes HA: Vitamin C—New tricks for an old dog. Am Rev Resp Dis 127:139–41, 1983.
7. Johnston CS, Retrum KR, and Srilakshmi JC: Antihistamine effects and complications of supplemental vitamin C. J Am Diet Assoc 92:988–9, 1992.
8. Foreman JC: Mast cells and the actions of flavonoids. J Allergy Clin Immunol 127:546–50, 1984.
9. Cody V, et al.: Plant Flavonoids in Biology and Medicine II—Biochemical, Pharmacological, and Structure-activity Relationships. Alan R Liss, New York, 1988.
10. Taussig S: The mechanism of the physiological action of bromelain. Med Hypoth 6:99–104, 1980.
11. Duke JA and Ayensu ES: Medicinal Plants of China. Reference Publications, Algonac, MI, 1985.
12. American Pharmaceutical Association: Handbook of Nonprescription Drugs, 8th edition. American Pharmaceutical Association, Washington, DC, 1986.
13. Tinkelman DG and Avner SE: Ephedrine therapy in asthmatic children. JAMA 237:553–7, 1977.

Bladder Infection

1. Sobota AE: Inhibition of bacterial adherence by cranberry juice: Potential use for the treatment of urinary tract infections. J Urol 131:1013–6, 1984.

2. Prodromos PN, et al.: Cranberry juice in the treatment of urinary tract infections. Southwestern Med 47:17, 1968.
3. Avorn J, et al.: Reduction of bacteriuria and pyuria after ingestion of cranberry juice. JAMA 271:751–4, 1994.

Boils

1. Altman PM: Australian teatree oil. Australian J Pharmacy 69:276–8, 1988.
   Feinblatt HM: Cajeput-type oil for the treatment of furunculosis. J Nat Med Assoc 52:32–4, 1960.
2. Body I: Treatment of recurrent faruncles with oral zinc. Lancet ii:1358, 1977.

Bronchitis and Pneumonia

1. Hahn FE and Ciak J: Berberine. Antibiotics 3:577–88, 1976.
   Amin AH, Subbaiah TV, and Abbasi KM: Berberine sulfate: Antimicrobial activity, bioassay, and mode of action. Can J Microbiol 15:1067–76, 1969.
2. Rimoldi R, Ginesu F, and Giura R: The use of bromelain in pneumological therapy. Drugs Exp Clin Res 4:55–66, 1978.
   Ryan R: A double-blind clinical evaluation of bromelain in the treatment of acute sinusitis. Headache 7:13–7, 1967.
   Taussig S and Batkin: Bromelain, the enzyme complex of pineapple (*Ananas comosus*) and its clinical application: An update. J Ethnopharmacol 22:191–203, 1988.
3. Neubauer R: A plant protease for the potentiation of and possible replacement of antibiotics. Exp Med Surg 19:143–60, 1961.
   Tinozzi S and Venegoni A: Effect of bromelain on serum and tissue levels of amoxycillin. Drugs Exp Clin Res 4:39–44, 1978.

Candidiasis

1. Truss O: The Missing Diagnosis. POB 26508, Birmingham, AL, 1983.
   Crook WG: The Yeast Connection, 2nd edition. Professional Books, Jackson, TN, 1984.
2. Kroker GF: Chronic candidiasis and allergy. In: Food Allergy and Intolerance. Brostoff J and Challacombe SJ (eds). Saunders, Philadelphia, 1987 pp. 850–72.
   Galland L: Nutrition and candidiasis. J Orthomol Psychiatry 15:50–60, 1985.
3. Rubinstein E, Mark Z, Haspel J, et al.: Antibacterial activity of the pancreatic fluid. Gastroenterol 88:927–32, 1985.
4. Pizzorno JE and Murray MT (eds): A Textbook of Natural Medicine. Bastyr College Publications, Seattle, 1992, Chapter IV, pp. 1–6.
5. Abe F, Nagata S, and Hotchi M: Experimental candidiasis in liver injury. Mycopathol 100:37–42, 1987.
6. Adetumbi MA and Lau BH: *Allium sativum* (garlic)—A natural antibiotic. Med Hypoth 12:227–37, 1983.
   Moore GS and Atkins RD: The fungicidal and fungistatic effects of an aqueous garlic extract on medically important yeast-like fungi. Mycol 69:341–8, 1977.
   Sandhu DK, Warraich MK, and Singh S: Sensitivity of yeasts isolated from cases of vaginitis to aqueous extracts of garlic. Mykosen 23:691–8, 1980.
   Prasad G and Sharma VD: Efficacy of garlic (*Allium sativum*) treatment against experimental candidiasis in chicks. Br Vet J 136:448–51, 1980.
7. Neuhauser I and Gustus EL: Successful treatment of intestinal moniliasis with fatty acid resin complex. Arch Intern Med 93:53–60, 1954.

Scwhabe AD, Bennett LR, and Bowman LP: Octanoic acid absorption and oxidation in humans. J Applied Physiol 19:335–7, 1964.

8. Collins EB and Hardt P: Inhibition of *Candida albicans* by *Lactobacillus acidophilus*. J Dairy Sci 63:830–2, 1980.

Canker Sores

1. Wray D, et al.: Recurrent aphthae: Treatment with vitamin B12, folic acid, and iron. Br Med J 2:490–3, 1975.

   Wray DW, et al.: Nutritional deficiencies in recurrent aphthae. J Oral Path 7:418–23, 1978.

2. Little JW: Food allergens and basophil histamine release in recurrent aphthous stomatitis. Oral Surg 54:388–95, 1982.

   Thomas HC, et al.: Food antibodies in oral disease: A study of serum antibodies to food proteins in aphthous ulceration and other oral diseases. J Clin Path 26:371–4, 1973.

   Wilson CWM: Food sensitivities, taste changes, aphthous ulcers and atopic symptoms in allergic disease. Ann Allergy 44:302–7, 1980.

   Rays RA, Hamerlinck F, and Cormane RH: Immunoglobulin-bearing lymphocytes and polymorphonuclear leukocytes in recurrent aphthous ulcers in man. Arch Oral Biol 22:147–53, 1977.

   Wray D: Gluten-sensitive recurrent aphthous stomatitis. Dig Dis Sci 26:737–40, 1981.

   Walker DM, et al.: Gluten hypersensitivity in recurrent aphthous ulceration. J Dent Res 58 (Special Issue C):1271, 1979.

3. Hay KD and Reade PC: The use of an elimination diet in the treatment of recurrent aphthous ulceration of the oral cavity. Oral Surg 57:504–7, 1984.

4. Das SK, et al.: Deglycyrrhizinated liquorice in apthous ulcers. JAPI 37:647, 1989.

Carpal Tunnel Syndrome

1. Ellis JM, et al.: Response of vitamin B6 deficiency and the carpal tunnel syndrome to pyridoxine. Proc Natl Acad Sci USA, 79:7494–8, 1982.

   Ellis J, et al.: Clinical results of a crossover treatment with pyridoxine and placebo of the carpal tunnel syndrome. Am J Clin Nutr 32:2040–6, 1979.

   Ellis JM, et al.: Survey and new data on treatment with pyridoxine of patients having a clinical syndrome including the carpal tunnel and other defects. Res Comm Clin Path Pharm 17:165–7, 1977.

2. Guzman FJL, et al.: Carpal tunnel syndrome and vitamin B6. Klin Wochenschr 67:38–41, 1989.

   Hamfelt, A: Carpal tunnel syndrome and vitamin B6 deficiency. Clin Chem, 28:721, 1982.

3. Phalen, G.S: The birth of a syndrome, or carpal tunnel syndrome revisited. J Hand Surg, 6:109–10, 1981.

4. Gaby, A: The Doctor's Guide to Vitamin B6. Rodale Press, Emmaus, PA, 1984.

Cataract

1. Taylor A: Cataract: Relationships between nutrition and oxidation. J Am Coll Nutr 12:138–46, 1993.

   Jacques PF and Chylack LT: Epidemiologic evidence of a role for the antioxidant vitamin and carotenoids in cataract prevention. Am J Clin Nutr 53:352S–5S, 1991.

   Taylor A: Associations between nutrition and cataract. Nutr Rev 47:225–33, 1989.

Jacques PF, et al.: Antioxidant status in persons with and without senile cataract. Arch Ophthalmol 106:337–40, 1988.

2. Atkinson D: Malnutrition as an etiological factor in senile cataract. Eye, Ear, Nose and Throat Monthly 31:79–83, 1952.

3. Ringvold A, Johnsen H and Blika S: Senile cataract and ascorbic acid loading. Acta Opthalmol 63:277–80, 1985.

Bouton S: Vitamin C and the aging eye. Arch Int Med 63:930–45, 1939.

Cerebral Vascular Insufficiency

1. Kleijnen J and Knipschild P: Drug profiles—*Ginkgo biloba*. Lancet 340:1136–9, 1993.

Kleijnen J and Knipschild P: *Ginkgo biloba* for cerebral insufficiency. Br J Clin Pharamacol 34:352–8, 1992.

Vorberg G: *Ginkgo biloba* extract (GBE): A long-term study of chronic cerebral insufficiency in geriatric patients. Clin Trials J 22:149–157, 1985.

2. Dion JE, et al.: Clinical events following neuroangiography: A prospective study. Stroke 18:997–1004, 1987.

3. Barnett HJM, Barnes RW, and Robertson JT: The uncertainties surrounding carotic endartectomy. JAMA 268:3120–1, 1992.

Fode NC, et al.: Multicenter retrospective review of results and complications of carotid endarterectomy. Stroke 17:370–6, 1986.

4. Winslow CM, et al.: The appropriateness of carotid endarterectomy. N Engl J Med 318:721–7, 1988.

5. NASCET collaborators: Beneficial effect of carotid endarterectomy in symptomatic patients with high-grade carotid stenosis. N Eng J Med 325:445–53, 1991.

European Carotid Surgery Trialists Collaborative Group. MRC European Surgery Trial: Interim results for symptomatic patients with severe (70–99%) or with mild (0–29%) carotid stenosis. Lancet 337:1235–43, 1991.

Easton JD and Wilterdink JL: Carotid endarterectomy: Trials and tribulations. Ann Neurol 35:5–17, 1994.

Cholesterol

1. National Research Council: Diet and Health. Implications for Reducing Chronic Disease Risk. National Academy Press, Washington, D.C., 1989.

2. Wilson PWF: High-density lipoprotein, low-density lipoprotein and coronary artery disease. Am J Cardiol 66:7A–10A, 1990.

3. The Expert Panel: Report of the National Cholesterol Education Program Expert Panel on detection, evaluation, and treatment of high cholesterol in adults. Arch Intern Med 148:136–69, 1988.

4. Stanto JL and Keast DR: Serum cholesterol, fat intake, and breakfast consumption in the United States adult population. J Am Coll Nutr 8:567–72, 1989.

5. Stamler J and Shekelle R: Dietary cholesterol and human coronary artery disease. Arch Pathol Lab Med 112:1032–40, 1988.

6. Booyens J and Van Der Merwe CF: Margarines and coronary artery disease. Med Hypoth 37:241–4, 1992.

Mensink RP and Katan MB: Effect of dietary trans fatty acids on high-density and low-density lipoprotein cholesterol levels in healthy subjects. New Engl J Med 323:439–45, 1990.

7. Schmidt EB and Dyerberg J: Omega-3 fatty acids: Current status in cardiovascular medicine. Drugs 47:405–24, 1994.

8. Cobias L, et al.: Lipid, lipoprotein, and hemostatic effects of fish vs fish oil w-3 fatty acids in mildly hyperlipidemic males. Am J Clin Nutr 53:1210–6, 1991.

9. Ripsin CM, Keenan JM, Jacobs DR, et al.: Oat products and lipid lowering: A meta-analysis. JAMA 267:3317–25, 1992.

10. Warshafsky S. et al.: Effect of garlic on total serum cholesterol. Ann Intern Med 119:599–605, 1993.

Jain AK, et al.: Can garlic reduce levels of serum lipids? A controlled clinical study. Am J Med 94:632–5, 1993.

Rotzch W, et al.: Postprandial lipaemia under treatment with *Allium sativum:* Controlled double-blind study in healthy volunteers with reduced HDL2-cholesterol levels. Arzneim-Forsch 42:1223–7, 1992.

11. Kiesewetter H, et al.: Effect of garlic on thrombocyte aggregation, microcirculation, and other risk factors. Int J Clin Pharmacol Ther Toxicol 29:151–5, 1991.

Legnani C et al.: Effects of dried garlic preparation on fibrinolysis and platelet aggregation in healthy subjects. Arzneim-Forsch 43:119–21, 1993.

Phelps S and Harris WS: Garlic supplementation and lipoprotein oxidation susceptibility. Lipids 28:475–7, 1993.

12. Sandvik L, et al.: Physical fitness as a predictor of mortality among healthy, middle-aged Norwegian men. New Engl J Med 328:533–7, 1993.

13. Paffenbarger RS, et al.: The association of changes in physical activity level and other lifestyle characteristics with mortality among men. New Engl J Med 328:538–545, 1993.

14. Kelley MD: Hypercholesterolemia: The cost of treatment in perspective. Southern Med J 83:1421–5, 1991.

15. The Coronary Drug Project Group: Clofibrate and niacin in coronary heart disease. JAMA 231:360–81, 1975.

16. Canner PL and the Coronary Drug Project Group: Mortality in Coronary Drug Project patients during a nine-year post-treatment period. J Am Coll Cardiol 8:1245–55, 1986.

17. Welsh AL and Ede M: Inositol hexanicotinate for improved nicotinic acid therapy. Int Record Med 174:9–15, 1961.

El-Enein AMA, et al.: The role of nicotinic acid and inositol hexaniacinate as anticholesterolemic and antilipemic agents. Nutr Rep Intl 28:899–911, 1983.

18. Sunderland GT, et al.: A double-blind, randomized, placebo-controlled trial of hexopal in primary Raynaud's disease. Clin Rheumatol 7:46–9, 1988.

19. Henkin Y, Johnson KC, and Segrest JP: Rechallenge with crystalline niacin after drug-induced hepatitis from sustained-release niacin. JAMA 264:241–3, 1990.

20. Satyavati GV: Gum guggul (*Commiphora mukul*)—The success story of an ancient insight leading to a modern discovery. Ind J Med Res 87:327–335, 1988.

Nityanand S, Srivastava JS, and Asthana OP: Clinical trials with gugulipid: A new hypolipidaemic agent. J Assoc Phys India 37:321–8, 1989.

21. Goa KL and Brogden RN: L-carnitine—A preliminary review of its pharmacokinetics and its therapeutic use in ischemic cardiac disease and primary and secondary carnitine deficiencies in relationship to its role in fatty acid metabolism. Drugs 34:1–24, 1987.

Chronic Fatigue Syndrome

1. Holmes GP, et al.: Chronic fatigue syndrome: A working case definition. Ann Intern Med 108:387–9, 1988.

2. Bates DW, et al.: Prevalence of fatigue and chronic fatigue syndrome in a primary care practice. Arch Int Med 2759–65, 1993.

3. Shafran SD: The chronic fatigue syndrome. Am J Med 90:731–9, 1991.

Kyle DV and Deshazo RD: Chronic fatigue syndrome: A conundrum. Am J Med Sci 303:28–34, 1992.

Caligiuri M, et al.: Phenotypic and functional deficiency of natural killer cells in patients with chronic fatigue syndrome. J Immunol 139:3306–13, 1987.

Gupta S and Vayuvegula B: A comprehensive immunological analysis in chronic fatigue syndrome. Scand J Immunol 33:319–27, 1991.

Demitrack MA: Chronic fatigue syndrome: A disease of the hypothalamic-pituitary-adrenal axis. Annals Med 26:1–3, 1994.

Cold Sores

1. Dimitrova Z, et al.: Antiherpes effect of *Melissa officinalis L.* extracts. Acta Microbiol Bulg 29:65–72, 1993.
   Cohen RA, Kucera LS, and Herrmann EC: Antiviral activity of *Melissa officinalis* (Lemon balm) extract. Proc Soc Exp Biol Med 117:431–4, 1964.
2. Wolbling RH and Milbradt R: Clinical therapy of Herpes simplex. Therapiewoche 34:1193–1200, 1984.
   Vogt, et al.: Melissa extract in herpes simplex: A double-blind, placebo-controlled study. Der Allgemeinarzt 13:832–41, 1991.

Common Cold

1. Sanchez A, et al.: Role of sugars in human neutrophilic phagocytosis. Am J Clin Nutr 26:1180–4, 1973.
2. Hemila H: Vitamin C and the common cold. Br J Nutr 67:3–16, 1992.
3. Eby GA, Davis DR, and Halcomb WW: Reduction in duration of common colds by zinc gluconate lozenges in a double-blind study. Antimicrob Agents Chemother 25:20–4, 1984.
4. Graham NMH, et al.: Adverse effects of aspirin, acetominophen, and ibuprofen on immune function, viral shedding, and clinical status in rhinovirus-infected volunteers. J Infect Dis 162:1277–82, 1990.

Constipation

1. Sonnenberg A and Koch TR: Epidemiology of constipation in the United States. Dis Colon Rectum 32:1–8, 1989.

Crohn's Disease and Ulcerative Colitis

1. Levi AJ: Diet in the management of Crohn's disease. Gut 26:985–8, 1985.
   Jarnerot J, Jarnmark I, and Nilsson K: Consumption of refined sugar by patients with Crohn's disease, ulcerative colitis, or irritable bowel syndrome. Scand J Gastroenterol 18:999–1002, 1983.
   Mayberry JF, Rhodes J, and Newcombe RG: Increased sugar consumption in Crohn's disease. Digestion 20:323–6, 1980.
   Grimes DS: Refined carbohydrate, smooth-muscle spasm and diseases of the colon. Lancet i:395–7, 1976.
   Thornton JR, Emmett PM, and Heaton KW: Diet and Crohn's disease: Characteristics of the pre-illness diet. Br Med J 279:762–4, 1979.
2. Morain CO, Segal AW, and Levi AJ: Elemental diet as primary treatment of acute Crohn's disease: A controlled trial. Br Med J 288:1859–62, 1984.
   Harries AD, et al.: Controlled trial of supplemented oral nutrition in Crohn's disease. Lancet i:887–90, 1983.
   Axelsson C and Jarnum S: Assessment of the therapeutic value of an elemental diet in chronic inflammatory bowel disease. Scand J Gastroenterol 12:89–95, 1977.
   Voitk AJ, et al.: Experience with elemental diet in the treatment of inflammatory bowel disease. Arch Surg 107:329–33, 1973.
   Workman EM, et al.: Diet in the management of Crohn's disease. Human Nutr: Applied Nutr 38A:469–73, 1984.
   Jones VA, et al.: Crohn's disease: Maintenance of remission by diet. Lancet ii:177–80, 1985.

Rowe A and Uyeyama K: Regional enteritis—Its allergic aspects. Gastroenterol 23:554–71, 1953.

3. Rosenberg IH, Bengoa JM, and Sitrin MD: Nutritional aspects of inflammatory bowel disease. Ann Rev Nutr 5:463–84, 1985.
4. Heaton KW, Tornton JR, and Emmett PM: Treatment of Crohn's disease with an un-refined-carbohydrate, fiber-rich diet. Br Med J 279:764–6, 1979.
5. Salyers AA, Kurtitza AP, and McCarthy RE: Influence of dietary fiber on the intestinal environment. Proc Soc Exp Biol Med 180:415–21, 1985.
6. Hawthorne AB, et al.: Treatment of ulcerative colitis with fish oil supplementation: A prospective 12-month randomized, controlled trial. Gut 33:922–8, 1992.

Depression

1. Null G: Prozac, Eli Lilly and the FDA. Towns Lett #115/116:134,178–87, 1993.
2. Daniel Carr, et al.: Physical conditioning facilitates the exercised-induced secretion of beta-endorphin and beta-lipoprotein in women. New Engl J Med 305:560–5, 1981.
3. Lobstein D, Mosbacher BJ, and Ismail AH: Depression as a powerful discriminator between physically active and sedentary middle-aged men. J Psychosom Res 27:69–76, 1983.
4. Werbach M: Nutritional Influences on Mental Illness: A Sourcebook of Clinical Research. Third Line Press, Tarzana, CA, 1991.
5. Mulder H and Zoller M: Antidepressive effects of a hypericum extract standardized to the active hypericine content. Arzneim-Forsch 34:918029, 1984.
6. Woelk H: Multicentric practice-study analyzing the functional capacity in depressive patients. Presented at The Fourth International Congress on Phytotherapy. Munich, Germany, September 10–13, 1992, abstract SL54.
   Sommer H: Improvement of psychovegetative complaints by hypericum. Presented at The Fourth International Congress on Phytotherapy. Munich, Germany, September 10–13, 1992, abstract SL55.

Diabetes

1. University Group Diabetes Program: A story of the effectiveness of hypoglycemic agents on vascular complications in patients with adult-onset diabetes. II. Mortality results. Diabetes 19:789–830, 1970.
2. Anderson J: Chapter 57: Nutrition management of diabetes mellitus. In: Modern Nutrition in Health and Disease. Goodhart R and Young VR (eds). Lea and Febiger, Philadelphia, 1988, pp. 1201–29.
3. Anderson JW and Ward K: High-carbohydrate, high-fiber diets for insulin-treated men with diabetes mellitus. Am J Clin Nutr 32:2312–21, 1979.
4. Simpson HCR, et al.: A high-carbohydrate leguminous fiber diet improves all aspects of diabetic control. Lancet i:1–5, 1981.
5. Amiel SA: Intensified insulin therapy. Diabetes Metab Rev 9:3–24, 1993.
6. Pocoit F, Reimers JI and Andersen HU: Nicotinamide—Biological actions and therapeutic potential in diabetes prevention. Diabetologia 36:574–6, 1993.
   Cleary JP: Vitamin B3 in the treatment of diabetes mellitus: Case reports and review of the literature. J Nutr Med 1:217–225, 1990.
7. Shanmugasundaram ERB, et al.: Use of *Gymnema sylvestre* leaf extract in the control of blood glucose in insulin-dependent diabetes mellitus. J Ethnopharmacol 30:281–94, 1990.
   Baskaran K, et al.: Antidiabetic effect of a leaf extract from *Gymnema sylvestre* in non-insulin-dependent diabetes mellitus patients. J Ethnopharmacol 30:295–305, 1990.

8. Cunningham J: Reduced mononuclear leukocyte ascorbic acid content in adults with insulin-depedent diabetes mellitus consuming adequate dietary vitamin C. Metabol 40:146–9, 1991.
9. Anderson RA: Chromium, glucose tolerance, and diabetes. Biol Trace Elem Res 32:19–24, 1992.
    Anderson RA, et al.: Effects of supplemental chromium on patients with symptoms of reactive hypoglycemia. Metabol 36:351–5, 1987.
10. Sancetta SM, Ayres PR, and Scott RW: The use of vitamin B12 in the management of the neurological manifestations of diabetes mellitus, with notes on the administration of massive doses. Ann Int Med 35:1028–48, 1951.
    Galli C and Socin A: Biological aspects and possible uses of vitamin E. Acta Vitaminol Enzymol 4:245–52, 1984.
    Vogelsang A: Vitamin E in the treatment of diabetes mellitus. Ann NY Acad Sci 52:406, 1949.
11. Jones CL and Gonzalez V: Pyridoxine deficiency: A new factor in diabetic neuropathy. J Am Pod Assoc 68:646–53, 1978.
    Solomon LR and Cohen K: Erythrocyte O2 transport and metabolism and effects of vitamin B6 therapy in type II diabetes mellitus. Diabetes 38:881–6, 1989.
12. White JR and Campbell RK: Magnesium and diabetes: A review. Ann Pharmacother 27:775–80, 1993.
13. Davie SJ, Gould BJ, and Yudkin JS: Effect of vitamin C on glycosylation of proteins. Diabetes 41:167–73, 1992.

Ear Infection

1. Willaims RL, et al.: Use of antibiotics in preventing recurrent otitis media and in treating otitis media with effusion. JAMA 270:1344–51, 1993.
    Bluestone CD: Otitis media in children: To treat or not to treat. NEJM 306:1399–404, 1982.
    Van Buchen FL, Dunk JH, and van Hof MA: Therapy of acute otitis media: Myringotomy, antibiotics, or neither? Lancet 2:883–7, 1981.
    Diamant M and Diamant B: Abuse and timing of use of antibiotics in acute otitis media. Arch Otol 100:226–32, 1974.
    Mygind N, et al.: Penicillin in acute otitis media: A double-blind, placebo-controlled trial. Clin Otol 6:5–13, 1981.
2. Kraemer MJ, Richardson MA, Weiss NS, et al.: Risk factors for persistent middle-ear effusion. JAMA 249:1022–5, 1983.
    Black N: The aetiology of glue ear: A case-control study. Int J Pediatr Otorhinolaryngol 9:121–33, 1985.
3. Etzel RA, et al.: Passive smoking and middle ear effusion among children in day care. Pediatrics 90:228–32, 1992.
4. Duncan B, et al.: Exclusive breast-feeding for at least four months protects against otitis media. Pediatrics 91:867–72, 1993.
    Saarinen UM: Prolonged breast-feeding as prophylaxis for recurrent otitis media. Acta Ped Scand 71:567–71, 1982.
    Editor: Breast-feeding prevents otitis media. Nutr Rev 41:241–2, 1983.
5. Viscomi GJ: Allergic secretory otitis media: An approach to management. Laryngoscope 85:751–8, 1975.
    Van Cauwenberge PB: The role of allergy in otitis media with effusion. Ther Umschau 39:1011–6, 1982.
    Bellionin P, Cantani A, and Salvinelli F: Allergy: A leading role in otitis media with effusion. Allergol Immunol 15:205–8, 1987.
6. McMahan JT, et al.: Chronic otitis media with effusion and allergy: Modified RAST analysis of 119 cases. Otol Head Neck Surg 89:427–31, 1981.

Eczema

1. Sloper KS, Wadsworth J, and Brostoff J: Children with atopic eczema. I. Clinical response to food elimination and subsequent double-blind food challenge. Quart J Med 80:677–93, 1991.
2. Biagi PL, et al.: A long-term study on the use of evening primrose oil (Efamol) in atopic children. Drugs Exptl Clin Res 4:285–90, 1988.
3. Evans FQ: The rational use of glycyrrhetinic acid in dermatology. Brit J Clin Prac 12:269–79, 1958.
4. Okimasa E, et al.: Inhibition of phospholipase A2 by glycyrrhizin: An anti-inflammatory drug. Acta Med Okayama 37:385–91, 1983.
   Mann C and Staba EJ: The chemistry, pharmacology, and commercial formulations of chamomile. Herbs, Spices, and Medicinal Plants 1:235–80, 1984.

Fibrocystic Breast Disease

1. Petrakis NL and King EB: Cytological abnormalities in nipple aspirates of breast fluid from women with severe constipation. Lancet 2:1203–5, 1981.
2. Hentges DJ: Does diet influence human fecal microflora composition? Nutr Rev 38:329–6, 1980.
3. Goldin B, et al.: Effect of diet on excretion of estrogens in pre- and postmenopausal women. Cancer Res 41:3771–3, 1981.
4. London RS, et al.: Endocrine parameters and alpha-tocopherol therapy of patients with mammary dysplasia. Cancer Res 41:3811–3, 1981.
   London RS, et al.: The effect of alpha-tocopherol on premenstrual symptomatology: A double-blind study. II. Endocrine correlates. J Am Col Nutr 3:351–6, 1984.
5. Sundaram GS, et al.: Serum hormones and lipoproteins in benign breast disease. Cancer Res 41:3814–6, 1981.
6. Boyle CA, et al.: Caffeine consumption and fibrocystic breast disease: A case-control epidemiologic study. JNCI 72:1015–9, 1984.
   Minton JP, et al.: Clinical and biochemical studies on methylxanthine-related fibrocystic breast disease. Surgery 90:299–304, 1981.
   Minton JP, et al.: Caffeine, cyclic nucleotides, and breast disease. Surgery 86:105–9, 1979.
7. Ernster VL, et al.: Effects of caffeine-free diet on benign breast disease: A random trial. Surgery 91:263–7, 1982.

Food Allergy

1. Brostoff J and Challacombe SJ (eds): Food Allergy and Intolerance. Saunders, Philadelphia, 1987.
2. Murray, MT: The Healing Power of Foods. Prima Publishing, Rocklin, CA, 1993.

Gallstones

1. Trowell H, Burkitt D, and Heaton K: Dietary Fibre, Fibre-depleted Foods and Disease. Academic Press, New York, 1985.
2. Pixley F, Wilson D, McPherson K, et al.: Effect of vegetariansim on development of gallstones in women. Brit Med J 291:11–2, 1985.
3. Breneman JC: Allergy elimination diet as the most effective gallbladder diet. Annals Allergy 26:83–7, 1968.

4. Nassauto G, et al.: Effect of silibinin on biliary lipid composition: Experimental and clinical study. J Hepatol 12:290–5, 1991.
5. Shandalik R, Gatti G, and Perucca E: Pharmacokinetics of silybin in bile following administration of silipide and silymarin in cholecystectomy patients. Arzneim-Forsch 42:964–8, 1992.

   Barzaghi N, et al.: Pharmacokinetic studies on IdB 1016, a silybin-phosphatidyl-choline complex, in healthy human subjects. Eur J Drug Metab Pharmacokinet 15:333–8, 1990.

Glaucoma

1. Virno M, Bucci M, Pecori-Giraldi J, and Missiroli A: Oral treatment of glaucoma with vitamin C. Eye, Ear, Nose, Throat Monthly 46:1502–8, 1967.

   Bietti G: Further contributions on the value of osmotic substances as means to reduce intraocular pressure. Trans Ophthamol Soc U.K. 86:247–54, 1966.

   Fishbein S and Goodstein S: The pressure-lowering effect of ascorbic acid. Ann Ophthamol 4:487–91, 1972.

   Linner E: The pressure-lowering effect of ascorbic acid in ocular hypertension. Acta Ophthamol 47:685–9, 1969.
2. Shen T and Yu M: Clinical evaluation of glycerin-sodium ascorbate solution in lowering intraocular pressure. Chinese Med J 1:64–8, 1975.
3. Stocker FW: New ways of influencing intraocular pressure. NY State Med J 49:58–63, 1949.
4. Raymond LF: Allergy and chronic simple glaucoma. Ann Allergy 22:146–50, 1964.

Gout

1. Blau LW: Cherry diet control for gout and arthritis. Texas Report on Biol and Med 8:309–11, 1950.
2. Lewis AS, Murphy L, McCalla C, et al.: Inhibition of mammalian xanthine oxidase by folate compounds and amethopterin. J Biol Chem 259:12–5, 1984.
3. Oster KA: Xanthine oxidase and folic acid. Ann Int Med 87:252, 1977.

Hayfever

1. Irving A and Jones W: Methods for testing impairment of driving due to drugs. Eur J Clin Pharmacol 43:61–6, 1992.
2. Kemp JP: Antihistamines—Is there anything safe to prescribe? Annals Allergy 69:276–80, 1992.

Headache

1. Brostoff J and Challacombe SJ (eds): Food Allergy and Intolerance. Saunders, Philadelphia, 1987.

   Mansfield LE, et al.: Food allergy and adult migraine: Double-blind and mediator confirmation of an allergic etiology. Ann Allergy 55:126–9, 1985.

   Carter CM, Egger J, and Soothill JF: A dietary management of severe childhood migraine. Hum Nutr: Appl Nutr 39A:294–303, 1985.

Hughes EC, et al.: Migraine: A diagnostic test for etiology of food sensitivity by a nutritionally supported fast and confirmed by long-term report. Ann Allergy 55:28–32, 1985.

Egger J, et al.: Is migraine food allergy? Lancet ii:865–9, 1983.

Monro J, et al.: Food allergy in migraine. Lancet ii:1–4, 1980

2. Swanson DR: Migraine and magnesium: Eleven neglected connections. Perspect Biol Med 31:526–57, 1988.

Ramadan NM, Halvorson H, Vande-Linde A, et al.: Low brain magnesium in migraine. Headache 29:590–3, 1989.

Galland LD, Baker SM, and McLellan RK: Magnesium deficiency in the pathogenesis of mitral valve prolapse. Magnesium 5:165–74, 1986.

3. Johnson ES, et al.: Efficacy of feverfew as prophylactic treatment of migraine. Br Med J 291:569–73, 1985.

4. Murphy JJ, Heptinstall S, and Mitchell JRA: Randomized double-blind, placebo-controlled trial of feverfew in migraine prevention. Lancet ii:189–92, 1988.

5. Johnson ES, et al.: Efficacy of feverfew as prophylactic treatment of migraine. Br Med J 291:569–73, 1985.

Makheja AM and Bailey JM: The active principle in feverfew. Lancet ii:1054, 1981.

Makheja AM and Bailey JM: A platelet phospholipase inhibitor from the medicinal herb feverfew (*Tanacetum parthenium*). Prostagland Leukotri Med 8:653–60, 1982.

Heptinstall S, et al.: Extracts of feverfew inhibit granule secretion in blood platelets and polymorphonuclear leukocytes. Lancet i:1071–4, 1985.

6. Murray MT: The Healing Power of Herbs. Prima Publishing, Rocklin, CA, 1991.

Heart Disease

1. Tsuyusaki T, Noro C, and Kikawada R: Mechanocardiography of ischemic or hypertensive heart failure. In: Biomedical and Clinical Aspects of Coenzyme Q10, vol. 2, Yamamura Y, Folkers K, Ito Y (eds). Elsevier/North-Holland Biomedical Press, Amsterdam, 1980. pp. 273–88.

2. Judy WV, et al.: Myocardial effects of Coenzyme Q10 in primary heart failure. In: Biomedical and Clinical Aspects of Coenzyme Q10, vol. 4. Folkers K, Yamamura Y (eds). Elsevier Science Publishers, Amsterdam, 1984. pp. 353–367.

Vanfraechem JHP, Picalausa C, and Folkers K. Coenzyme Q10 and physical performance in myocardial failure. In: Biomedical and Clinical Aspects of Coenzyme Q10, vol. 4. Folkers K, Yamamura Y (eds). Elsevier Science Publishers, Amsterdam, 1984. pp. 281–90.

3. Langsjoen PH, Vadhanavikit S, and Folkers K: Response of patients in classes III and IV of cardiomyopathy to therapy in a blind and crossover trial with coenzyme Q10. Proc Natl Acad Sci 82:4240, 1985.

4. Gaby AR: Coenzyme Q10. In: A Textbook of Natural Medicine. Pizzorno JE and Murray MT (eds). Bastyr College Publications, Seattle, 1989.

5. Ammon HPT and Handel M: Crataegus, toxicology and pharmacology, Part I: Toxicity. Planta Med 43:105–20, 1981; Part II: Pharmacodynamics. Planta Med 43:209–39, 1981; Part III: Pharmacodynamics and pharmacokinetics. Planta Med 43:313–22, 1981.

Leuchtgens H: Crataegus Special Extract WS 1442 in NYHA II heart failure: A placebo-controlled, randomized, double-blind study. Fortschr Med 111(20–21): 352–4, 1993.

O'Conolly VM, et al.: Treatment of cardiac performance (NYHA stages I to II) in advanced age with standardized crataegus extract. Fortschr Med 104:805–8, 1986.

Wolkerstorfer H: Treatment of heart disease with a digoxin-crataegus combination. Munch Med Wochenschr 108(8):438–41, 1966.

6. Murray MT: The Healing Power of Herbs. Prima Publishing, Rocklin, CA, 1991.

Hemorrhoids

1. Trowell H, Burkitt D, and Heaton K: Dietary Fibre, Fibre-Depleted Foods and Disease. Academic Press, London, UK, 1985.
2. Moesgaard F, Nielsen ML, Hansen JB, and Knudsen JT: High-fiber diet reduces bleeding and pain in patients with hemorrhoids. Dis Colon Rectum 25:454–6, 1982.
   Webster DJ, Gough DC, and Craven JL: The use of bulk evacuation in patients with hemorrhoids. Br J Surg 65:291–2, 1978.

Hepatitis

1. Cathcart RF: The method of determining proper doses of vitamin C for the treatment of disease by titrating to bowel tolerance. J Orthomol Psychiatry 10:125–32, 1981.
2. Klenner FR: Observations on the dose of administration of ascorbic acid when employed beyond the range of a vitamin in human pathology. J Applied Nutr 23:61–88, 1971.
   Baetgen D: Results of the treatment of epidemic hepatitis is children with high doses of ascorbic acid for the years 1957–1958. Medizinische Monatchrift 15:30–6, 1961.
   Baur H and Staub H: Treatment of hepatitis with infusions of ascorbic acid: Comparison with other therapies. JAMA 156:565, 1954.
3. Murata A: Viricidal activity of vitamin C: Vitamin C for prevention and treatment of viral diseases. In: Process First Intersectional Congress International Association Microbiology Society, vol. 3. Hasegawa T. Tokyo U Press, 1975. pp. 432–42.
4. Schandalik R, Gatti G, Perucca E: Pharmacokinetics of silybin in bile following administration of silipide and silymarin in cholecystectomy patients. Arzneim-Forsch 42:964–8, 1992.
   Barzaghi N, et al.: Pharmacokinetic studies on IdB 1016, a silybin-phosphatidylcholine complex, in healthy human subjects. Eur J Drug Metab Pharmacokinet 15:333–8, 1990.
5. Mascarella S et al.: Therapeutic and antilipoperoxidant effects of silybin-phosphatidylcholine complex in chronic liver disease: Preliminary results. Curr Ther Res 53(1):98–102, 1993.
   Vailati A, et al.: Randomized open study of the dose-effect relationship of a short course of IdB 1016 in patients with viral or alcoholic hepatitis. Fitoterapia 44:219–28, 1993.
6. Kouttab NM, Prada M, and Cazzola P: Thymomodulin: Biological properties and clinical appliactions. Med Oncol and Tumor Pharmacother 6:5–9, 1989.
   Galli M, et al.: Attempt to treat acute type B hepatitis with an orally administered thymic extract (Thymomodulin): Preliminary results. Drugs Exptl Clin Res 11:665–9, 1985.
   Bortolotti F, et al.: Effect of an orally administered thymic derivative, Thymodulin, in chronic type B hepatitis in children. Curr Ther Res 43:67–72, 1984.
7. Burgstiner CB: Cure for hepatitis? "Physician, heal thyself," and he did. J Med Assoc Georgia 80:21–2, 1991.

Herpes

1. Griffith R, DeLong D, and Nelson J: Relation of arginine-lysine antagonism to herpes simplex growth in tissue culture. Chemother 27:209–13, 1981.
2. Griffith RS, et al.: Success of L-lysine therapy in frequently recurrent herpes simplex infection. Dermatol 175:183–90, 1987.

High Blood Pressure

1. Veterans Administration Cooperative Study Group on Antihypertensive Agents. Effects of treatment on morbidity in hypertension. II. Results of patients with diastolic blood pressure averaging 90 through 114 millimeters hydrargyrum. JAMA 213:1143–51, 1970.

    U.S. Public Health Service Hospitals Cooperative Study Group. Treatment of mild hypertension: Results of a ten-year intervention trial. Circ Res 40 (supplement I): I98–I105, 1977.

    Helgeland A: Treatment of mild hypertension: A five-year controlled drug trial: The Oslo study. Am J Med 69:725–32, 1980.
2. Freis ED: Rationale against the drug treatment of marginal diastolic systemic hypertension. Am J Cardiol 66:368–71, 1990.
3. Multiple Risk Factor Intervention Trial Research Group: Baseline rest electrocardiographic abnormalities, antihypertensive treatment, and mortality in the Multiple Risk Factor Intervention Trial. Am J Cardiol 55:1–15, 1985.

    Miettinen TA: Multifactorial primary prevention of cardiovascular diseases in middle-aged men: Risk factor changes, incidence, and mortality. JAMA 254:2097–2102, 1985.

    Medical Research Council Working Party on Mild Hypertension. MRC trial of treatment of mild hypertension: Principal results. Br Med J 291:97–104, 1980.

    Report by the Management Committee. The Australian therapeutic trial in mild hypertension. Lancet i:1261–7, 1980.
4. Kaplan NM: Non-drug treatment of hypertension. Ann Int Med 102:359–73, 1985.
5. Alderman MH: Which antihypertensive drugs first—and why! JAMA 267:2786–7, 1992.

Hives

1. Czarnetzki BM: Urticaria. Springer-Verlag, New York, 1986.
2. Pachor ML, et al.: Elimination diet and challenge test in diagnosis of food intolerance. Italian J Med 2:1–6, 1986.
3. Winkelmann RK: Food sensitivity and urticaria or vasculitis. In: Food Allergy and Intolerance. Brostoff J and Challacombe SJ (eds). Saunders, Philadelphia, 1987. pp. 602–17.
4. Ormerod AD, Reid TMS, and Main RA: Penicillin in milk—Its importance in urticaria. Clin Allergy 17:229–34, 1987.

    Wicher K and Reisman RE: Anaphylactic reaction to penicillin in a soft drink. J Allergy Clin Immunol 66:155–7, 1980.

    Schwartz HJ and Sher TH: Anaphylaxis to penicillin in a frozen dinner. Ann Allergy 52:342–3, 1984.
5. Boonk WJ and Van Ketel WG: The role of penicillin in the pathogenesis of chronic urticaria. Br J Derm 106:183–90, 1982.

Hyperactivity and Learning Disorders

1. Feingold N: Why Your Child is Hyperactive. Random House, New York, 1975.
2. Rowe K: Food additives. Aust Paediatr J 20:171–4, 1984.

    Swanson J and Kinsbourne M: Food dyes impair performance of children on a laboratory learning task. Science 207:1485–7, 1980.

    Weiss B, Williams J, Margen S, et al.: Behavioral responses to artificial food colours. Science 207:1487–9, 1980.

    Weiss B: Food additives and environmental chemicals as sources of childhood behavior disorders. J Am Acad Child Psychiatry 21:144–152, 1982.

Schauss A: Nutrition and behavior: Complex interdisciplinary research. Nutr Health 3:9–37, 1984.

Rippere V: Food additives and hyperactive children: A critique of Conners. Br J Clin Psych 22:19–32, 1983.

Cook P and Woodhill J: The Feingold dietary treatment of the hyperkinetic syndrome. Med J Aust 2:85–90, 1976.

Salzman L: Allergy testing, psychological assessment and dietary treatment of the hyperactive child syndrome. Med J Aust 2:248–251, 1976.

3. Furia T (ed): CRC Handbook of Food Additives, vols. 1 and 2. CRC Press, Boca Raton, Fl, 1980.

4. Conners C, et al.: Food additives and hyperkinesis: A double-blind experiment. Pediatrics 58:154–166, 1976.

Goyette C, et al.: Effects of artificial colors on hyperkinetic children: A double-blind challenge study. Psychopharmacol Bull 14:39–40, 1978.

Conners C: Food Additives and Hyperactive Children. Plenum Press, New York, 1980.

Harley J, et al.: Hyperkinesis and food additives: Testing the Feingold hypothesis. Pediatrics 61:811–7, 1978.

Rowe K, Hopkins I, and Lynch B: Artificial food colourings and hyperkinesis. Aust Paediatr J 15:202, 1979.

Levy F, Dumbrell S, Hobbes G, et al.: Hyperkinesis and diet: A double-blind crossover trial with tartrazine challenge. Med J Aust 1:61–4, 1978.

5. Mattes J: The Feingold diet: A current reappraisal. J Learn Disabil 16:319–323, 1983.

Rimland B: The Feingold diet: An assessment of the reviews by Mattes, by Kavale and Forness and others. J Learn Disabil 16:331–3, 1983.

6. Werbach MR: Nutritional Influences on Mental Illness. Third Line Press, Tarzana, CA, 1991.

Tseng R, Mellon J, and Bammer K: The Relationship Between Nutrition and Student Achievement, Behavior, and Health—A Review of the Literature. California State Department of Education, Sacramento, CA, 1980.

7. Benton D and Roberts G: Effect of vitamin and mineral supplementation on intelligence of a sample of schoolchildren. Lancet i:140–3, 1988.

8. Marlowe M, et al: Hair mineral content as a predictor of learning disabilities. J Learn Disabil 17:418–421, 1977.

Pihl R and Parkes M: Hair element content in learning disabled children. Science 198:204–6, 1977.

9. David O, Clark J, and Voeller K: Lead and hyperactivity. Lancet ii:900–3, 1972.

David O, Hoffman S, and Sverd J: Lead and hyperactivity. Behavioral response to chelation: A pilot study. Am J Psychiatry 133:1155–1188, 1976.

Benignus V, et al.: Effects of age and body lead burden on CNS function in young children. EEG spectra. EEG and Clin Neurophys 52:240–8, 1981.

Rimland B and Larson G: Hair mineral analysis and behavior: An analysis of 51 studies. J Learn Disabil 16:279–285, 1983.

Bryce-Smith D: Lead-induced disorders of mentation in children. Nutr Health 1:179–184, 1983.

Hypoglycemia

1. Winokur A, et al.: Insulin resistance after glucose tolerance testing in patients with major depression. Am J Psychiatry 145:325–30, 1988.

Wright JH, et al.: Glucose metabolism in unipolar depression. Br J Psychiatry 132:386–93, 1978.

2. Schauss AG: Nutrition and behavior: Complex interdisciplinary research. Nutr Health 3:9–37, 1984.

Benton D: Hypoglycemia and aggression: A review. Int J Neurosci 41:163–8, 1988.

Virkkunen M: Reactive hypoglycemic tendency among arsonists. Acta Psychiatr Scan 69:445–52, 1984.

Schoenthaler SJ: Diet and crime: An empirical examination of the value of nutrition in the control and treatment of incarcerated juvenile offenders. Int J Biosoc Res 4:25–39, 1983.

Schoenthaler SJ: The northern California diet-behavior program: An empirical evaluation of 3,000 incarcerated juveniles in Stanislaus County Juvenile Hall. Int J Biosoc Res 5:99–106, 1983.

3. Abraham GE: Nutritional factors in the etiology of the premenstrual tension syndromes. J Repro Med 28:446–64, 1983.

Walsh CH and O'Sullivan DJ: Studies of glucose tolerance, insulin and growth hormone secretion during the menstrual cycle in healthy women. Irish J Med Sci 144:18–24, 1975.

4. Critchley M: Migraine. Lancet i:123–6, 1933.

Dexter JD, Roberts J, and Byer JA: The five-hour glucose tolerance test and effect of low-sucrose diet in migraine. Headache 18:91–4, 1978.

5. Hanson M, Bergentz SE, Ericsson BF, et al.: The oral glucose tolerance test in men under 55 years of age with intermittent claudication. Angiol June:469–73, 1987.

6. Bansal S, Toh SH, and LaBresh KA: Chest pain as a presentation of reactive hypoglycemia. Chest 84:641–2, 1983.

7. Chalew SA, et al.: The use of the plasma epinephrine response in the diagnosis of idiopathic postprandial syndrome. JAMA 251:612–5, 1984.

Hadji-Georgopoulus A, et al.: Elevated hypoglycemic index and late hyperinsulinism in symptomatic postprandial hypoglycemia. J Clin Endocrinol Metabol 50:371–6, 1980.

Fabrykant M: The problem of functional hyperinsulinism on functional hypoglycemia attributed to nervous causes. 1. Laboratory and clinical correlations. Metabol 4:469–79, 1955.

8. Jenkins DJA, et al.: Glycemic index of foods: a physiological basis for carbohydrate exchange. Amer J Clin Nutr 24:362–6, 1981.

9. Truswell AS: Glycemic index of foods. European J Clin Nutr 46(Suppl. 2):S91–101, 1992.

10. Anderson RA, et al.: Effects of supplemental chromium on patients with symptoms of reactive hypoglycemia. Metabol 36:351–5, 1987.

Hypothyroidism

1. Barnes BO and Galton L: Hypothyroidism: The Unsuspected Illness. Thomas Crowell, New York, 1976.

Langer SE and Scheer JF: Solved: The Riddle of Illness. Keats, New Canaan, CT, 1984.

Gold M, Pottash A, and Extein I: Hypothyroidism and depression, evidence from complete thyroid function evaluation. JAMA 245:1919–22, 1981.

Impotence

1. NIH Consensus Conference Panel on Impotence: Impotence. JAMA 270:83–90, 1993.

Lerner SE, Melman A, and Christ GJ: A review of erectile dysfunction: New insights and more questions. J Urol 149:1246–55, 1993.

Morley JE: Management of impotence. Postgrad Med 93:65–72, 1993.

2. White JR, et al.: Enhanced sexual behavior in exercising men. Arch Sex Behav 19:193–209, 1990.

3. Shibata S, et al.: Chemistry and pharmacology of Panax. Econ Med Plant Res 1:217–84, 1985.

4. Susset JG, et al.: Effect of yohimbine hydrochloride on erectile impotence: A double-blind study. J Urol 141:1360–3, 1989.

Morales A, et al.: Is yohimbine effective in the treatment of organic impotence? Results of a controlled trial. J Urol 137:1168–72, 1987.
5. Waynberg J: Aphrodisiacs: Contribution to the clinical validation of the traditional use of *Ptychopetalum guyanna*. Presented at The First International Congress on Ethnopharmacology, Strasbourg, France, June 5–9, 1990.
6. Sikora R, et al.: *Ginkgo biloba* extract in the therapy of erectile dysfunction. J Urol 141:188A, 1989

Insomnia

1. Lindahl O and Lindwall L: Double-blind study of a valerian preparation. Pharmacol Biochem Behav 32:1065–6, 1989.
2. Leathwood P, et al.: Aqueous extract of valerian root (*valeriana officinalis L.*) improves sleep quality in man. Pharmacol Biochem Behav 17:65–71, 1982.
3. Leathwood PD and Chauffard F: Aqueous extract of valerian reduces latency to fall asleep in man. Planta Med 54:144–8, 1985.

Irritable Bowel Syndrome

1. Jones V, et al.: Food intolerance: A major factor in the pathogenesis of irritable bowel syndrome. Lancet ii:1115–8, 1982.
   Petitpierre M, Gumowski P, and Girard J: Irritable bowel syndrome and hypersensitivity to food. Ann Allergy 54:538–40, 1985.
2. Somerville K, Richmond C, and Bell G: Delayed release peppermint oil capsules (Colpermin) for the spastic colon syndrome: A pharmacokinetic study. Br J Clin Pharmacol 18:638–40, 1984.
   Rees W, Evans B, and Rhodes J: Treating irritable bowel syndrome with peppermint oil. Br Med J ii:835–6, 1979.

Kidney Stones

1. National Institute of Health: Prevention and treatment of kidney stones. National Institute Health Consensus Development Conference Consensus Statement 7:1–8, 1988.
2. Curhan GC, et al.: A prospective study of dietary calcium and other nutrients and the risk of symptomatic kidney stones. N Engl J Med 328:833–8, 1993.
   Massey LK, Roman-Smith H, and Sutton RA: Effect of dietary oxalate and calcium on urinary oxalate and risk of formation of calcium oxalate kidney stones. J Am Diet Assoc 93:901–6, 1993.
3. Johansson G, et al.: Biochemical and clinical effects of the prophylactic treatment of renal calcium stones with magnesium hydroxide. J Urol 124:770–4, 1980.
   Wunderlich W: Aspects of the influence of magnesium ions on the formation of calcium oxalate. Urol Res 9:157–60, 1981.
   Hallson P, Rose G, and Sulaiman M: Magnesium reduces calcium oxalate crystal formation in human whole urine. Clin Sci 62:17–9, 1982.
   Gershoff S and Prien E: Effect of daily MgO and Vitamin B6 administration to patients with recurring calcium oxalate stones. Amer J Clin Nutr 20:393–9, 1967.
4. Prien E and Gershoff S: Magnesium oxide-pyridoxine therapy for recurrent calcium oxalate calculi. J Urol 112:509–12, 1974.
5. Vahlensieck W: Review: The importance of diet in urinary stones. Urol Res 14:283–8, 1986.

6. Robertson W, Peacock M, and Marshall D: Prevalence of urinary stone disease in vegetarians. Eur Urol 8:334–9, 1982.
    Rose G and Westbury E: The influence of calcium content of water, intake of vegetables and fruit and of other food factors upon the incidence of renal calculi. Urol Res 3:61–66, 1975.
7. Shaw P, Williams G, and Green N: Idiopathic hypercalciuria: Its control with unprocessed bran. Br J Urol 52:426–9, 1980.
8. Ulmann A, Aubert J, Bourdeau A, et al.: Effects of weight and glucose ingestion on urinary calcium and phosphate excretion: Implications for calcium urolithiasis. J Clin Endo Metab 54:1063–7, 1982.
    Rao N, et al.: Are stone formers maladaptive to refined carbohydrates? Br J Urol 54:575–7, 1982.
9. Giannini S, et al.: Possible link between vitamin D and hyperoxaluria in patients with renal stone disease. Clin Sce 84:51–4, 1993.
10. Pak CYC and Fuller C: Idiopathic hypocitraturic calcium-oxalate nephrolithiasis successfully treated with potassium citrate. Ann Int Med 104:33–7, 1986.

Macular Degeneration

1. Eye Disease Case-Control Study Group: Antioxidant status and neovascular age-related macular degneration. Arch Ophthalmol 111:104–9, 1993.
    Goldberg J, et al.: Factors associated with age-related macular degeneration: An analysis of data from the First National Health and Nutrition Examination Survey. Am J Epidemiol 128:700–10, 1988.
2. Newsome DA, et al.: Oral zinc in macular degeneration. Arch Ophthalmol 106:192–8, 1988.
3. Lebuisson DA, Leroy L, and Rigal G: Treatment of senile macular degeneration with Ginkgo biloba extract: A preliminary double-blind, drug versus placebo study. Presse Med 15:1556–8, 1986.
4. Scharrer A and Ober M: Anthocyanosides in the treatment of retinopathies. Klin Monatsbl Augenheilkd 178:386–9, 1981.
    Caselli L: Clinical and electroretinographic study on the activity of anthocyanosides. Arch Med Int 37:29–35, 1985.

Menopause

1. Wilson RA: Feminine Forever. Evans, New York, 1966.
2. Armstrong BK: Oestrogen therapy after the menopause: Boon or bane? Med J Austral 148:213–4, 1988.
    DuPont WD and Page DL: Menopausal estrogen replacement therapy and breast cancer. Arch Int Med 151:67–72, 1991.
    Steinberg KK, et al.: A meta-analysis of the effect of estrogen replacement therapy on the risk of breast cancer. JAMA 265:1985–90, 1991.
    Henrich JB: The postmenopausal estrogen/breast cancer controversy. JAMA 268:1900–2, 1992.
3. Session DR, et al.: Current concepts in estrogen replacement therapy in the menopause. Fertil Steril 59:277–84, 1993.
    Birkenfeld A and Kase NG: Menopause medicine: Current treatment options and trends. Comprehen Ther 17:36–45, 1991.
4. Hammar M, et al.: Does physical exercise influence the frequency of postmenopausal hot flushes. Acta Obstet Gynecol Scand 69:409–12, 1990.
5. Messina M and Barnes S: The role of soy products in reducing risk of cancer. J Natl Cancer Inst 83:541–6, 1991.
    Messina M and Messina V: Increasing the use of soyfoods and their potential role in cancer prevention. J Am Diet Assoc 91:836–40, 1991.

6. Kaldas RS and Hughes CL: Reproductive and general metabolic effects of phytoe-strogens in mammals. Reprod Toxicol 3:81–9, 1989.
7. Albert-Puleo M: Fennel and anise as estrogenic agents. J Ethnopharmacol 2:337–344, 1980.
8. Christy CJ: Vitamin E in menopause. Am J Ob Gyn 50:84–7, 1945.
   McLaren HC: Vitamin E in the menopause. Br Med J ii:1378–81, 1949.
   Finkler RS: The effect of vitamin E in the menopause. J Clin Endocrinol Metab 9:89–94, 1949.
9. Rose DP: Dietary fiber, phytoestrogens, and breast cancer. Nutr 8:47–51, 1992.
   Adlercreutz H, et al.: Determination of urinary lignans and phytoestrogen metabo-lites, potential antiestrogens and anticarcinogens, in urine of women on various ha-bitual diets. Steroid Biochem 25:791–7, 1986.
10. Murase Y and Iishima H: Clinical studies of oral administration of gamm-oryzanol on climacteric complaints and its syndrome. Obtet Gynecol Prac 12:147–9, 1963.
11. Ishihara M: Effect of gamma-oryzanol on serum lipid peroxide levels and climac-teric disturbances. Asia Oceania J Obstet Gynecol 10:317, 1984.

Multiple Sclerosis

1. Swank RL: Multiple sclerosis: Fat-oil relationship. Nutr 7:368–76, 1991.
   Swank RL and Pullen MH: The Multiple Sclerosis Diet Book. Doubleday, Garden City, NY, 1977.
2. Millar ZHD, Zilkha KJ, Langman MJS, et al.: Double-blind trial of linolate supple-mentation of the diet in multiple sclerosis. Br Med J i:765–8, 1973.
   Bates D, Fawcett PRW, Shaw DA, and Weightman D: Polyunsaturated fatty acids in treatment of acute remitting multiple sclerosis. Br Med J ii:1390–1, 1978.
   Paty DW, Cousin HK, Read S, and Adlakkha K: Linoleic acid in multiple sclerosis: Failure to show any therapeutic benefit. Acta Neurol Scand 58:53–8, 1978.
3. Ransberger K: Enzyme treatment of immune complex diseases. Arthr Rheuma 8:16–9, 1986.
   Ransberger K and van Schaik W: Enzyme therapy in multiple sclerosis. Der Kasse-narzt 41:42–5, 1986.

Osteoarthritis

1. Brooks PM, Potter SR and Buchanan WW: NSAID and osteoarthritis—Help or hin-drance? J Rheumatol 9:3–5, 1982.
   Shield MJ: Anti-inflammatory drugs and their effects on cartilage synthesis and renal function. Eur J Rheum Inflam 13:7–16, 1993.
   Newman NM and Ling RSM: Acetabular bone destruction related to non-steroidal anti-inflammatory drugs. Lancet ii:11–13, 1985.
   Solomon L: Drug-induced arthropathy and necrosis of the femoral head. J Bone Joint Surg 55B:246–51, 1973.
2. Ronningen H and Langeland N: Indomethacin treatment in osteoarthritis of the hip joint. Acta Orthop Scand 50:169–74, 1979.
3. Vaz AL: Double-blind clinical evaluation of the relative efficacy of ibuprofen and glucosamine sulfate in the management of osteoarthrosis of the knee in out-patients. Curr Med Res Opin 8:145–9, 1982.
   Crolle G and D'este E: Glucosamine sulfate for the management of arthrosis: a con-trolled clinical investigation. Curr Med Res Opin 7:104–14, 1981.
   Tapadinhas MJ, Rivera IC, and Bignamini AA: Oral glucosamine sulfate in the management of arthrosis: report on a multi-centre open investigation in Portugal. Pharmatherapeutica 3:157–68, 1982.
   D'Ambrosia ED, et al.: Glucosamine sulphate: A controlled clinical investigation in arthrosis. Pharmatherapeutica 2:504–8, 1982.

4. Setnikar I, Pacini A, and Revel L: Antiarthritic effects of glucosamine sulfate studied in animal models. Arzneim-Forsch 41:542–5, 1991.
5. Travers RL, Rennie GC, and Newnham RE: Boron and arthritis: The results of a double-blind pilot study. J Nutr Med 1:127–32, 1990.

Osteoporosis

1. Pocock NA, et al.: Physical fitness is the major determinant of femoral neck and lumbar spine density. J Clin Invest 78:618–21, 1986.

   Krolner B, et al.: Physical exercise as prophylaxis against involutional vertebral bone loss: A controlled trial. Clin Sci 64:541–6, 1983.

   Yeater R and Martin R: Senile osteoporosis: The effects of exercise. Postg Med 75:147–9, 1984.

   Marcus R, et al.: Osteoporosis and exercise in women. Med Sci Sports Exer 24:S301–7, 1992.
2. Donaldson C, et al.: Effect of prolonged bed rest on bone mineral. Metabol 19:1071–84, 1970.
3. Ellis F, Holesh S, and Ellis J: Incidence of osteoporosis in vegetarians and omnivores. Am J Clin Nutr 25:55–8, 1972.

   Marsh A, et al.: Bone mineral mass in adult lactoovovegetarian and omnivorous adults. Am J Clin Nutr 37:453–6, 1983.
4. Licata A, et al.: Acute effects of dietary protein on calcium metabolism in patients with osteoporosis. J Geron 36:14–9, 1981.
5. Thom J, et al.: The influence of refined carbohydrates on urinary calcium excretion. Br J Urol 50:459–64, 1978.
6. Aloia JF, et al.: Risk factors for postmenopausal osteoporosis. Am J Med 78:95–100, 1985.
7. Dempster DW and Lindsay R: Pathogenesis of osteoporosis. Lancet 341:797–805, 1993.

   Lee CJ, Lawler GS, and Johnson GH: Effects of supplementation of the diets with calcium and calcium-rich foods on bone density of elderly females with osteoporosis. Am J Clin Nutr 34:819–23, 1981.

   Gaby AR: Preventing and Reversing Osteoporosis. Prima Publishing, Rocklin, CA, 1994.
8. Cohen L and Kitzes R: Infrared spectroscopy and magnesium content of bone mineral in osteoporotic women. Isr J Med Sci 17:1123–5, 1981.
9. Rude RK, Adams JS, Ryzen E, et al.: Low serum concentration of 1,25-dihydroxyvitamin D in human magnesium deficiency. J Clin Endo Metabol 61:933–40, 1985.
10. Seelig MS: Magnesium deficiency with phosphate and vitamin D excess: Role in pediatric cardiovascular nutrition. Cardio Med 3:637–50, 1978.
11. Newcomer A, et al.: Lactase deficiency: Prevalence in osteoporosis. Ann Int Med 89:218–20, 1978.
12. Brattstrom LE, Hultberg BL and Hardebo JE: Folic acid responsive postmenopausal homocysteinemia. Metabol 34:1073–7, 1985.
13. Neilsen FH, Hunt CD, Mullen LM, and Hunt JR: Effect of dietary boron on mineral, estrogen, and testosterone metabolism in postmenopausal women. FASEB J 1:394–7, 1987.
14. Block G: Dietary guidelines and the results of food consumption surveys. Am J Clin Nutr 53:356S–7S, 1991.
15. Nielsen FH, Gallagher SK, Johnson LK, and Nielsen EJ: Boron enhances and mimics some of the effects of estrogen therapy in postmenopausal women. J Trace Elem Exp Med 5:237–46, 1992.

Premenstrual Syndrome

1. Barr W: Pyridoxine supplements in the premenstrual syndrome. Practitioner 228:425–7, 1984.

2. Brush MG, Bennett T, and Hansen K: Pyridoxine in the treatment of premenstrual syndrome: A retrospective survery in 630 patients. Br J Clin Pract 42:448–52, 1988.

3. Abraham GE and Hargrove JT: Effect of vitamin B6 on premenstrual symptomatology in women with premenstrual tension syndromes: A double-blind crossover study. Infert 3:155–65, 1980.

4. Berman MK, et al.: Vitamin B6 in premenstrual syndrome. J Am Diet Assoc 90:859–61, 1990.

   Kliejnen J, Ter Riet G, and Knipschild P: Vitamin B6 in the treatment of premenstrual syndrome—A review. Br J Obstet Gynaecol 97:847–52, 1990.

   Stokes J and Mendels J: Pyridoxine and premenstrual tension. Lancet i:1177, 1972.

5. Abraham GE and Lubran MM: Serum and red cell magnesium levels in patients with premenstrual tension. Am J Clin Nutr 34:2364–6, 1981.

6. Abraham GE: Nutritional factors in the etiology of the premenstrual tension syndromes. J Repro Med 28:446–64, 1983.

   Piesse JW: Nutritional factors in the premenstrual syndrome. Int Clin Nutr Rev 4:54–81, 1984.

7. Fachinetti F, et al.: Oral magnesium successfully relieves premenstrual mood changes. Obstet Gynecol 78:177–81, 1991.

8. London RS, Sundaram GS, Murphy L, and Goldstein PJ: Evaluation and treatment of breast symptoms in patients with the premenstrual syndrome. J Reprod Med 28:503–8, 1983.

Prostate Enlargement (BPH)

1. Fahim M, et al.: Zinc treatment for the reduction of hyperplasia of the prostate. Fed Proc 35:361, 1976.

   Hart JP and Cooper WL: Vitamin F in the treatment of prostatic hyperplasia. Report Number 1, Lee Foundation for Nutritional Research, Milwaukee, WI, 1941.

2. Boccafoschi and Annoscia S: Comparison of *Serenoa repens* extract with placebo by controlled clinical trial in patients with prostatic adenomatosis. Urol 50:1257–68, 1983.

   Cirillo-Marucco E, et al.: Extract of *Serenoa repens* (Permixon) in the early treatment of prostatic hypertrophy. Urol 5:1269–77, 1983.

   Tripodi V, et al.: Treatment of prostatic hypertrophy with *Serenoa repens* extract. Med Praxis 4:41–6, 1983.

   Emili E, Lo Cigno M, and Petrone U: Clinical trial of a new drug for treating hypertrophy of the prostate (Permixon). Urol 50:1042–8, 1983.

   Greca P and Volpi R: Experience with a new drug in the medical treatment of prostatic adenoma. Urol 52:532–5, 1985.

   Duvia R, Radice GP, and Galdini R: Advances in the phytotherapy of prostatic hypertrophy. Med Praxis 4:143–8, 1983.

   Tasca A, et al.: Treatment of obstructive symptomatology caused by prostatic adenoma with an extract of *Serenoa repens:* Double-blind clinical study versus placebo. Minerva Urol Nefrol 37:87–91, 1985.

   Crimi A and Russo A: Extract of *Serenoa repens* for the treatment of the functional disturbances of prostate hypertrophy. Med Praxis 4:47–51, 1983.

   Champlault G, Patel JC, and Bonnard AM: A double-blind trial of an extract of the plant *Serenoa repens* in benign prostatic hyperplasia. Br J Clin Pharmacol 18:461–2, 1984.

   Mattei FM, Capone M, and Acconcia A.: *Serenoa repens* extract in the medical treatment of benign prostatic hypertrophy. Urol 55:547–52, 1988.

Prostatitis

1. Purvis K and Christiansen E: Review: Infection in the male reproductive tract: Impact, diagnosis and treatment in relation to male infertility. Int J Androl 16:1–13, 1993.

2. Luerti M and Vignali M: Influence of bromelain on penetration of antibiotics in uterus, salpinx and ovary. Drugs Exp Clin Res 4:45–8, 1978.

Tinozzi S and Venegoni A: Effect of bromelain on serum and tissue levels of amoxycillin. Drugs Exp Clin Res 4:39–44, 1978.

Neubauer R: A plant protease for the potentiation of and possible replacement of antibiotics. Exp Med Surg 19:143–60, 1961.

3. Amin AH, Subbaiah TV, and Abbasi KM: Berberine sulfate: Antimicrobial activity, bioassay, and mode of action. Can J Microbiol 15:1067–76, 1969.

Johnson CC, Johnson G, and Poe CF: Toxicity of alkaloids to certain bacteria. Acta Pharmacol Toxicol 8:71–8, 1952.

Hahn FE and Ciak J: Berberine. Antibiotics 3:577–88, 1976.

4. Sun D, Courtney HS, and Beachey EH: Berberine sulfate blocks adherence of *Streptococcus pyogenes* to epithelial cells, fibronectin, and hexadecane. Antimicrobial Agents and Chemother 32:1370–4, 1988.

5. Kumazawa Y, Itagaki A, Fukumoto M, et al.: Activation of peritoneal macrophages by berberine alkaloids in terms of induction of cytostatic activity. Int J Immunopharmacol 6:587–92, 1984.

6. Babbar OP, Chatwal VK, Ray IB, and Mehra MK: Effect of berberine chloride eye drops on clinically positive trachoma patients. Ind J Med Res 76(Suppl):83–8, 1982.

Mohan M, Pant CR, Angra SK, and Mahajan VM: Berberine in trachoma. Ind J Opthalmol 30:69–75, 1982.

7. Ask-Upmark E: Prostatitis and its treatment. Acta Med Scand 181:355–7, 1967.

8. Ohkoshi M, Kawamura N, and Nagakubo I: Clinical evaluation of Cernilton in chronic prostatitis. Jap J Clin Urol 21:73–85, 1967.

Buck AC, Rees RWM, and Ebeling L: Treatment of chronic prostatitis and prostadynia with pollen extract. Br J Urol 64:496–9, 1989.

Psoriasis

1. Proctor M, et al.: Lowered cutaneous and urinary levels of polyamines with clinical improvement in treated psoriasis. Arch Dermatol 115:945–9, 1979.

2. Maurice PDL, et al.: The effects of dietary supplementation with fish oil in patients with psoriasis. Brit J Dermatol 1117:599–606, 1987.

3. Lithell H, et al.: A fasting and vegetarian diet treatment trial on chronic inflammatory disorders. Acta Derm Vener (StockH) 63:397–403, 1983.

Bittiner SB, et al.: A double-blind, randomized, placebo-controlled trial of fish oil in psoriasis. Lancet i:378–80, 1988.

4. Rosenberg E and Belew P: Microbial factors in psoriasis. Arch Dermatol 118:1434–44, 1982.

5. Monk BE and Neill SM: Alcohol consumption and psoriasis. Dermatol 173:57–60, 1986.

6. Weber G and Galle K: The liver, a therapeutic target in dermatoses. Med Welt 34:108–11, 1983.

Rheumatoid Arthritis

1. Heliovaara M, et al.: Serum antioxidants and risk of rheumatoid arthritis. Ann Rheum Dis 53:51–3, 1994.

2. Jenkins R, Rooney P, Jones D, et al.: Increased intestinal permeability in patients with rheumatoid arthritis: A side effect of oral nonsteroidal anti-inflammatory drug therapy? Br J Rheum 26:103–07, 1987.

3. Fries JF, Miller SR, Spitz PW, et al.: Toward an epidemiology of gastropathy associated with nonsteroidal anti-inflammatory drug use. Gastroenterol 96:647–55, 1989.

4. Scott DL, Coulton BL, Symmons DPM and Popert AJ: Long-term outcome of treating rheumatoid arthritis: Results after 20 years. Lancet i:1108–11, 1989.

5. Kjeldsen-Kragh J, Haugen M, Borchgrevink CF, et al.: Controlled trial of fasting and one-year vegetarian diet in rheumatoid arhtritis. Lancet 338:899–902, 1991.
6. Skoldstam L, Larsson L, and Lindstrom FD: Effects of fasting and lactovegetarian diet on rheumatoid arthritis. Scand J Rheumatol 8:249–55, 1979.

   Kroker GP, et al.: Fasting and rheumatoid arthritis: A multicenter study. Clin Ecol 2:137–44, 1984.

   Hafstrom I, et al.: Effects of fasting on disease activity, neutrophil function, fatty acid composition, and leukotriene biosynthesis in patients with rheumatoid arthritis. Arthr Rheum 31:585–92, 1988.
7. Darlington LG, Ramsey NW and Mansfield JR: Placebo-controlled, blind study of dietary manipulation therapy in rheumatoid arthritis. Lancet i:236–8, 1986.

   Hicklin JA, McEwen LM, and Morgan JE: The effect of diet in rheumatoid arthritis. Clin Allergy 10:463–7, 1980.

   Panush RS: Delayed reactions to foods. Food allergy and rheumatic disease. Ann Allergy 56:500–3, 1986.

   Van de Laar MAFJ and Ander Korst JK: Food intolerance in rheumatoid arthritis. I. A double-blind, controlled trial of the clinical effects of elimination of milk allergens and azo dyes. Ann Rheum Dis 51:298–302, 1992.
8. Ransberger K: Enzyme treatment of immune complex diseases. Arthr Rheum 8:16–9, 1986.

   Steffen C, et al.: Enzyme therapy in comparison with immune complex determinations in chronic polyarteritis. Rheumatol 44:51–6, 1985.

   Ransberger K and van Schaik W: Enzyme therapy in multiple sclerosis. Der Kassenarzt 41:42–5, 1986.
9. De Witte TJ, et al.: Hypochlorhydria and hypergastrinemia in rheumatoid arthritis. Ann Rheumatic Dis 38:14–7, 1979.

   Henriksson K, et al.: Gastrin, gastric acid secretion, and gastric microflora in patients with rheumatoid arthritis. Ann Rheumatic Dis 45:475–83, 1986.
10. Kremer J, Michaelek AV, Lininger L, et al.: Effects of manipulation of dietary fatty acids on clinical manifestation of rheumatoid arthritis. Lancet i:184–7, 1985.

    Lee TH and Arm JP: Prospects for modifying the allergic response by fish oil diets. Clin Allergy 16:89–100, 1986.

    Magaro M, et al.: Influence of diet with different lipid composition on neutrophil composition on neutrophil chemiluminescence and disease activity in patients with rheumatoid arthritis. Ann Rheum Dis 47:793–6, 1988.

    Darlington LG: Do diets rich in polyunsaturated fatty acids affect disease activity in rheumatoid arthritis? Ann Rheum Dis 47:169–72, 1988.

    Hansen TM, et al.: Treatment of rheumatoid arthritis with prostaglandin E1 precursors as cis-linoleic acid and gamma-linolenic acid. Scand J Rheumatol 12:85–8, 1983.

    Belch JJF, et al.: Effects of altering dietary essential fatty acid on requirements for non-steroidal anti-inflammatory drugs in patients with rheumatoid arthritis: A double-blind placebo-controlled study. Ann Rheum Dis 4:96–104, 1988.
11. Deodhar SD, Sethi R and Srimal RC: Preliminary studies on antirheumatic activity of curcumin (*diferuloyl methane*). Ind J Med Res 71:632–4, 1980.
12. Deal CL, et al.: Treatment of arthritis with topical capsaicin: A double-blind trial. Clin Ther 13(3):383–95, 1991.

Sinus Infection

1. Dohlman AW, et al.: Subacute sinusitis: Are antimicrobials necessary? J Aller Clin Immunol 91:1015–23, 1993.

Stroke

1. Dyken ML, et al.: Low-dose aspirin and stroke. "It ain't necessarily so." Stroke 23:1395–1403, 1992.

2. Anadere I, Chmiel H, and Witte S: Hemorrheological findings in patients with completed stroke and the influence of *Ginkgo biloba* extract. Clin Hemorheo 4:411–20, 1985.

   DeFeudis FV (ed): *Ginkgo biloba* extract (Egb 761): Pharmacological activities and clinical applications. Elsevier, Paris, France, 1991.

Ulcer

1. Andre C, Moulinier B, Andre F, and Daniere S: Evidence for anaphylactic reactions in peptic ulcer and varioliform gastritis. Ann Allergy 51:325–8, 1983.
2. Siegel J: Immunologic approach to the treatment and prevention of gastrointestinal ulcers. Ann Allergy 38:27–9, 1977.
3. Kumar N, Kumar A, Broor SL, et al.: Effect of milk on patients with duodenal ulcers. Brit Med J 293:666, 1986.
4. Kassir ZA: Endoscopic controlled trial of four drug regimens in the treatment of chronic duodenal ulceration. Irish Med J 78:153–6, 1985.
5. Glick L: Deglycyrrhizinated licorice in peptic ulcer. Lancet ii:817, 1982.

   Tewari SN and Wilson AK: Deglycyrrhizinated licorice in duodenal ulcer. Practitioner 210:820–5, 1972.

   Morgan Ag, et al.: Comparison between cimetidine and Caved-S in the treatment of gastric ulceration, and subsequent maintenance therapy. Gut 23:545–51, 1982.

   Turpie AG, Runcie J and Thomson TJ: Clinical trial of deglycyrrhizinated licorice in gastric ulcer. Gut 10:299–303, 1969.

Vaginitis

1. Ratzen J: Monilial and trichomonal vaginitis—Topical treatment with povidone iodine treatments. Cal Med 110:24–7, 1969.
2. Shook D: A clinical study of a povidone iodine regimen for resistant vaginitis. Curr Ther Res 5:256–63, 1963.

   Maneksha S: Comparison of povidone iodine (Betadine) vaginal pessaries and lactic acid pessaries in the treatment of vaginitis. J Int Med Res 2:236–9, 1974.

   Reeve P: The inactivation of *Chlamydia trachomatis* by povidone iodine. J Antimicrob Chemo 2:77–80, 1976.

   Mayhew S: Vaginitis: A study of the efficacy of povidone iodine in unselected cases. J Int Med Res 9:157–9, 1981.

   Gershenfeld L: Povidone iodine as a trichomoniacide. Am J Pharm 134:324–31, 1962.

   Gershenfeld L: Povidone iodine as a vaginal microbicide. Am J Pharm 134:278–91, 1962.

   Singha H: The use of a vaginal cleansing kit in non-specific vaginitis. Practitioner 223:403–4, 1979.
3. Swate T and Weed J: Boric acid treatment of vulvovaginal candidiasis. Ob Gyn 43:894–5, 1974.

   Keller Van Slyke K: Treatment of vulvovaginal candidiasis with boric acid powder. Am J Ob Gyn 141:145–8, 1981.
4. Altman PM: Australian teatree oil. Australian J Pharm 69:276–8, 1988.

   Essential Oils Data Search: *Melaleuca alternifolia*. Vancouver, WA, 1985.
5. Pena EF: *Maleluca alternafolia* oil: Its use for trichomonal vaginitis and other vaginal infections. Ob Gyn 19:793–5, 1962.

Varicose Veins

1. Trowell H, Burkitt D, and Heaton K: Dietary Fibre, Fibre-Depleted Foods and Disease. Academic Press, London, UK, 1985.
   Vahouny G and Kritchevsky D: Dietary Fiber in Health and Disease. Plenum Press, New York, 1982.
2. Latto C, Wilkinson RW, and Gilmore OJA: Diverticular disease and varicose veins. Lancet i:1089–90, 1973.
3. Allegra C: Comparative capillaroscopic study of certain bioflavonoids and total triterpenic fractions of *Centella asiatica* in venous insufficiency. Clin Terap 110:550–5, 1984.
   Pointel JP, et al.: Titrated extract of *Centella asiatica* (TECA) in the treatment of venous insufficiency of the lower limbs. Angiol 38:46–50, 1987.
   Cesarone MR, et al.: Activity of *Centella asiatica* in venous insufficiency. Minerva Cardioangiol 40:137–43, 1992.
   Montecchio GP, et al.: Centella asiatica triterpenic fraction (CATTF) reduces the number of circulating endothelial cells in subjects with post-phlebitic syndrome. Haematol 76:256–9, 1991.
   Cappelli R, Nicora M, Di Perri T: Use of extract of *Ruscus aculeatus* in venous disease in the lower limbs. Drugs Exp Clin Res 14:277–83, 1988.
   Hitzenberger G: The therapeutic effectiveness of chestnut extract. Wien Med Wochenschr 139(17):385–9, 1989.
   Bisler H, et al.: Effects of horse-chestnut seed extract on transcapillary filtration in chronic venous insufficiency. Dtsch Med Wochenschr 111(35):1321–9, 1986.
4. Masquelier J. Procyanidolic oligomers (leucocyanidins). Parfums Cosmet Arom 95:89–97, 1990.
   Masquelier J. Pycnogenols: Recent advances in the therapeutic activity of procyanidins. In: Natural Products as Medicinal Agents, vol. 1. Hippokrates Verlag, Stuttgart, 1981, pp. 243–56.
5. Kreysel HW, Nissen HP, and Enghoffer E: A possible role of lysosomal enzymes in the pathogenesis of varicosis and the reduction in their serum activity by venostasin. VASA 12:377–82, 1983.
6. Visudhiphan S, et al.: The relationship between high fibrinolytic activity and daily capsicum ingestion in Thais. Am J Clin Nutr 35:1452–8, 1982.
   Bordia AK, Josh HK, and Sanadhya YK: Effect of garlic oil on fibrinolytic activity in patient with CHD. Atherosclerosis 28:155–9, 1977.
   Baghurst KI, Raj MJ, and Truswell AS: Onions and platelet aggregation. Lancet i:101, 1977.
   Srivastava K: Effects of aqueous extracts of onion, garlic and ginger on the platelet aggregation and metabolism of arachidonic acid in the blood vascular system: In vitro study. Prost Leukotri Med 13:227–35, 1984.
7. Ako H, Cheung A, and Matsura P: Isolation of a fibrinolysis enzyme activator from commercial bromelain. Arch Int Pharmacodyn 254:157–67, 1981.
   Taussig S and Batkin S: Bromelain, the enzyme complex of pineapple (*Ananas comosus*) and its clinical application: An update. J Ethnopharmacol 22:191–203, 1988.
8. Taussig S and Nieper H: Bromelain: Its use in prevention and treatment of cardiovascular disease. Present status. J Int Assoc Prev Med 6:139–51, 1979.
   Seligman B: Oral bromelains as adjuncts in the treatment of acute thrombophlebitis. Angiol 20:22–6, 1969.
   Giacca S: Clinical experiments with bromelain in peripheral venous diseases and chronic bronchitis. Minerva Med 56(Suppl.98):3925–32, 1965.
9. Durant JH and Waibel PP: Prevention of hematoma in surgery of varices. Praxis 61:950–1, 1972.

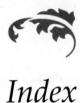

Index

Drugs (prescription) (*continued*)
  rising costs of, 5–6
  as toxins, 76
  for ulcers, 347–348
Dunner, David, 219
Duodenal ulcers, 346–350
Duodenum, 69
Dyazide, 5
Dymelor, 224–226, 234

Ear infection, 234–239
Ear Oil, 238–239
Echinacea, 118–120
EchinaFresh, 119
EchinaGuard, 119
Eczema, 50, 239–240
Edison, Thomas A., 315–316
EDTA (edetate calcium disodium)
  eight-hour mobilization test, 78
  intravenous EDTA chelation
    therapy, 145, 146, 150–155,
    189–191
E-guggulsterone, 201
Eicosapentaenoic acid (EPA), 50, 51
Eight-hour mobilization test, 78
Elavil, 218, 220
Elderly as drug company targets, 5
Electrolytes, 44
Eleutherococcus senticosis (Siberian
  ginseng), 107–108
Elimination. *See also* Bowels
  colon malfunction, 72–73
  constipation, 56, 72, 73, 210–213
  diarrhea, 43, 71–72
  hemorrhoids, 56, 263–265
Elimination diet, 245
ELISA (enzyme-linked immunosor-
  bent assay), 245
Ellis, John, 186
E-mergen-C, 48
Emphysema, 29
EMS (eosinophilia-myalgia
  syndrome), 17
Encyclopedia of Natural Medicine, 169
Endarterectomy, 190
Endogenous opiates, 304
Endorphins, 219, 301, 304–305
Enema, 342
Enteric-coated peppermint oil, 295

Enteric coating of enzymes, 70–71
Environmental medicine, 76–77
EnzyDophilus, 184
Enzymatic Therapy, 60
Enzyme-linked immunosorbent
  assay (ELISA), 245
Enzymes
  enteric coating, 70–71
  pancreatic enzymes and
    digestion, 69–72
  and zinc deficiency, 91
Eosinophilia-myalgia syndrome
  (EMS), 17
EPA (eicosapentaenoic acid),
  50, 51
Ephedra and asthma, 169–170
Ephedrine, 135–136, 169–170
Epidemiology and the optimal diet,
  55–56
Ergoloid mesylates (Hydergine),
  95
Escalation, 135–136
Essential fatty acids, 49, 240. *See also*
  Omega-3 fatty acids
Estrogen replacement therapy, 301,
  302–304, 320
Eustachian tube problems, 235
Evening primrose oil, 50, 51. *See
  also* Gamma-linoleic acid
  (GLA)
Exercise
  benefits of, 31–32
  and cholesterol, 197–198
  and endorphins, 304–305
  and fasting, 82
  and hot flashes, 304–305
  and impotence, 286–287
  natural approach with, 139
  and osteoporosis, 316
  recommendations, 32
  and varicose veins, 355–356
  and weight loss, 131–132
Exhaustion stage of General Adaptation Syndrome, 102
Expectorants, 169, 170
Eye diseases
  cataracts, 42, 43, 187–188
  glaucoma, 251–252
  macular degeneration, 299–300